Key Topics in Otolaryngology

Key Topics in Otolaryngology

Edited by Adrien Butler

AMERICAN
MEDICAL PUBLISHERS
www.americanmedicalpublishers.com

American Medical Publishers,
41 Flatbush Avenue,
1st Floor, New York,
NY 11217, USA

Visit us on the World Wide Web at:
www.americanmedicalpublishers.com

ISBN: 978-1-63927-410-9

Cataloging-in-Publication Data

Key topics in otolaryngology / edited by Adrien Butler.
p. cm.
Includes bibliographical references and index.
ISBN 978-1-63927-410-9
1. Otolaryngology. 2. Otolaryngology--Practice. 3. Otolaryngology--Diagnosis. I. Butler, Adrien.
RF46 .K49 2022
617.51--dc23

Table of Contents

Preface

This book has been an outcome of determined endeavour from a group of educationists in the field. The primary objective was to involve a broad spectrum of professionals from diverse cultural background involved in the field for developing new researches. The book not only targets students but also scholars pursuing higher research for further enhancement of the theoretical and practical applications of the subject.

Otolaryngology is a subfield in medicine that focuses on the conditions of the ear, nose and throat. It also deals with the conditions of other related structures of head and neck. It is concerned with the surgical management of cancers and benign tumors of the head and the neck. The most important procedures of otolaryngology are free muscle and bone transfer, free skin and fat transfer as well as microvascular reconstruction repair. In free muscle surgery, a muscle is collected from the back or abdominal region to reconstruct the skull or cranial vault. Whereas the free bone transfers deal with the bone defects. Bone transfers are used for the mandibular reconstruction. This book contains some path-breaking studies in the field of otolaryngology. It presents researches and studies performed by experts across the globe. The readers would gain knowledge that would broaden their perspective about otolaryngology.

It was an honour to edit such a profound book and also a challenging task to compile and examine all the relevant data for accuracy and originality. I wish to acknowledge the efforts of the contributors for submitting such brilliant and diverse chapters in the field and for endlessly working for the completion of the book. Last, but not the least; I thank my family for being a constant source of support in all my research endeavours.

Editor

1

Diagnosis and Surgical Management of Congenital Intranasal Teratoma in a Newborn

W. X. Yeo and K. K. Tan

Department of Otolaryngology, KK Women's and Children's Hospital, Singapore

Correspondence should be addressed to W. X. Yeo; yeoweixin@hotmail.com

Academic Editor: Rong-San Jiang

Teratomas are the most common germ cell tumors of childhood. Head and neck teratomas, however, account for less than five percent of all teratomas. Considered rare at an incidence of 1 in 20,000 to 40,000 live births, they may occur in the cervical region, nasopharynx, brain, orbit, or oropharynx. Teratoma presenting as an isolated intranasal mass is extremely rare. In this report, we describe a case of a mature teratoma arising from the roof of the nasal cavity presenting as an isolated intranasal mass, the first of its kind from our literature review. The tumor was resected endoscopically with no recurrence detected.

1. Introduction

Teratomas are the most common germ cell tumors of childhood [1], consisting of tissues from each of the three embryonic germ layers (ectoderm, mesoderm, and endoderm). They are mostly benign [2], although malignant transformation has been infrequently described [3, 4]. Teratomas of the head and neck account for less than five percent of all teratomas [5, 6], occurring in about 1 in 20,000 to 1 in 40,000 live births [7]. They are most commonly found in the cervical region and the nasopharynx [8, 9], areas which may result in respiratory distress or issues. Occurrences have also been described in other head and neck regions such as the brain [2], orbit [10], and oropharynx [11]. Teratoma presenting as an isolated intranasal mass is extremely rare. In this report, we describe a case of a mature teratoma arising from the roof of the nasal cavity presenting as an isolated intranasal mass, the first of its kind from our literature review. The tumor was successfully resected endoscopically.

2. Case Report

A full-term newborn boy presented with noisy breathing and mild subcostal retractions at birth. There was no stridor or desaturations on room air. On examination, there were no external nasal deformities or swellings. Bedside nasoendoscopy revealed a soft fleshy mass occupying the left nasal cavity. An attempt to pass a 6-French catheter beyond the mass into the nasopharynx was successful, which suggested that there was no associated choanal atresia. Examination of the right nasal cavity, apart from a septal deviation as a result of mass effect from the left nasal mass, was otherwise unremarkable. The oral cavity and oropharynx were also clear with no evidence of cleft palate.

Computed tomography (CT) and magnetic resonance imaging (MRI) scanning of the nose were performed, which revealed a left nasal mass lesion arising from the roof of the nasal cavity with extension into the posterior choana (Figure 1). There were no underlying bony skull base defects, nor any herniation of intracranial structures to suggest a nasal encephalocele. In view of the presence of an isolated intranasal mass, the differential diagnoses considered at the time of presentation were congenital midline nasal mass (e.g., nasal glioma) and nasal tumor (e.g., nasal chondromesenchymal hamartoma, or nasal teratoma).

The patient subsequently underwent an examination of the nose and endoscopic resection of the nasal mass under general anesthesia. Intraoperatively, a large left nasal mass was noted (Figure 2(a)), which extended anteriorly to

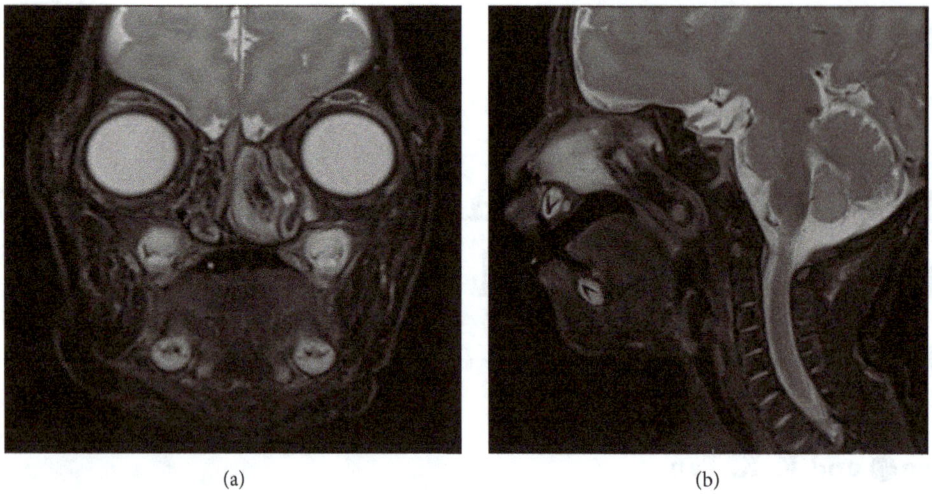

Figure 1: MRI T2-weighted axial (a) and sagittal (b) images depicting a left nasal mass arising from the roof of the nasal cavity and extending to the posterior choana, with no intracranial extension seen.

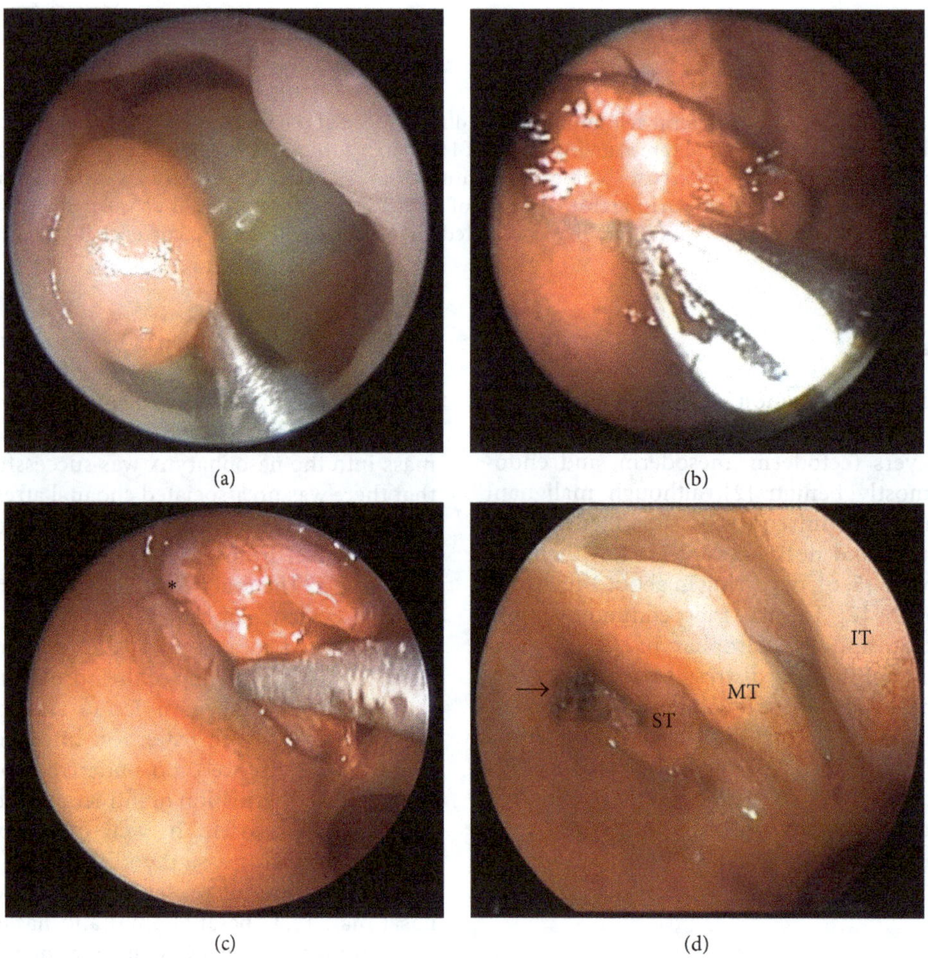

Figure 2: Intraoperative images depicting a large fleshy left nasal mass (a), which was endoscopically debulked with a microdebrider (Skimmer) (b). The stalk of the teratoma (asterisk) was revealed to be arising from the roof of the nasal cavity (c). Postresection image (d) showing the site of tumor origin (arrow) in relation to the turbinates. ST, superior turbinate; MT, middle turbinate; IT, inferior turbinate.

the nasal vestibule and posteriorly to the posterior choana. An incisional biopsy was performed, and intraoperative frozen section revealed a "stratified squamous epithelium, fat, and skeletal muscle lesion—in keeping with a teratoma." The tumor was gradually debulked and removed endoscopically with a microdebrider (Skimmer®) (Figure 2(b)). The stalk of the tumor was traced to be arising from the roof of the nasal cavity medial to the superior turbinate (Figures 2(c) and 2(d)). Nearing the skull base, the stalk of the tumor was carefully removed with Tru-Cut blades. Any visible remnant tumor tissue was cauterized with suction diathermy to ensure complete removal of the tumor. Care was taken at this point to prevent any breach of the skull base which might have otherwise resulted in a cerebrospinal fluid (CSF) leak.

Postoperatively, the patient had an uneventful recovery and was discharged well on postoperative day 3. Final histology confirmed the diagnosis of a mature teratoma, with presence of tissues from all three germ layers (e.g., stratified squamous epithelium with adnexal structures (ectoderm), skeletal muscle (mesoderm), and ciliated respiratory epithelium (endoderm)). On follow-up at three weeks and three months postresection, there was no evidence of tumor recurrence on examination under general anesthesia (which allowed for optimal examination of the nasal cavity). The patient is currently being followed up every six months.

3. Discussion

The nasopharynx is a common site of origin for congenital head and neck teratomas, which is often associated with cleft palate formation [12]. In comparison, congenital teratomas arising from the nasal cavity are much rarer. A handful of cases have been described arising from the nasal septum [13–16], either with or without an associated cleft palate. One case described a congenital teratoma arising from the nasal vestibule [17]. To the best of our knowledge, this is the first report of a congenital teratoma arising from the roof of the nasal cavity.

An intranasal mass in a newborn often triggers the consideration of a congenital midline nasal mass such as a nasal encephalocele or a nasal glioma [18]. This is especially so when the mass is seen arising from the roof of the nasal cavity, as with this case. Preoperative imaging with MRI and CT is therefore essential to assess for any intracranial extensions or bony skull base defects suggestive of a nasal encephalocele [19, 20]. This is because treatment is vastly different and would require a multidisciplinary team involving the expertise of a neurosurgeon [21]. Apart from congenital midline nasal masses, tumors have to be considered as well. Tumors may be benign or malignant [22], of which teratoma is one of the diagnoses.

As this was an isolated intranasal teratoma, resection was performed via an endoscopic approach. A Skimmer microdebrider was chosen for its small size, which permitted the debulking of the teratoma within the confines of a neonatal nasal cavity. Similar successful cases of endoscopic resection have also been previously described for nasopharyngeal [23] and nasal septum teratoma [15], although the choice of surgical approach (open versus endoscopic) is usually dictated by the location and extent of the disease. Other surgical modalities have also been described, including radiofrequency coblation of a nasopharyngeal teratoma [24] and CO_2-laser resection of an extensive nasopharyngeal and oral teratoma [25].

In general, the long-term prognosis of head and neck teratomas following surgery is excellent [3], as teratomas are mostly benign tumors with low recurrence rates so long as resection is complete. Routine follow-up for recurrence should include physical examination and imaging studies when appropriate [26]. Periodic measurements of serum alpha-fetoprotein (AFP) levels may also be performed, as teratoma recurrences have been detected by elevations of AFP levels after resection [27, 28].

In summary, we report the first case of a congenital teratoma arising from the roof of the nasal cavity that has been successfully resected via an endoscopic approach.

Conflicts of Interest

The authors declare that they have no conflicts of interest.

References

[1] U. Göbel, G. Calaminus, J. Engert et al., "Teratomas in infancy and childhood," *Medical and Pediatric Oncology*, vol. 31, no. 1, pp. 8–15, 1998.

[2] P. J. Anderson and D. J. David, "Teratomas of the head and neck region," *Journal of Cranio-Maxillofacial Surgery*, vol. 31, no. 6, pp. 369–377, 2003.

[3] V. R. C. Alexander, J. G. Manjaly, C. M. Pepper, S. N. Ifeacho, R. J. Hewitt, and B. E. Hartley, "Head and neck teratomas in children–a series of 23 cases at Great Ormond Street Hospital," *International Journal of Pediatric Otorhinolaryngology*, vol. 79, no. 12, pp. 2008–2014, 2015.

[4] T. Touran, H. Applebaum, D. B. Frost, R. Richardson, P. Taber, and J. Rowland, "Congenital metastatic cervical teratoma: diagnostic and management considerations," *Journal of Pediatric Surgery*, vol. 24, no. 1, pp. 21–23, 1989.

[5] A. Chakravarti, T. B. Shashidhar, S. Naglot, and J. K. Sahni, "Head and neck teratomas in children: a case series," *Indian Journal of Otolaryngology and Head & Neck Surgery*, vol. 63, no. 2, pp. 193–197, 2011.

[6] M. A. Rothschild, P. Catalano, M. Urken et al., "Evaluation and management of congenital cervical teratoma. Case report and review," *Archives of Otolaryngology-Head and Neck Surgery*, vol. 120, no. 4, pp. 444–448, 1994.

[7] R. G. Azizkhan, G. M. Haase, H. Applebaum et al., "Diagnosis, management, and outcome of cervicofacial teratomas in neonates: a Childrens Cancer Group study," *Journal of Pediatric Surgery*, vol. 30, no. 2, pp. 312–316, 1995.

[8] R. F. Ward and M. M. April, "Teratomas of the head and neck," *Otolaryngologic Clinics of North America*, vol. 22, no. 3, pp. 621–629, 1989.

[9] S. E. Kountakis, A. M. Minotti, A. Maillard, and C. M. Stiernberg, "Teratomas of the head and neck," *American Journal of Otolaryngology*, vol. 15, no. 4, pp. 292–296, 1994.

[10] D. S. Morris, T. Fayers, and P. J. Dolman, "Orbital teratoma: case report and management review," *Journal of American*

Association for Pediatric Ophthalmology and Strabismus, vol. 13, no. 6, pp. 605–607, 2009.
[11] M. Bahgat, Y. Bahgat, and A. Bahgat, "Oropharyngeal teratoma, a rare cause of airway obstruction in neonates," *BMJ Case Reports*, vol. 2012, 2012.
[12] D. S. Chauhan, Y. Guruprasad, and S. Inderchand, "Congenital nasopharyngeal teratoma with a cleft palate: case report and a 7 year follow up," *Journal of Maxillofacial and Oral Surgery*, vol. 10, no. 3, pp. 253–256, 2011.
[13] A. Veyssière, L. Streit, H. Traoré, and H. Bénateau, "Cleft palate caused by congenital teratoma," *Paediatrics and International Child Health*, vol. 37, no. 1, pp. 66–69, 2017.
[14] X. Pang, H. J. Kwon, B. Shi, and C. Li, "A rare nasopharyngeal teratoma arising from the vomer," *Journal of Craniofacial Surgery*, vol. 27, no. 2, pp. e165–e166, 2016.
[15] M. E. Huth, S. Heimgartner, I. Schnyder, and M. D. Caversaccio, "Teratoma of the nasal septum in a neonate: an endoscopic approach," *Journal of Pediatric Surgery*, vol. 43, no. 11, pp. 2102–2105, 2008.
[16] T. S. Ibekwe, D. D. Kokong, B. A. Ngwu, O. A. Akinyemi, O. G. Nwaorgu, and E. E. Akang, "Nasal septal teratoma in a child," *World Journal of Surgical Oncology*, vol. 5, p. 58, 2007.
[17] S. C. Shetty, S. Gupta, M. Cherian, G. Chary, and S. Shariff, "Mature teratoma of the nasal vestibule: a case report," *Ear, Nose, and Throat Journal*, vol. 79, no. 8, pp. 620–623, 2000.
[18] R. Van Wyhe, E. Chamata, and L. Hollier, "Midline craniofacial masses in children," *Seminars in Plastic Surgery*, vol. 30, no. 4, pp. 176–180, 2016.
[19] M. Tirumandas, A. Sharma, I. Gbenimacho et al., "Nasal encephaloceles: a review of etiology, pathophysiology, clinical presentations, diagnosis, treatment, and complications," *Child's Nervous System*, vol. 29, no. 5, pp. 739–744, 2013.
[20] A. J. Barkovich, P. Vandermarck, M. S. Edwards, and P. H. Cogen, "Congenital nasal masses: CT and MR imaging features in 16 cases," *American Journal of Neuroradiology*, vol. 12, no. 1, pp. 105–116, 1991.
[21] E. Adil, C. Robson, A. Perez-Atayde et al., "Congenital nasal neuroglial heterotopia and encephaloceles: An update on current evaluation and management," *Laryngoscope*, vol. 126, no. 9, pp. 2161–2167, 2016.
[22] F. C. Holsinger, A. C. Hafemeister, M. J. Hicks, M. Sulek, W. W. Huh, and E. M. Friedman, "Differential diagnosis of pediatric tumors of the nasal cavity and paranasal sinuses: a 45-year multi-institutional review," *Ear, Nose, and Throat Journal*, vol. 89, no. 11, pp. 534–540, 2010.
[23] R. Kim, S. John, A. Law, C. Barber, and R. Douglas, "Endoscopic resection of neonatal nasopharyngeal teratoma," *ANZ Journal of Surgery*, vol. 82, no. 1-2, pp. 80-81, 2012.
[24] S. Y. Hwang, N. Jefferson, A. Mohorikar, and I. Jacobson, "Radiofrequency coblation of congenital nasopharyngeal teratoma: a novel technique," *Case Reports in Otolaryngology*, vol. 2015, Article ID 634958, 3 pages, 2015.
[25] A. R. Gunkel, G. M. Sprinzl, F. K. Pühringer, H. Fischer, B. Simma, and W. F. Thumfart, "Microendoscopic transoral CO_2-laser resection of an extensive nasopharyngeal and oral teratoma," *American Journal of Otolaryngology*, vol. 18, no. 2, pp. 140–144, 1997.
[26] M. M. April, R. F. Ward, and J. M. Garelick, "Diagnosis, management, and follow-up of congenital head and neck teratomas," *Laryngoscope*, vol. 108, no. 9, pp. 1398–1401, 1998.
[27] D. F. Billmire and J. L. Grofeld, "Teratomas in childhood: analysis of 142 cases," *Journal of Pediatric Surgery*, vol. 21, no. 6, pp. 548–551, 1986.
[28] A. Aubin, S. Pondaven, D. Bakhos, H. Lardy, A. Robier, and E. Lescanne, "Oropharyngeal teratomas in newborns: management and outcome," *European Annals of Otorhinolaryngology, Head and Neck Diseases*, vol. 131, no. 5, pp. 271–275, 2014.

2

Nasopharyngeal Pleomorphic Adenoma

Serdal Celik,[1] Osman Kilic,[1] Tulay Zenginkinet,[2] and M. Tayyar Kalcioglu[1]

[1]*Istanbul Medeniyet University, Faculty of Medicine, Department of Otorhinolaryngology, Goztepe Training and Research Hospital, Istanbul, Turkey*
[2]*Istanbul Medeniyet University, Goztepe Training and Research Hospital, Department of Pathology, Istanbul, Turkey*

Correspondence should be addressed to M. Tayyar Kalcioglu; mtkalcioglu@hotmail.com

Academic Editor: Abrão Rapoport

Salivary gland tumors are rare among all head and neck tumors. Pleomorphic adenoma (PA) is the most commonly seen subtype, and 85% of the cases are located in the parotid gland. PA may very rarely be seen in minor salivary glands. Minor salivary gland PAs are mostly located in the hard and soft palates. Nasopharyngeal PA is very rare, and a total of 8 cases have been published to date. In this case report, a 51-year-old female patient who had nasopharyngeal PA with chondroid metaplasia is presented, and we review the relevant literature.

1. Introduction

Salivary gland tumors are rare and constitute less than 5% of all head and neck tumors [1]. Pleomorphic adenoma (PA), also known as benign mixed tumor, is the most common type among benign tumors of salivary glands. PA usually occurs in the 4th to 5th decades of life. It is located on the parotid gland, mainly on the superficial lobe, in 85% of cases. Even though PA rarely locates in the minor salivary glands, it is the most commonly seen minor salivary gland tumor and is most commonly located in hard and soft palates. These locations are followed by the upper lip in frequency [2–4]. PA originating from the nasopharynx is very rare, and only 8 cases have been reported in the literature to date [5–11]. In this case report, a 51-year-old female with nasopharyngeal PA is presented, and we review the relevant literature.

2. Case Presentation

A 51-year-old female patient came to our clinic with postnasal drainage and intermittent nasal obstruction. Oropharynx examination was normal. There were no features on anterior rhinoscopic examination. On nasopharyngeal endoscopic examination, there was an approximately 1 × 1 cm mass with a smooth surface on the posterior wall of the nasopharynx (Figure 1). There were no other abnormal features on ENT examination. The nasopharyngeal mass was completely removed with the pedicle under local anesthesia. Pathologic evaluation of the specimen was reported as "pleomorphic adenoma showing chondroid metaplasia" (Figure 2). Complementary surgery was offered, but the patient did not accept additional intervention. Follow-up with endoscopic examination was performed every 3 months. No recurrence was seen during postoperative 1-year endoscopic follow-up (Figure 3). No additional masses were found in any head or neck region during the period of follow-up.

3. Discussion

When a nasopharyngeal mass is detected in an adult patient, nasopharyngeal malignancy is usually suspected. Most common types of nasopharyngeal cancer are keratinising squamous cell carcinoma, nonkeratinising carcinoma, and basaloid squamous cell carcinomas [12, 13]. Malignant diseases arising in the nasopharynx are asymptomatic in the early stage. They may be confused with other benign lesions. Therefore, diagnosis of nasopharyngeal malignancy is usually delayed [13]. Although the adenoid tissue usually

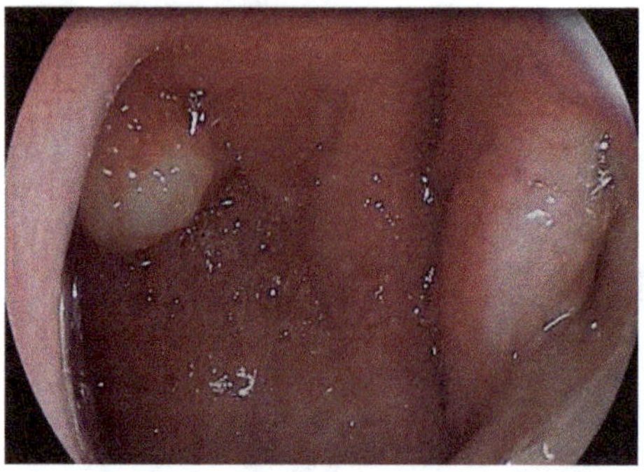

FIGURE 1: Preoperative nasopharyngeal endoscopy. The nasopharynx is seen in the posterior wall with a stalk-shaped mass and a 1 × 1 cm mass lesion.

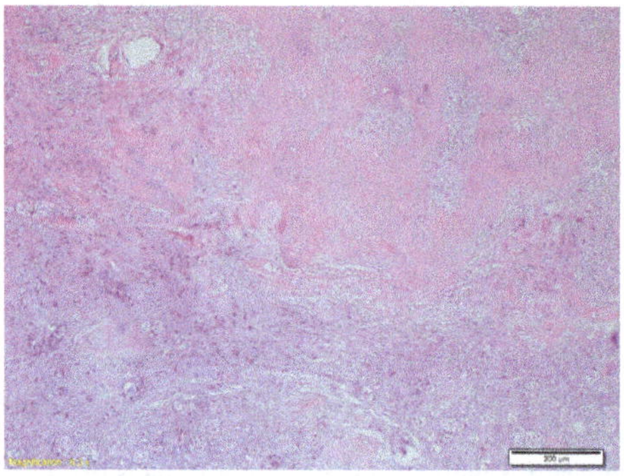

FIGURE 2: Pathologic specimen image. Pleomorphic adenoma showing chondroid metaplasia (10 H&E).

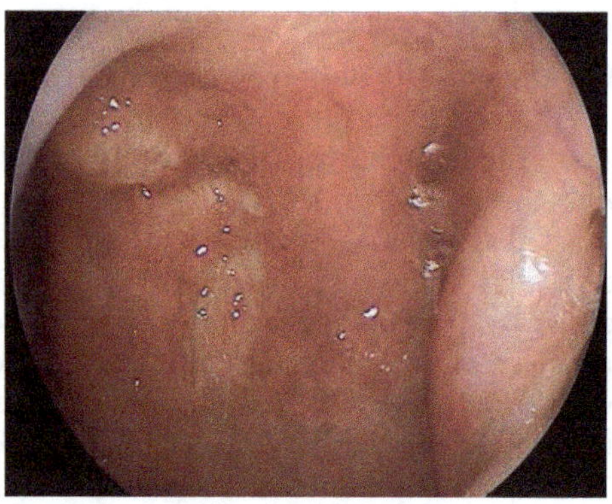

FIGURE 3: Postoperative 1st year image after punch biopsy. There was no significant difference between this and the appearance in the early postoperative period.

shrinks in adolescence, it may be a cause of nasal masses in adults [12]. Benign lesions in the nasopharynx of adults also include cystic lesions such as branching cleft cyst, Tornwaldt cyst, and mucus retention cyst [14, 15].

PAs are the most common salivary gland tumors and comprise 45–70% of all salivary gland tumors [16, 17]. They are most commonly seen in the parotid gland and comprise 65% of all neoplasms originating from the parotid [17]. PAs, also known as benign mixed tumors, have various morphologic patterns and subtypes and comprise myoepithelial and epithelial cells. Macroscopically, a PA has a capsule. However, this is not a real capsule. The compressed normal salivary gland tissue takes the form of a false capsule. These tissues often show finger-like (pseudopod) extensions into the normal tissue [4]. The recurrence rate in cases of enucleation due to focal infiltrations of the tumor capsule and pseudopods of the pleomorphic adenoma is 20–45% [3]. No recurrence was observed during the 1-year follow-up period in our case.

PA is typically located in the parotid lower pole or the superficial lobe. Deep lobe localization is rare [3]. PA is usually a slow-growing asymptomatic mass, seen between the 4th and 5th decades of life [18]. The patients are usually females (64.5%). The current case was a 51-year-old female with characteristics similar to those described in the literature.

Nasopharyngeal PA is seen very rarely. According to the sources available to us, there have been only 8 cases reported in the literature [5–11]. Detailed demographic and clinical characteristics of these 8 cases are given in Table 1. PA cases with nasopharyngeal locations usually are referred to clinics because of nasal obstruction, nasal bleeding, dysphagia, and serous otitis-induced hearing loss due to Eustachian tube dysfunction. Serous otitis media (SOM) was detected in 5 of these 8 cases [5, 6, 9–11]. Some other pathologies such as adenoid vegetation or nasopharyngeal carcinoma can also cause SOM. SOM can also be seen in benign pathologies such as choanal polyps that can grow to cause obstruction at the entrance of the Eustachian tube [17]. All possible masses should be kept in mind if the patient has SOM. In the current case, because of the location and size of the tumor, it was clear that the patient did not have SOM.

Pleomorphic adenoma-related squamous cell carcinoma (SCC) has been detected in 3 of 8 cases published in the literature [5, 7]. In two of these cases, total surgical excision was performed by the authors, and no recurrence was observed during 20 months of follow-up [5]. In another case report by Furukawa et al., recurrence was not observed during 2 years of follow-up of a patient who underwent radiotherapy after total excision [7]. In order to be able to say something definite in this regard, a histopathological evaluation of the tissue is necessary. In the current case, the follow-up was only made with endoscopic examinations because the patient did not allow any additional interventions. According to our endoscopic examinations in the current case, neither malignant transformation nor recurrence was observed during 1 year of follow-up.

Surgical procedures such as lateral rhinotomy and transnasal endoscopic approaches used for the other nasopharyngeal benign tumors can be used for this mass [18]. In a case report published by Martínez-Capoccioni et al., excision of the posterior nasal septum was performed with a transnasal endoscopic approach, and the mass was totally excised with a better surgical view [9]. Surgically, total excision is the preferred method of reducing the risk of recurrence [19]. In our case, total excision of the mass with transnasal endoscopic approach was performed.

In conclusion, very rarely seen nasopharyngeal PAs should be kept in mind in the differential diagnosis of nasopharyngeal masses. The gold standard for treatment of PA is total surgical excision of the mass.

TABLE 1: Nasopharyngeal pleomorphic adenoma cases in the literature.

	Age	Sex	Treatment	Follow-up duration (months)	Recurrence	Multiple location	Complaint	Size (cm)	Malignancy
Ryu et al. [5]	57	M	Surgery	12	No	No	Nasal obstruction	3.3	SCC
Ryu et al. [5]	37	M	Surgery	6	No	No	SOM	3.5	SCC
Lee et al. [6]	78	M	Surgery	20	No	No	Tinnitus, SOM	N/A	No
Furukawa et al. [7]	51	F	Surgery + RT	20	No	No	Nasal obstruction	N/A	SCC
Berrettini et al. [8]	51	F	Surgery	6	No	No	Nasal obstruction	4	No
Martínez-Capoccioni et al. [9]	52	F	Surgery	52	No	No	SOM	2	No
Maruyama et al. [11]	80	F	Surgery	24	No	No	SOM	2	No
Yazıcı et al. [10]	62	M	Surgery	12	No	No	SOM	2	No
Current case	51	F	Surgery	12	No	No	Nasal obstruction	1	No

SCC: squamous cell carcinoma; SOM: serous otitis media; RT: radiotherapy; M: male; F: female.

Disclosure

This study was presented in the 40th Turkish National Otorhinolaryngology and Head and Neck Surgery Congress, 7th-11th December, 2018, Antalya, Turkey.

Conflicts of Interest

The authors declare that they have no conflicts of interest.

References

[1] C. A. Waldron, S. K. El-Mofty, and D. R. Gnepp, "Tumors of the intraoral minor salivary glands: a demographic and histologic study of 426 cases," *Oral Surgery, Oral Medicine, Oral Pathology*, vol. 66, no. 3, pp. 323–333, 1988.

[2] P. J. Bradley, "Pleomorphic salivary adenoma of the parotid gland: which operation to perform?," *Current Opinion in Otolaryngology and Head and Neck Surgery*, vol. 12, no. 2, pp. 69-70, 2004.

[3] E. Stennert, O. Guntinas-Lichius, J. P. Klussmann, and G. Arnold, "Histopathology of pleomorphic adenoma in the parotid gland: a prospective unselected series of 100 cases," *The Laryngoscope*, vol. 111, no. 12, pp. 2195–2200, 2001.

[4] O. M. Ayoub, K. Bhatia, and R. K. Mal, "Pleomorphic adenoma of the parotid gland: is long-term follow-up needed?," *Auris Nasus Larynx*, vol. 29, no. 3, pp. 283–285, 2002.

[5] G. Ryu, S. D. Hong, and S. Chung, "Nasopharyngeal pleomorphic adenoma mimicking squamous cell carcinoma: report of 2 cases and review of the literatüre," *Journal of Korean Skull Base Society*, vol. 13, no. 1, pp. 44–48, 2018.

[6] S. L. Lee, C. Y. Lee, S. M. Silver, and S. Kuhar, "Nasopharyngeal pleomorphic adenoma in the adult," *The Laryngoscope*, vol. 116, no. 7, pp. 1281–1283, 2006.

[7] M. Furukawa, H. Suzuki, K. Matsuura, E. Takahashi, H. Suzuki, and F. Tezuka, "Carcinoma ex pleomorphic adenoma of the palatal minor salivary gland with extension into the nasopharynx," *Auris Nasus Larynx*, vol. 28, no. 3, pp. 279–281, 2001.

[8] S. Berrettini, S. Fortunato, A. De Vito, and L. Bruschini, "A rare case of nasopharyngeal pleomorphic adenoma," *Case Reports in Otolaryngology*, vol. 2013, Article ID 712873, 3 pages, 2013.

[9] G. Martínez-Capoccioni, C. Martín-Martín, and F. Espinosa-Restrepo, "Transnasal endoscopic resection of a nasopharyngeal pleomorphic adenoma: a rare case report," *European Archives of Oto-Rhino-Laryngology*, vol. 269, no. 8, pp. 2009–2013, 2012.

[10] Z. M. Yazici, Y. Yegin, O. Erdur, M. Celik, and F. T. Kayhan, "Management of pleomorphic adenoma in the nasopharynx: a case report," *Balkan Medical Journal*, vol. 32, no. 1, pp. 118–120, 2015.

[11] A. Maruyama, A. Tsunoda, M. Takahashi, S. Kishimoto, and M. Suzuki, "Nasopharyngeal pleomorphic adenoma presenting as otitis media with effusion: case report and literature review," *American Journal of Otolaryngology*, vol. 35, no. 1, pp. 73–76, 2014.

[12] R. H. Kamel and E. A. Ishak, "Enlarged adenoid and adenoidectomy in adults: endoscopic approach and histopathological study," *Journal of Laryngology and Otology*, vol. 104, no. 12, pp. 965–967, 2007.

[13] S. B. Hopping, M. L. Goodman, J. D. Keller, and W. W. Montgomery, "Nasopharyngeal masses in adults," *Annals of Otology, Rhinology and Laryngology*, vol. 92, no. 2, pp. 137–140, 2016.

[14] E. T. Chang and H.-O. Adami, "The enigmatic epidemiology of nasopharyngeal carcinoma," *Cancer Epidemiology Biomarkers and Prevention*, vol. 15, no. 10, pp. 1765–1777, 2006.

[15] K. Sekiya, M. Watanabe, R. N. Nadgir et al., "Nasopharyngeal cystic lesions," *Journal of Computer Assisted Tomography*, vol. 38, no. 1, pp. 9–13, 2014.

[16] M. N. de Silva, K. M. S. Kosgoda, W. M. Tilakaratne, and P. Murugadas, "A case of giant pleomorphic adenoma of the parotid gland," *Oral Oncology Extra*, vol. 40, no. 3, pp. 43–45, 2004.

[17] T. Sumi, A. Tsunoda, S. Shirakura, and S. Kishimoto, "Mechanical obstruction of the eustachian tube by the benign tumor of the parapharyngeal space does not cause otitis media with effusion," *Otology and Neurotology*, vol. 28, no. 8, pp. 1072–1075, 2007.

[18] M. M. Ardehali, S. H. Samimi Ardestani, N. Yazdani, H. Goodarzi, and S. Bastaninejad, "Endoscopic approach for excision of juvenile nasopharyngeal angiofibroma: complications and outcomes," *American Journal of Otolaryngology*, vol. 31, no. 5, pp. 343–349, 2010.

[19] S. Kariya, M. Kosaka, Y. Orita, H. Akagi, and K. Nishizaki, "Adenocarcinoma ex pleomorphic adenoma of the head and neck: report of five cases," *Auris Nasus Larynx*, vol. 33, no. 1, pp. 43–46, 2006.

3

Palatine Tonsil Stenting of the Airway as Determined by Drug-Induced Sleep Endoscopy

Habib G. Zalzal and Steven Coutras

Department of Otolaryngology-Head and Neck Surgery, West Virginia University School of Medicine, Morgantown, WV, USA

Correspondence should be addressed to Habib G. Zalzal; hgzalzal@hsc.wvu.edu

Academic Editor: M. Tayyar Kalcioglu

Objective. To demonstrate lateral pharyngeal wall collapse and increased apnea-hypopnea index in a child posttonsillectomy. *Background.* Some children have worsening of their sleep symptoms after tonsillectomy for obstructive sleep apnea. This case report demonstrates an open airway on drug-induced sleep endoscopy (DISE) in a child with tonsillar hypertrophy followed by more pronounced airway obstruction related to lateral pharyngeal wall collapse after tonsillectomy. *Case Presentation.* A 7-year-old boy presented with obstructive sleep apnea and underwent workup with DISE. Following adenotonsillectomy and subsequent lingual tonsillectomy with epiglottopexy, the patient's sleep apnea symptoms and polysomnogram results worsened. Subsequent DISE showed a more narrowed oropharyngeal airway space as compared to his preoperative DISE. *Discussion.* Palatine tonsillar tissue may splint open the airway and prevent airway obstruction in a subset of pediatric patients. Further clinical studies are necessary to determine which children experience this phenomenon. Clinical examination using DISE can be useful in making clinical decisions prior to tonsillectomy.

1. Introduction

Drug-induced sleep endoscopy (DISE) enables exploration of a patient's airway and is used particularly in patients with obstructive sleep apnea (OSA). First described in 1991, the pediatric procedure involves a flexible endoscope inserted through the nose of a sedated child [1, 2]. The endoscope is positioned at different upper airway levels to detect mechanisms and sites of obstruction [1, 2]. At present, DISE is restricted to children without hypertrophic tonsils and to those with persistent OSA following tonsillectomy and adenoidectomy (T&A) [2].

OSA affects up to 5.7% of all children and is widely recognized as a cause of significant morbidity [2–4]. Polysomnography is the most comprehensive method for diagnosis and evaluation of OSA severity [2, 4]. Adenotonsillar hypertrophy is an undisputed major contributor towards OSA in otherwise healthy children, such that the American Academy of Pediatrics recommends T&A as first-line therapy [2–4]. However, previous meta-analyses have noted 18%–33.7% of children who do not experience resolution of sleep apnea after this surgery, thus questioning the common attitude to systematically perform T&A in affected children [5, 6].

At our institution, we noted a few of our pediatric patients had worsened apnea-hypopnea index (AHI) on polysomnogram following T&A (Table 1). For one such patient described in this case report, we theorize a phenomenon that allows for hypertrophied tonsils to be nonobstructive, as the tonsils could instead splint or stent the airway open. This lends to the controversial belief that there may be a positive benefit for leaving tonsils in place.

2. Case Presentation

A 7-year-old boy presented to the otolaryngology sleep medicine clinic after being referred by his neurologist for OSA (Video 1). His past medical history was significant for a traumatic brain injury suffered after a dog attack during infancy, resulting in neurologic developmental delay,

Table 1: Characteristics of pediatric patients with worsened obstructive sleep apnea after tonsillectomy.

Patient (age/sex)	Comorbidities	Pre-DISE AHI	Procedures between polysomnogram	Recent AHI	Tonsil size (Brodsky scale)
7M[†]	ADHD, traumatic brain injury	1.7	Tonsillectomy and adenoidectomy; epiglottopexy; lingual tonsillectomy	4.5	3
7M	ADHD, fragile X	5.2	Tonsillectomy and adenoidectomy	9.4	3
7F	ADHD, Down's syndrome	4.9	Tonsillectomy and adenoidectomy; turbinate reduction	8.1	2

DISE, drug-induced sleep endoscopy; AHI, apnea-hypopnea index; ADHD, attention deficit hyperactivity disorder. [†]This individual was the first patient noted to have had tonsillar splinting after review of sleep endoscopy posttonsillectomy.

posttraumatic stress disorder, and attention deficit hyperactivity disorder. He underwent a polysomnogram prior to evaluation, which showed mild OSA with an AHI of 1.7, rapid eye movement (REM) AHI of 6.3, and a low oxygen saturation of 92%. On clinical examination, his tonsils were noted to be a +3 size (75% of oropharyngeal airway) on the Brodsky scale, but there was clinical concern that there may be additional sites of obstruction. He underwent a DISE with T&A one month later, and on postoperative follow-up, his mother did not believe his snoring had improved.

A few months later, based on initial DISE findings of a retroflexed epiglottis with lingual tonsil hypertrophy, he underwent an epiglottopexy with lingual tonsillectomy. A postoperative sleep study performed three months after that surgery (and five months after T&A) was concerning for worsening OSA (AHI 4.5; REM AHI 12.1; low O_2 saturation 94%). He underwent a second postoperative DISE four months after that polysomnogram, which showed complete collapse of the base of the tongue against the posterior pharynx. When compared to his preoperative DISE prior to T&A, it became apparent that the tonsils were likely not obstructing at the time, but splinting the airway open. The patient was scheduled for a posterior midline glossectomy but was lost to follow-up.

3. Discussion

With the advent of DISE, the complexity of pediatric OSA has recognized that adenotonsillar hypertrophy is not the sole cause of sleep apnea [3]. Tonsil size itself has been shown to not be a predictor of OSA severity, as even hypertrophied tonsils do not result in worse sleep apnea for pediatric patients [7]. A 2009 meta-analysis by Friedman et al. showed that treatment success of T&A was only 66.3%. Although one out of every three children failed to have complete resolution of sleep apnea following T&A, the surgery still reduced AHI significantly for the majority of patients and thus was recommended as first-line therapy [6].

Additionally, children with small tonsils may not experience the same benefit of T&A compared to those with larger tonsils based on the Brodsky standardized system [8, 9]. A 2016 study by Miller et al. established the Chan–Parikh system of classifying tonsillar obstruction via DISE. Their study concluded that a Brodsky score of +1 tonsils did not consistently demonstrate lateral pharyngeal wall collapse based on their new DISE-based scoring system [9].

Much is known about small tonsils not causing oropharyngeal obstruction, but little has been written on hypertrophied tonsils doing the same. Hypertrophied tonsils have been known to cause velopharyngeal insufficiency in certain patients due to posterior placement of the upper poles of the tonsils into the oropharyngeal and nasopharyngeal airway [10–12]. However, to our knowledge, there are no recorded reports in the literature of enlarged tonsils splinting the airway open to allow for an improved airway during sleep. It can be surmised that if tonsils are large enough to create enough space within the velopharynx, then perhaps it can do the same for the oropharynx along the base of the tongue. In addition to the case report described above, several other patients in our clinic were found to have similar instances of this tonsillar physiology (Video 2). It is the author's expectation that our video imaging of this stenting phenomenon may explain one possible mechanism as to why some patients with large tonsils do not improve following tonsillectomy.

4. Conclusion

While splinting of the tonsils to open the airway may not be a common pathology, patient characteristics should always be addressed before performing a T&A. If there is concern that the tonsils are not the obvious source of obstruction on physical examination, a preoperative DISE may assess whether a tonsillectomy is the correct surgery for this patient. While there is no identifying characteristics at this time for who may have this tonsil-splinting phenomenon, our hope is that our case presentation and video imaging sheds light as to why some patients may not improve after tonsillectomy for pediatric OSA.

Conflicts of Interest

The authors declare that there are no conflicts of interest associated with this research study.

Supplementary Materials

Video 1: this video begins with tonsillar-splinting phenomenon in the case report of the patient. Preoperatively, the tonsils are stenting the oropharyngeal airway and remain in a static nonobstructing position throughout respiration. The epiglottis represents main source of obstruction. The latter half of the video shows postoperative airway after tonsillectomy and epiglottopexy. There is now collapse of the tongue base only months after initial surgery when the previous tonsillar positioning would prevent such obstruction by splinting the airway open. Video 2: Patient #1 shows static, splinting tonsils throughout respiration with obstruction secondary to retroflexed epiglottis. Patient #2 shows splinting tonsils preventing further collapse of the posterior base of the tongue against the epiglottis. Patient #3 shows enlarged tonsils preventing obstruction of the tongue against the retroflexed epiglottis. Subsequent endoscopy after lingual tonsillectomy and epiglottopexy shows continued tonsillar splinting, but obstruction now due to arytenoid collapse. (*Supplementary Materials*)

References

[1] C. B. Croft and M. Pringle, "Sleep nasendoscopy: a technique of assessment in snoring and obstructive sleep apnea," *Clinical Otolaryngology*, vol. 16, no. 5, pp. 504–509, 1991.

[2] F. Galluzzi, L. Pignataro, and R. M. Gaini, "Drug induced sleep endoscopy in the decision-making process of children with obstructive sleep apnea," *Sleep Medicine*, vol. 16, no. 3, pp. 331–335, 2015.

[3] C. Guilleminault, J. H. Lee, and A. Chan, "Pediatric obstructive sleep apnea syndrome," *Archives of Pediatrics & Adolescent Medicine*, vol. 159, no. 8, pp. 775–785, 2005.

[4] C. L. Marcus, L. J. Brooks, K. A. Draper et al., "Diagnosis and management of childhood obstructive sleep apnea syndrome," *Pediatrics*, vol. 130, no. 3, pp. 576–584, 2012.

[5] S. Brietzke and D. Gallagher, "The effectiveness of tonsillectomy and adenoidectomy in the treatment of pediatric obstructive sleep apnea/hypopnea syndrome: a meta-analysis Otolaryngol head," *Otolaryngology-Head and Neck Surgery*, vol. 134, no. 6, pp. 979–984, 2006.

[6] M. Friedman, M. Wilson, H. C. Lin et al., "Updated systematic review of tonsillectomy and adenoidectomy for treatment of pediatric obstructive sleep apnea/hypopnea syndrome," *Otolaryngology-Head and Neck Surgery*, vol. 140, no. 6, pp. 800–808, 2009.

[7] A. Tang, J. R. Benke, A. P. Cohen, and S. L. Ishman, "Influence of tonsillar size on OSA improvement in children undergoing adenotonsillectomy," *Otolaryngology-Head and Neck Surgery*, vol. 153, no. 2, pp. 281–285, 2015.

[8] M. Imanguli and S. O. Ulualp, "Risk factors for residual obstructive sleep apnea after adenotonsillectomy in children," *The Laryngoscope*, vol. 126, no. 11, pp. 2624–2629, 2016.

[9] C. Miller, P. L. Purcell, J. P. Dahl et al., "Clinically small tonsils are typically not obstructive in children during drug-induced sleep endoscopy," *The Laryngoscope*, vol. 127, no. 8, pp. 1943–1949, 2017.

[10] R. J. Shprintzen, A. E. Sher, and C. B. Croft, "Hypernasal speech caused by tonsillar hypertrophy," *International Journal of Pediatric Otorhinolaryngology*, vol. 14, no. 1, pp. 45–56, 1987.

[11] K. MacKenzie-Stepner, M. A. Witzel, D. A. Stringer, and R. Laskin, "Velopharyngeal insufficiency due to hypertrophic tonsils. A report of two cases," *International Journal of Pediatric Otorhinolaryngology*, vol. 14, no. 1, pp. 57–63, 1987.

[12] A. W. Kummer, D. A. Billmire, and C. M. Myer, "Hypertrophic tonsils: the effect on resonance and velopharyngeal closure," *Plastic and Reconstructive Surgery*, vol. 91, no. 4, pp. 608–611, 1993.

4

Ear Prosthesis for Postburn Deformity

Alagesan Chinnasamy,[1] Vidhya Gopinath,[2] and Ashish R. Jain[2]

[1]*Melbourne Dental School, The University of Melbourne, Melbourne, VIC, Australia*
[2]*Department of Prosthodontics, Saveetha Dental College and Hospitals, Saveetha University, Chennai, India*

Correspondence should be addressed to Ashish R. Jain; dr.ashishjain_r@yahoo.com

Academic Editor: Luis M. J. Gutierrez

Prosthodontics is not just confined to replacement of missing teeth but beyond one's scope. The fabrication of any extraoral maxillofacial prosthesis presents the prosthodontist with several phenomenal challenges. Psychologically, these patients are severely affected either by congenital absence or loss of ear due to trauma or burns. Replacement or reconstruction can be done by surgical or prosthetic approach. However, not all situations are favourable to surgical reconstruction. This article emphasises on the steps in fabrication of ear prosthesis for burn deformity.

1. Introduction

Loss of external ear can be congenital or acquired due to accidental trauma or malignant disease. Congenital anomaly of the external ear may be termed as "microtia." It includes a spectrum of deformities from a grossly normal but small ear to the absence of the entire external ear. These deformities account for three in every 10,000 births, with bilaterally missing ears seen in fewer than 10% of all cases [1–3]. The patient presented in this article had a unilateral acquired missing ear due to burn deformity. Leading life with this kind of physical deformity is very stressful and often depressing for the patient. It directly affects the patient's mental, social, and psychological well-being. Acceptable aesthetics in restoring a prominent facial defect, such as malformed ear, is a challenging task for a maxillofacial prosthodontist. Maxillofacial training is an essential part of postgraduate curriculum in prosthodontics. Oral malignancy, facial tumours, trauma, and burns most of the time require rehabilitation either by surgery or prosthetic approach [4–8]. Poly(methyl methacrylate), poly(vinyl chloride), polyurethane, and silicone are the materials of choice for prosthetic rehabilitation as they are biologically accepted. However, silicones are preferred due to its flexibility, light weight, and lifelike appearance. A surgical approach may not be a treatment of choice most of the time due to certain constrains. In the face of these deformities and limitations, the surgical goals of reconstruction vary and can be very challenging, and this article presents a simple procedure for reconstruction of missing ear due to burns. A prosthetic ear is an artificial ear that is usually made of silicone from a mould that is prepared using the opposite ear (or a parent's ear in bilateral cases) as a template [9–13]. The prosthesis can either be held onto the head with adhesive or using magnets or clips (requires minor surgical procedure) or can be attached to the spectacle. The function of the prosthetic ear shape is not just confined to cosmetic reconstruction but it also directs the sound waves into the auditory canal and to maintain a proper environment for the inner ear membranes. It normally improves hearing by about 20%. The prosthetic ear will retain eyeglasses and retain a hearing aid if needed. It also serves as a great psychological benefit in the rehabilitation of the patient's social, physical, and mental well-being [14, 15].

2. Case Report

A 28-year-old male patient who lost his right ear in an electric burn reported to the Department of Prosthodontics, Saveetha Dental College and Hospital, for further treatment. Examination and history revealed that the patient had suffered from electric burns with scar formation, but some

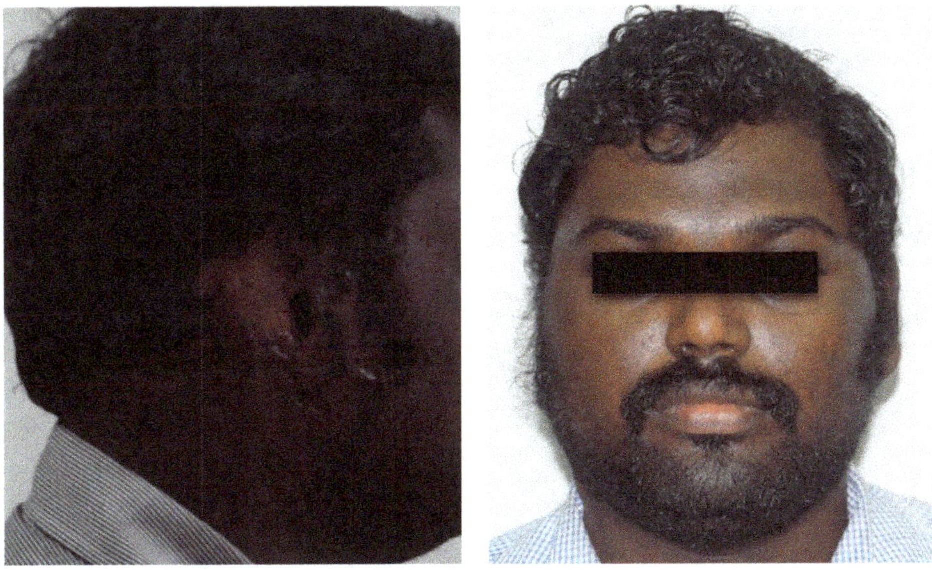

(a) (b)

Figure 1: Profile and frontal photographs of patient missing ear.

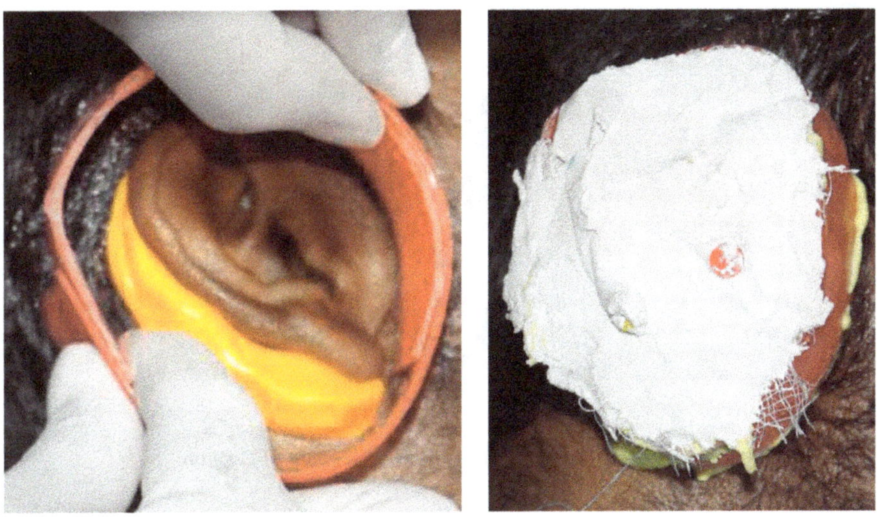

(a) (b)

Figure 2: Impression of donor ear using irreversible hydrocolloid.

rudimentary ear was present in the tragus region of missing right ear (Figure 1). Hearing capability was not compromised on both sides. A prosthetic reconstruction was decided to fulfil the patient's desire of cosmetic correction without surgery.

2.1. Impression Procedures. Examination of the defect showed healthy tissue with scar formation and rudimentary tissue tag at the height of the tragus, and the contralateral ear was normal. Before the impression making, three horizontal markings are made on the normal ear at the junction of helix with the side of the head as the first marking, the second at the middle of the tragus, and the last one at the junction of the ear lobe with the side of the head. Similar markings were made on the defective side, so that these markings were accurately transferred to the working cast. The borders were confined and closed by hair and smeared with vaseline. While making an impression, the external auditory canal was blocked with a cotton plug and the impression was made by irreversible hydrocolloid and with the gauge in between, and backing is done by quick-setting plaster to provide support for the impression (Figure 2). The impression of the donor ear was made with light body additional silicone, and the impression was poured with the dental stone to get the master cast of the defect site and the cast of the normal ear (Figure 3).

2.2. Sculpting. The prosthesis should have a lifelike appearance, so sculpting was done with utmost care to complement the aesthetics. The prosthesis can be sculpted from

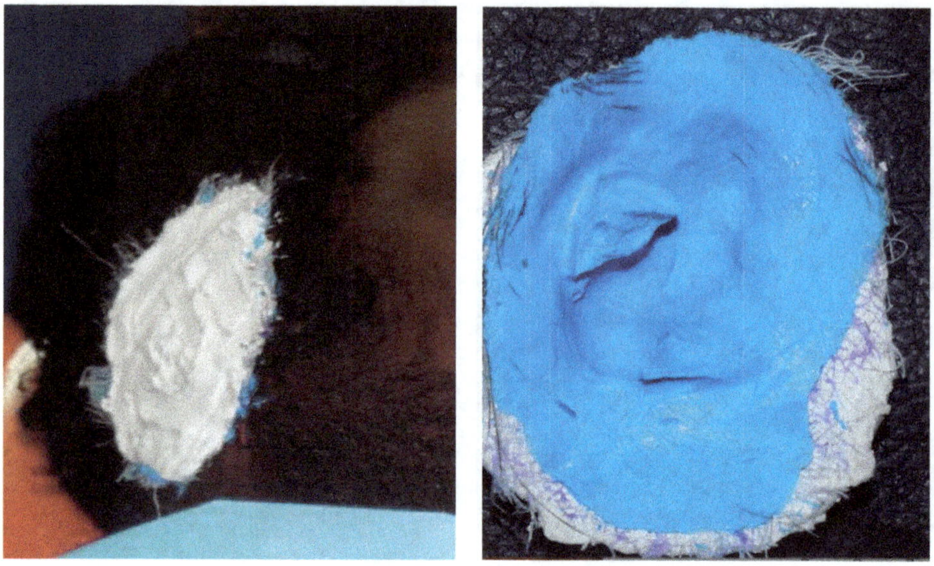

(a) (b)

FIGURE 3: Impression of missing ear using polyvinylsiloxane.

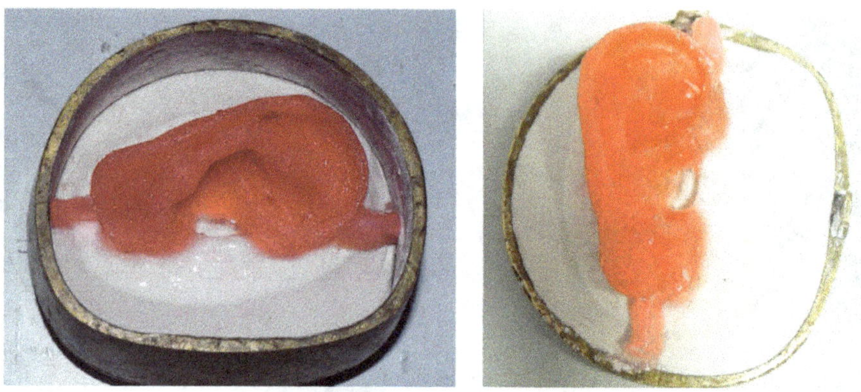

(a) (b)

FIGURE 4: Fabrication using three piece mould system.

the beginning or the donor technique may be used. The donor ear can be selected from a sibling or from any person whose ear matches with the patient's ear. For this patient, the donor technique was used and the impression was made and filled with modelling wax and later retrieved from the impression (Figure 4(a)).

2.3. Surface Die Fabrication: Three Piece Die. After the wax pattern try-in was done, it was oriented on the master cast using the markings placed on the defect site and necessary modification was done to match the contralateral ear. The wax pattern was then sealed in position on the master cast and leading edges were thinned as much as possible so as to allow the silicone edges to feather into the natural skin and when used in conjunction with adhesive they disappear. A three piece mould was fabricated for easy placement of silicone in the mould. To get the three piece mould, top portion of the dental flask was used as the base, the master cast along with the wax ear pattern was placed on this top portion of the flask, and dental plaster was poured to flush with the surface of the cast leaving no undercuts (Figure 4). Once set, two grooves were created on the plaster at the back portion of the ear to reorient the piece of mould. Separating media was applied as a separating agent and the dental stone was mixed and filled on the back side of the ear wax pattern to flush just underneath the superior margin of the helix extending till the base of the helix and junction of the lobe with the side of the head without leaving any undercut. Once the second pour was set, similar grooving procedure was carried out and the third pour was done using plaster, and the lid was placed and clamped and allowed to set.

2.4. Packing. Dewaxing was done in the usual manner. After keeping the flask in hot water for fifteen minutes, the flask was opened carefully and all three pieces of mould were thoroughly cleaned with hot water to remove traces of

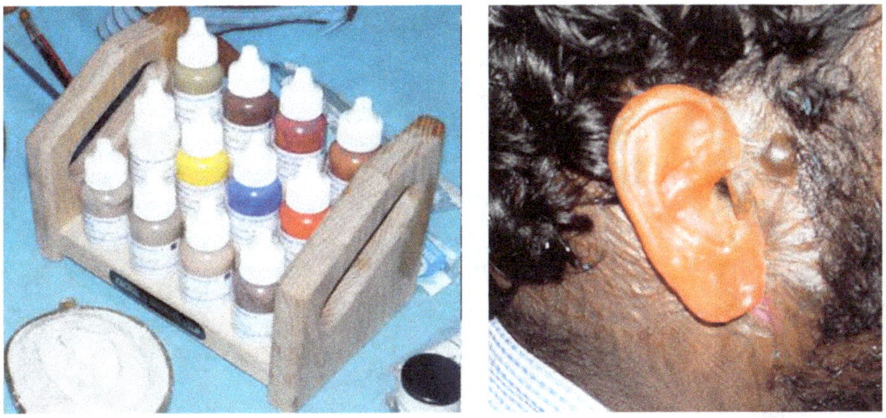

(a) (b)

FIGURE 5: Colour matching using intrinsic factor II stain.

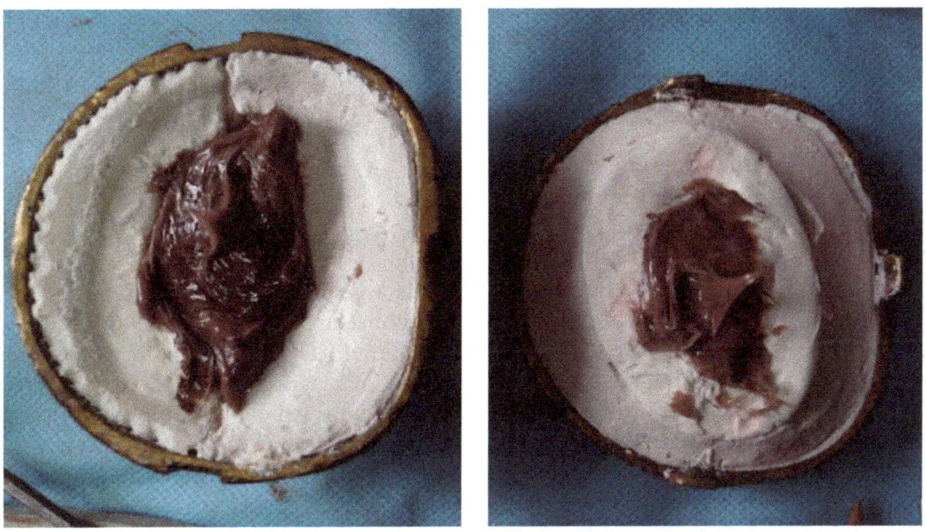

(a) (b)

FIGURE 6: Packing using dark and light shades of RTV silicones.

petroleum jelly and wax. Cold mould seal was diluted with water in 1 : 1 ratio and applied. The moulds were allowed to dry completely as traces of vaseline, wax, or water will interfere with setting of silicone and the prosthesis will have the tacky surface that will invite catching of dust at a later date. The three piece mould was now ready for silicone packing. Medical-grade factor-II room temperature vulcanising (RTV) silicone was used and was mixed as per the manufacturer's instruction. Thixo was added to prevent porosity in the prosthesis. To fabricate a lifelike silicone prosthesis, the patient must always be present for the colour match. It requires great care and patience from the doctor along with an understanding of colour matching for a successful result. As the silicone is translucent, desired skin colour can be obtained using primary colours in proper proportions. Using red, yellow, and blue primary colours of intrinsic colouring system, the first base shade was prepared, and then as per the requirement, additional shades were prepared. Care was taken while adding colour, as colour loading will lead to opacity and lifeless appearance (Figure 5). To match with the patient's normal ear, the dark and light shade silicone was poured in the mould. To create the characteristics, red flocks were placed on the surface layer and the mould was packed and allowed for bench curing for 24 hours. Cured prosthesis was retrieved from the mould, cleaned thoroughly with soap, and the excess silicone flesh was trimmed from the margins (Figure 6). The prosthesis was tried on the patient and margins were trimmed as per requirement, and then the prosthesis was attached to the spectacle frame and placed in position (Figure 7).

2.5. Retention and Care. An instruction leaflet with "Do's and Dont's" explained in it was given to the patient with an instruction that the prosthetic ear should be replaced every few years as the old one wears off. The skin surface should be maintained clean.

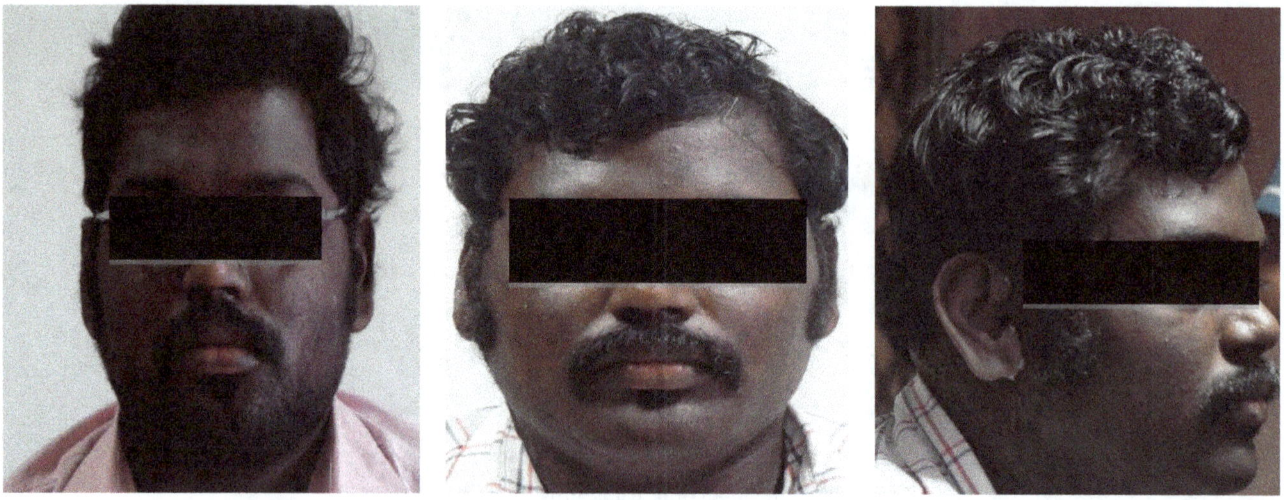

(a) (b) (c)

FIGURE 7: Frontal and profile photographs after insertion of ear prosthesis.

3. Discussion

The choice between surgical reconstruction and prosthetic restoration of facial defects is a difficult decision. As consistent good results have not been demonstrated in staged surgical ear reconstruction, the prosthetic restoration is the preferred option. There are various techniques for fabrication of ear prosthesis: conventional technique, shaper/tracer technique, photocopying technique, computerised tomography (CT) scanning, magnetic resonance imaging (MRI), 3-D laser scanning, computer numerically controlled (CNC) milling, rapid prototyping, and stereolithography [4–9]. The prosthesis made by CAD/CAM techniques is better than that fabricated by conventional methods. Unfortunately, taking into account the complexity and the high cost of the equipment needed, these techniques can only be used in well-developed establishments and an academic institution which makes us rely on more conventional techniques for the fabrication of extraoral maxillofacial prosthesis. The application of osseointegrated ear implants has changed the patient perception about facial prosthesis because of effective retention and improved aesthetics. However, it requires sufficient healthy bone at the defect site for implant placement, surgical intervention, cost involvement, and usually a time interval between implant placement and prosthetic rehabilitation. On the contrary, adhesive-retained prosthesis can be placed immediately on a healthy tissue bed, without surgery and is cost-effective [11–13]. Many techniques are in use for fabrication of wax pattern for adhesive-retained silicone ear prosthesis. One among them is sculpting the pattern by carving the wax. The second is a slicing technique in which the wax pattern is made using slices of wax pattern of normal ear and placing them in opposite directions [14, 15]. The technique used in this methodology was modification of donor ear which allows easy, quick incorporation of finer anatomical details making it more lifelike appearance. With the advancement in technologies, CAD/CAM is also being used for scanning and three dimensional reconstruction of ear, but it requires special armamentarium which may not be freely accessible and not cost-effective.

4. Conclusion

This article presents an outline of the fabrication procedure in constructing an ear prosthesis with three piece stone mould for processing silicone. Medical-grade silicone maxillofacial prosthetic material has the ability to match any skin colour using intrinsic and extrinsic colour system and is colour stable, has rubbery consistency to match the elasticity of the skin, is biologically inert, and is thus biocompatible. An aesthetic spectacle retained ear prosthesis was made by a meticulous step-by-step procedure using donor ear for fabrication of wax pattern. Rehabilitation of a patient with missing ear due to any condition can be achieved by restoring the defect and fulfilling the objective of maintaining patient comfort, aesthetics, and bringing the patient back to the society to lead a normal life.

Conflicts of Interest

The authors declare that they have no conflicts of interest.

References

[1] C. J. Venkata Krishnan, S. M. Balaji, and A. R. Jain, "A simple ear splint for microtia patients," *Indian Journal of Dental Research*, vol. 26, no. 2, pp. 220-221, 2015.

[2] J. F. Wolfaardt and P. Coss, "An impression and cast construction technique for implant-retained auricular prostheses," *Journal of Prosthetic Dentistry*, vol. 75, no. 1, pp. 45–49, 1996.

[3] A. C. Cheng, D. Morrison, R. S. Cho, and D. Archibald, "Vacuum-formed matrix as a guide for the fabrication of craniofacial implant tissue bar-retained auricular prostheses," *Journal of Prosthetic Dentistry*, vol. 79, no. 6, pp. 711–714, 1998.

[4] A. J. Godoy, J. C. Lemon, S. H. Nakamura, and G. E. King, “A shade guide for acrylic resin facial prostheses,” *Journal of Prosthetic Dentistry*, vol. 68, no. 1, pp. 120–122, 1992.

[5] R. R. Wang and C. J. Andres, “Hemifacial microsomia and treatment options for auricular replacement: a review of the literature,” *Journal of Prosthetic Dentistry*, vol. 82, no. 2, pp. 197–204, 1999.

[6] J. C. Lemon and M. S. Chambers, “Locking retentive attachment for an implant-retained auricular prosthesis,” *Journal of Prosthetic Dentistry*, vol. 87, no. 3, pp. 336–338, 2002.

[7] A. Tjellström, “Osseointegrated implants for replacement of absent or defective ears,” *Clinics in Plastic Surgery*, vol. 17, no. 2, pp. 355–366, 1990.

[8] R. F. Wright, J. J. Wazen, E. S. Asher, and J. H. Evans, “Multidisciplinary treatment for an implant retained auricular prosthesis rehabilitation,” *New York State Dental Journal*, vol. 65, no. 7, pp. 26–31, 1999.

[9] J. Beumer, T. A. Curtis, and M. T. Marunick, *Maxillofacial rehabilitation. Restoration of Facial Defects*, Medico Dental Media International, Inc., St. Louis, MO, USA, 1st edition, 1996.

[10] K. F. Thomas, *Prosthetic Rehabilitation*, Quintessence Publishing Co., Ltd., London, UK, 1st edition, 1994.

[11] T. D. Taylor, *Clinical Maxillofacial Prosthetics*, Quintessence Publishing Co. Inc, Hanover Park, IL, USA, 1st edition, 2000.

[12] J. C. Lemon, M. S. Chambers, P. J. Wesley, and J. W. Martin, “Technique for fabricating a mirror-image prosthetic ear,” *Journal of Prosthetic Dentistry*, vol. 75, no. 3, pp. 292-293, 1996.

[13] E. Sivayoham and T. J. Woolford, “Current opinion on auricular reconstruction,” *Current Opinion in Otolaryngology and Head and Neck Surgery*, vol. 20, no. 4, pp. 287–290, 2012.

[14] K. Storck, R. Staudenmaier, M. Buchberger et al., “Total reconstruction of the auricle: our experiences on indications and recent techniques,” *BioMed Research International*, vol. 2014, Article ID 373286, 15 pages, 2014.

[15] M. O. Karatas, E. D. Cifter, D. O. Ozenen, A. Balik, and E. B. Tuncer, “Manufacturing implant supported auricular prostheses by rapid prototyping techniques,” *European Journal of Dentistry*, vol. 5, no. 4, pp. 472–477, 2011.

5

A Case of Invasive Sinonasal Carcinosarcoma: The Importance of Early Detection

Jason Yuen,[1] **Vinay Varadarajan**,[2] **Marios Stavrakas**,[2] **Samiul Muquit**,[1] **and Hisham Khalil**[2]

[1]*South West Neurosurgery Centre, Derriford Hospital, Plymouth PL6 8DH, UK*
[2]*Department of Ear, Nose and Throat, Derriford Hospital, Plymouth PL6 8DH, UK*

Correspondence should be addressed to Hisham Khalil; hisham.khalil@plymouth.ac.uk

Academic Editor: Kamal Morshed

Sinonasal carcinosarcomas represent rare neoplasms, with aggressive character and unfavourable prognosis. We present a case of extensive sinonasal carcinosarcoma extending into the anterior cranial fossa and into the orbit and also a review of the current international literature regarding this rare yet aggressive neoplasm. There is currently a lack of specific guidelines on the optimal management of sinonasal carcinosarcoma and the treatment represents a challenge for the clinician. The key message that we would like to disseminate to our colleagues is the importance of suspicion and early detection, as well as the necessity to adopt a holistic approach when counselling patients.

1. Introduction

A malignant biphasic neoplasm consisting of an epithelial (squamous) element and mesenchymal component is known as a carcinosarcoma (also known as pleomorphic carcinoma, spindle cell carcinoma, pseudosarcoma, and pseudosarcomatous squamous cell carcinoma) [1, 2] although the exact nomenclature and subclassifications are variable [3]. It is classified under squamous cell carcinoma by the World Health Organization (WHO) [4].

Carcinosarcoma may arise from any squamous epithelium (e.g., salivary glands, respiratory tract, upper aerodigestive tract, and female reproductive organs) [5], but its occurrence in the sinonasal region is extremely rare [1]. There is very little evidence available about its best management.

2. Case Presentation

A 75-year-old gentleman first presented to primary care with a three month history of left-sided headaches and diplopia. He also complained of altered taste sensation and paraesthesia in the left maxillary region. There was no history of epistaxis. The patient attended his general practitioner on multiple occasions and was given sinusitis treatment until a CT scan was finally performed due to persistence of symptoms, upon which the patient was then referred to the ENT service.

He has a background history of fast atrial flutter (on bisoprolol), hypertension, polymyalgia rheumatica, benign prostatic hyperplasia, and previously excised papillary squamous cell carcinoma in the left thigh. He quit smoking 40 years prior to presentation. Otherwise, he had lived independently with WHO performance status of 1 (Karnofsky status 90).

The patient underwent complete head and neck examination including flexible nasoendoscopy. There was no discreet neck lymphadenopathy. Nasoendoscopy revealed a mass down to the left inferior turbinate obscuring the left nasal cavity. He complained of diplopia on the left side on the lateral gaze with proptosis of approximately 3 mm compared to the contralateral side. Vision was 6/30 bilaterally with glasses. There was no relative afferent pupillary defect or papilloedema.

2.1. Investigations. Initial CT scan revealed an aggressive lesion in left ethmoidal and frontal sinuses, invading the left orbit and anterior cranial fossa. CT neck and thorax showed no cervical or chest lymphadenopathy.

Subsequent MRI imaging also showed evidence of bone erosion with breaching of the dura in the vicinity of the left orbitofrontal cortex although there was no signal change in the brain to suggest brain invasion (Figure 1). There was destruction of left lamina papyracea. An incidental right anterior cranial fossa meningioma, distant from sinonasal lesion was also identified. This pathologic finding did not have any significant clinical relevance with the primary disease.

A staged whole body positron-emission tomography (PET) scan showed no other distant lesions but confirmed lesion progression through the frontal sinus.

Our initial differential diagnoses were squamous cell carcinoma, carcinosarcoma, lymphoma, teratocarcinosarcoma, olfactory neuroblastoma, small cell carcinoma and alveolar rhabdomyosarcoma.

2.2. Treatment. After the diagnostic workup, the patient underwent endoscopic examination of the nose and biopsy of the lesion under general anaesthesia. Extensive disease was noted at the ipsilateral maxillary antrum. Histology revealed an extensive necrotic biphasic epithelioid, spindled malignant neoplasm in keeping with carcinosarcoma. Immunohistochemistry afterwards showed no loss of DNA mismatch repair (MMR) protein expression.

2.3. Outcome. After a successful biopsy and radiological investigative workup, the patient was discharged home. Unfortunately in the community, his preexisting comorbidities worsened, and he developed poorly controlled fast atrial flutter and urosepsis with E. Coli bacteraemia. He was readmitted for antimicrobial and supportive treatment. The patient eventually recovered and was discharged.

Discussion was undertaken at the multidisciplinary meeting and with international experts in the field. The consensus is that although the disease can potentially be resected with major surgery such as craniofacial resection, due to its location and size, surgical treatment would have significant risk of bleeding, cerebrospinal fluid (CSF) leak, and meningitis. After detailed consultation and discussion about the possible treatment options including the risks of such procedures with the patient and his family, he was not keen to proceed and opted for palliative radiotherapy and symptomatic management.

The radiotherapy dose delivered was 20 Gy in five days, then a two-week break and finally another 20 Gy in five days. One year after diagnosis, patient tolerated the radiotherapy and continued to lead an independent life.

3. Discussion

In the head and neck area, carcinosarcomas most frequently occur in the larynx and oral cavity, followed by the skin, tonsils, sinonasal tract, pharynx and hypopharynx [6, 7]. Histologically, they have been classified as part of a spectrum

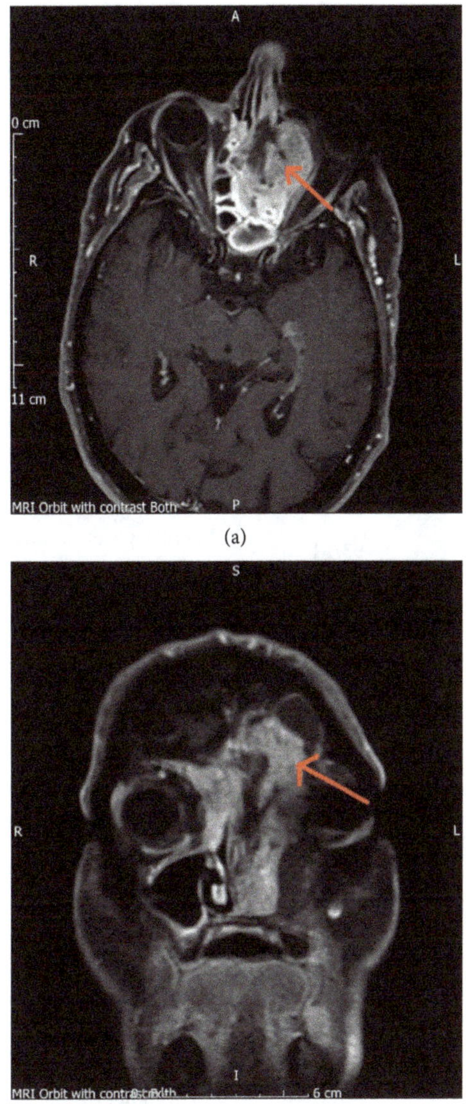

(a)

(b)

Figure 1: MRI head scan shows breaching of dura mater. Red arrow denotes lesion of interest. (a) Axial slide. (b) Coronal slide.

of sarcomatoid carcinomas, most of which present in late middle-aged men with a long history of tobacco use. They consist of foci of overt carcinoma admixed with areas of divergent differentiation into mesenchymal tissues [8]. Spindle cell formation is also typical in the sarcomatous component. A recent study suggested that a MET protooncogene mutation may be a prerequisite event in its pathogenesis [9].

Presenting symptoms of sinonasal carcinosarcomas typically include nasal obstruction, epistaxis, facial pain, and headache [10, 11]. These are rather nonspecific to the disease. They tend to grow rapidly, with extensive local destruction. Therefore, early diagnosis and aggressive therapy are necessary to improve the often dismal prognosis [2, 8].

In a Japanese case report of maxillary carcinosarcoma, the patient died despite intensive radiochemotherapy and total maxillectomy due to rapid tumour recurrence and metastasis. However, it appeared the carinomatous component

Table 1: Cases of sinonasal carcinosarcoma that are reported in the literature.

Number	Age (years)/sex	Location	Stage	Treatment	Outcome	Author, year
1	62/F	Maxillary sinus	ND	RT	No marked improvement of the tumor, DWD	Meyer and Shklar, 1957 [24]
2	71/M	Maxillary + ethmoid sinuses	T4aN0M0	Preoperative RT + TM + RE	ND about postoperative tumor condition, death due to intracerebral abscess at postoperative period	Feinmesser et al., 1982 [16]
3	65/F	Maxillary sinus	ND	TM + RT	LR, DWD 8 months later	Ampil, 1985 [14]
4	57/F, (postradiation)	Nasoethmoid sinus	ND	Tumor excision, ethmoidectomy and turbinectomy	LR 5 months after surgery, outcome uncertain	Hafiz et al., 1987 [17]
5	60/M	Nasomaxillary sinus	T3N0M0	TM + RT + CT	LR, DWD 2 months later (diffuse metastasis in lung and brain)	Sonobe, 1989 [11]
6	53/M	Maxillary + ethmoid sinuses	T4aN0M0	TM + craniofacial resection + RT + CT	Disease free after 9 months	Shindo et al., 1990 [2]
7	81/F	Maxillary sinus	T3N0M0	TM + RT + 2nd operation	LR, DWD 3 months after second operation	Sanabre et al., 1998 [27]
8	47/M	Maxillary sinus	ND	PM+RT	LR, DWD after 1 year	Furuta et al., 2001 [10]
9	54/M	Maxillary sinus	T3N3M0	RT + CT	DWD 4 months; possibly from lung metastasis	Howard et al., 2007 [19]
10 case series (19 cases)	Mean age at diagnosis 54 (range, 42–66) Male 11 Female 8	Sinonasal track, unclear exact locations	T1/2 3 T3/4 16 N0 19 M0 19	Surgery alone 2 Surgery and RT 7, RT alone 2 CT + RT 2	Mean follow-up 38 months (6–40) 5 with disease at last follow-up 0 death at follow-up	Doshi et al., 2010 [15]
11	75/M	Nasal cavity	T4N0M0	Surgery + CT + RT	Disease-free after 5 years	Terada and Kawasaki, 2011 [30]
12	60/M	Maxillary sinus and nasal cavity	Unclear	CT + RT	DWD after 9 months	Terada, 2011 [29]
13	29/F	Nasopharyngeal	T1N2cM0	RT	Clinically free-of-disease 2 months after RT	Lim et al., 2012 [22]
14	60/M	Maxillary + ethmoid sinuses	T3N0M0	TM + RT + CT	LR, FL	Moon, 2013 [1]
15	29/M	Nasal cavity	T2N0M0	Surgery	Disease-free after 6 months	Gupta, 2013 [32]
16	52/M	Frontal, sphenoid, ethmoid, and maxillary sinuses	T4aN0M0	TM + RT + CT	LR	Alem and AlNoury, 2014 [13]
17	61/M	Maxillary sinus	T4aN2cM1	TM with modified neck dissection	DWD shortly after surgery with sternal metastasis	Cheong et al., 2014 [12]
18 case series (15 cases)	Mean age at diagnosis 60.3 (SD, ±21.3) Male 6 Female 9	Nasal cavity 7 Maxillary sinus 5 Ethmoid sinus 1 Frontal sinus 1 Sphenoid sinus 1	T1/2 3 T3/4 10 TX 2 N0 9 N+ 0 NX 6 M0 14 M1 0 MX 1	Surgery alone 3 surgery and RT 7 RT alone 4 No therapy 1	Five-year disease-specific survival of 48.5%	Patel et al., 2015 [5]
19	66/M	Maxillary sinus	T3N0M0	PM + RT + CT	LR, DWD 10 months after initial presentation	Ando et al., 2015 [9]
20	78/F	Ethmoid sinus	T4N0M0	Surgery + RT	Disease-free after 36 months	Iqbal et al., 2015 [20]

TABLE 1: Continued.

Number	Age (years)/sex	Location	Stage	Treatment	Outcome	Author, year
21	66/M	Maxillary sinus	Recurrence	Palliative	DWD after 12 months	
22	68/M	Maxillary sinus	Recurrence	Palliative	DWD after 1 month	
23	46/M	Maxillary sinus	T4N0M0	Palliative	DWD after 5 months	
24	54/M	Sphenoid sinus	T4 N and M unclear	Surgery + CT + RT	DWD after 12 months	Liu et al., 2016 [23]
25	55/M	Maxillary sinus	T4aN0M0	RT	No significant effect, died 4 months after initial examination	Hasnaoui et al., 2017 [18]
26	35/F	Maxillary sinus	T4N0M0	PM + CT + RT	DWD after 12 months	Soltani et al., 2018 [28]
27	75/M	Ethmoid + frontal sinuses	T4aN0M0	RT	Remained independent after 12 months	Our case, 2018

ND, not described; RT, radiation therapy; DWD, dead with disease; TM, total maxillectomy; RE, removal of eye; LR, local recurrence; CT, chemotherapy; PM, partial maxillectomy; FL, follow-up loss; LNs, lymph nodes.

responded to the radiochemotherapy but that was not the case with the sarcomatous component [11].

Nonetheless, aggressive treatment may not cease disease progression and improve survival. Cheong et al. [12] reported on a 61-year-old male patient who underwent total maxillectomy and modified radical neck dissection and died shortly afterwards with sternal metastasis, despite having had extensive surgery with curative intent.

Table 1 shows the similar cases of sinonasal carcinosarcoma reported in the literature [1, 2, 9–31]. The optimal treatment of this disease remains undetermined. It is difficult to ascertain the effectiveness of the treatment modalities (a combination of surgery, radiotherapy, and chemotherapy) from the small number of cases available in the literature. They generally confer a poor outcome and a high recurrence rate. A recent large case-control analysis of 15 sinonasal patients in America showed an average five-year disease-specific survival of 48.5%, which is significantly poorer than controls with carcinosarcoma at other anatomical sites [5]. Therefore we advocate, when patients are operatively fit with resectable disease, they should undergo aggressive surgical treatment with adjuvant radiotherapy as an attempt to improve outcome. This is because radiotherapy alone tends to convey a less favourable outcome, and the role of chemotherapy is unclear.

Since the optimal management of carcinosarcoma remains uncertain, it is intuitive to study a related but separate (also highly aggressive) entity known as teratocarcinosarcoma [26, 33–35]. This tumour type also includes a component of neuroectodermal tissue and is much more prevalent in the medical literature. According to a recent systemic review of 49 patients, it is recommended that optimal treatment involves radical surgical resection followed by radiation therapy [25].

If more doctors are aware of this condition and the associated presenting symptoms, perhaps earlier diagnoses can be made. Therefore, patients may potentially get the option of a curative total resection, since the invasion of the skull base and surrounding structures is a poor prognostic factor.

In conclusion, sinonasal carcinosarcomas represent rare neoplasms, with aggressive character and unfavourable prognosis. Here we present a case of extensive sinonasal carcinosarcoma extending into the anterior cranial fossa and into the orbit and also a review of the current international literature regarding this rare yet aggressive neoplasm. There is currently a lack of specific guidelines on the optimal management of sinonasal carcinosarcoma, and the treatment represents a challenge for the clinicians. The key message that we would like to disseminate to our colleagues is the importance of suspicion and early detection, as well as the necessity to adopt a holistic approach when counselling patients.

Conflicts of Interest

The authors declare that there are no conflicts of interest regarding the publication of this article.

References

[1] J. K. Moon, A. Y. Kim, D. S. Chang, and K. Y. Park, “Carcinosarcoma of the maxillary sinus,” *Clinical and Experimental Otorhinolaryngology*, vol. 6, no. 2, pp. 114–116, 2013.

[2] M. L. Shindo, R. B. Stanley Jr., and M. T. Kiyabu, “Carcinosarcoma of the nasal cavity and paranasal sinuses,” *Head and Neck*, vol. 12, no. 6, pp. 516–519, 1990.

[3] J. G. Batsakis, ““Pseudosarcoma” of the mucous membranes in the head and neck,” *Journal of Laryngology and Otology*, vol. 95, no. 3, pp. 311–316, 1981.

[4] IARC, *World Health Organization Classification of Tumours-Pathology and Genetics of Head and Neck Tumours*, IARC Press, Lyon, France, 2005.

[5] T. D. Patel, A. Vazquez, M. A. Plitt, S. Baredes, and J. A. Eloy, “A case-control analysis of survival outcomes in sinonasal carcinosarcoma,” *American Journal of Otolaryngology*, vol. 36, no. 2, pp. 200–204, 2015.

[6] A. Cardesa, P. J. Slootweg, and SpringerLink (Online Service), *Pathology of the Head and Neck*, Springer-Verlag, Berlin, Heidelberg, Germany, 2006.

[7] T. Y. Kaminota, H. Yamada, and N. Hato, “A case of spindle cell carcinoma of the hypopharynx,” *Practica Oto-Rhino-Laryngologica*, vol. 145, p. 92, 2016.

[8] O. Nappi and M. R. Wick, "Sarcomatoid neoplasms of the respiratory tract," *Seminars in Diagnostic Pathology*, vol. 10, no. 2, pp. 137–147, 1993.
[9] M. Ando, Y. Saito, T. Morikawa et al., "Maxillary carcinosarcoma: identification of a novel MET mutation in both carcinomatous and sarcomatous components through next generation sequencing," *Head and Neck*, vol. 37, no. 12, pp. E179–E185, 2015.
[10] Y. Furuta, T. Nojima, N. Terakura, S. Fukuda, and Y. Inuyama, "A rare case of carcinosarcoma of the maxillary sinus with osteosarcomatous differentiation," *Auris, Nasus, Larynx* vol. 28, pp. S127–S129, 2001.
[11] H. Sonobe, K. Hayashi, K. Takahashi et al., "True carcinosarcoma of the maxillary sinus," *Pathology-Research and Practice*, vol. 185, no. 4, pp. 488–492, 1989.
[12] J. P. Cheong, S. Rahayu, A. Halim, A. Khir, and D. Noorafidah, "Report of a rare case of carcinosarcoma of the maxillary sinus with sternal metastasis," *Ear, Nose, and Throat Journal*, vol. 93, no. 6, pp. E1–E4, 2014.
[13] H. B. Alem and M. K. AlNoury, "Management of spindle cell carcinoma of the maxillary sinus: a case report and literature review," *American Journal of Case Reports*, vol. 15, pp. 454–458, 2014.
[14] F. L. Ampil, "The controversial role of radiotherapy in spindle cell carcinoma (pseudosarcoma) of the head and neck," *Radiation Medicine*, vol. 3, no. 4, pp. 225–229, 1985.
[15] D. V. Doshi, U. Tripathi, R. I. Dave, S. J. Pandya, H. K. Shukla, and B. C. Parikh, "Rare tumors of sinonasal track," *Indian Journal of Otolaryngology and Head and Neck Surgery*, vol. 62, no. 2, pp. 111–117, 2010.
[16] R. Feinmesser, J. Wiesel, E. Deutsch, M. Sela, and I. Gay, "Carcinosarcoma of the nose and paranasal sinuses-a case report," *Rhinology*, vol. 20, no. 3, pp. 167–170, 1982.
[17] M. A. Hafiz, J. Mira, and C. Toker, "Postirradiation carcinosarcoma of the nasal cavity," *Otolaryngology–Head and Neck Surgery*, vol. 97, no. 3, pp. 319–321, 1987.
[18] J. Hasnaoui, S. Anajar, M. Tatari et al., "Carcinosarcoma of the maxillary sinus: a rare case report," *Annals of Medicine and Surgery*, vol. 19, pp. 41–44, 2017.
[19] S. N. Howard, W. R. Bond, I. S. Hong, and R. D. Foss, "Right maxillary sinus sarcomatoid carcinoma (sarcomatoid/spindle cell carcinoma)," *Otolaryngology–Head and Neck Surgery*, vol. 137, no. 2, pp. 355–357, 2007.
[20] M. S. Iqbal, V. Paleri, J. Brown et al., "Spindle cell carcinoma of the head and neck region: treatment and outcomes of 15 patients," *Ecancermedicalscience*, vol. 9, p. 594, 2015.
[21] B. Lichtiger, B. Mackay, and C. F. Tessmer, "Spindle-cell variant of squamous carcinoma: a light and electron microscopic study of 13 cases," *Cancer*, vol. 26, no. 6, pp. 1311–1320, 1970.
[22] A. L. Lim, Z. Zahirrudin, and K. C. Pua, "A rare case of nasopharyngeal carcinosarcoma," *Medical Journal of Malaysia*, vol. 67, no. 4, pp. 428-429, 2012.
[23] T. W. Liu, S. H. Hung, and P. Y. Chen, "Sinonasal spindle cell carcinoma presenting with bilateral visual loss: A case report and review of the literature," *Oncology Letters*, vol. 12, no. 1, pp. 401–404, 2016.
[24] I. Meyer and G. Shklar, "Carcinosarcoma of the maxillary sinus; report of a case," *Oral Surgery, Oral Medicine, and Oral Pathology*, vol. 10, no. 10, pp. 1065–1074, 1957.
[25] P. Misra, Q. Husain, P. F. Svider, S. Sanghvi, J. K. Liu, and J. A. Eloy, "Management of sinonasal teratocarcinosarcoma: a systematic review," *American Journal of Otolaryngology*, vol. 35, no. 1, pp. 5–11, 2014.
[26] S. Mohanty, L. Somu, and M. Gopinath, "Sino nasal teratocarcinosarcoma—an interesting clinical entity," *Indian Journal of Surgery*, vol. 75, no. S1, pp. 141-142, 2013.
[27] A. A. Sanabre, J. Gonzalez-Lagunas, P. H. Redecilla, and G. R. Martin, "Carcinosarcoma of the maxillary sinus: a case report," *Journal of Oral and Maxillofacial Surgery*, vol. 56, no. 12, pp. 1456–1460, 1998.
[28] M. Soltani, P. Deyhimi, M. H. S. Najafabadi, S. Pourarz, N. A. Moghaddam, and M. Fayazi-Boroujeni, "A report of spindle cell carcinoma in maxillary sinus: diagnosis and management," *International Journal of Cancer Management*, vol. 11, no. 1, p. w9676, 2018.
[29] T. Terada, "Pure sarcomatoid carcinoma of maxillary sinus and nasal cavity simulating malignant fibrous histiocytoma," *American Journal of Clinical Pathology*, vol. 135, no. 1, pp. 128–131, 2011.
[30] T. Terada and T. Kawasaki, "Spindle cell carcinoma of the nasal cavity," *International Journal of Clinical Oncology*, vol. 16, no. 2, pp. 165–168, 2011.
[31] S. Viswanathan, K. Rahman, S. Pallavi et al., "Sarcomatoid (spindle cell) carcinoma of the head and neck mucosal region: a clinicopathologic review of 103 cases from a tertiary referral cancer centre," *Head and Neck Pathology*, vol. 4, no. 4, pp. 265–275, 2010.
[32] S. Gupta, D. Santoriello, R. Wieczorek, and M. D. De Lacure, "Spindle cell carcinoma of the nasal cavity," *Rare Tumors*, vol. 5, no. 10, pp. 38–40, 2013.
[33] S. Chakraborty, A. R. Chowdhury, and G. Bandyopadhyay, "Sinonasal teratocarcinosarcoma: case report of an unusual neoplasm," *Journal of Oral and Maxillofacial Pathology*, vol. 20, no. 1, pp. 147–150, 2016.
[34] D. J. Kurmi, R. S. Mittal, A. Sharma, A. Gandhi, and S. Singhvi, "Sinonasal teratocarcinosarcoma involving nasal cavity, nasopharynx, and all paranasal sinuses with bilateral orbital and intracranial extension: a rare case report," *Asian Journal of Neurosurgery*, vol. 12, no. 2, pp. 232–240, 2017.
[35] M. Sable, A. Kakkar, K. Garg, and V. Suri, "Sinonasal teratocarcinosarcoma: an underdiagnosed entity posing diagnostic challenges," *Turkish Neurosurgery*, vol. 27, no. 3, pp. 468–471, 2017.

6

Ectopic Intratracheal Thyroid: A Rare Cause of Airway Obstruction

Waheed Rahman, Nafil Ishaq Arimbrathodi, Faisal Abdulkader, Hussain Al-Enazi, and Zeynel A. Dogan

Department of Otolaryngology, Head and Neck Surgery, Hamad Medical Corporation, Doha, Qatar

Correspondence should be addressed to Nafil Ishaq Arimbrathodi; nafil42@gmail.com

Academic Editor: Gianluca Donatini

Ectopic intratracheal thyroid tissue (EITT) is a rare abnormality with only limited cases reported so far. The presenting symptoms can be very similar to those of bronchial asthma. We discuss the case of a 29-year-old man with subglottic ectopic thyroid, with a history of thyroid surgery for goiter, which has been managed with laser-assisted endoscopic approach. We have also included presenting symptoms, pathophysiology, diagnosis, and management of EITT. We aim to include EITT in the differentials of airway obstruction, particularly in those patients who have goiter or previous thyroid surgeries.

1. Introduction

Ectopic thyroid tissue (ETT) is a rare entity, which can be seen anywhere in the midline from the base of the tongue to mediastinum. Among them, the laryngotracheal region has the rarest occurrence that can cause upper airway obstruction. Since ectopic intratracheal thyroid tissue (EITT) is a rare condition, its symptoms can easily be mistaken for those of asthma. An associated hypothyroid level can lead to enlargement of EITT and worsening of symptoms. We are discussing EITT-causing stridor in a young man with a history of thyroid surgery who missed thyroxine therapy.

2. Case Report

A 29-year-old male, nonsmoker, presented to the emergency department with breathing difficulty. He had increasing dyspnea since few months, for which his general practitioner had treated him for asthma. Five years earlier, the patient had undergone thyroid surgery for goiter with subsequent thyroxine replacement therapy. But the patient missed the course and follow-up.

During the current presentation, fiber optic endoscopy showed bilateral mobile vocal cords and narrow infraglottic trachea with a right-sided subglottic mass.

CT showed subglottic soft tissue mass of about $4 \times 4.7 \times 2.4$ cm in the craniocaudal, anteroposterior, and transverse dimensions, respectively, extending at the level of C4, C5, C6, and C7 vertebrae, and it causes marked narrowing of the airways (Figures 1(a) and 1(b)).

On admission, TSH was 7.82 mIU/L (normal range 0.5–5.0 mIU/L) and free T4 was 13.31 mcg/dl (normal range 7.0–14.0 mcg/dl).

The patient underwent emergency tracheobronchoscopy which showed subglottic mass (Figure 2). Biopsy of mass done and the patient was tracheostomised. The histopathology and immunostain study result confirmed multinodular goiter associated with hyperplastic nodules with no evidence of malignancy.

We have done microlaryngoscopic excision of the subglottic mass utilizing CO_2 laser. The histopathology confirmed ectopic thyroid tissue (Figures 3–5). The patient weaned from tracheostomy tube and discharged on thyroxin supplement, and regular follow-up with ENT and endocrinology was given.

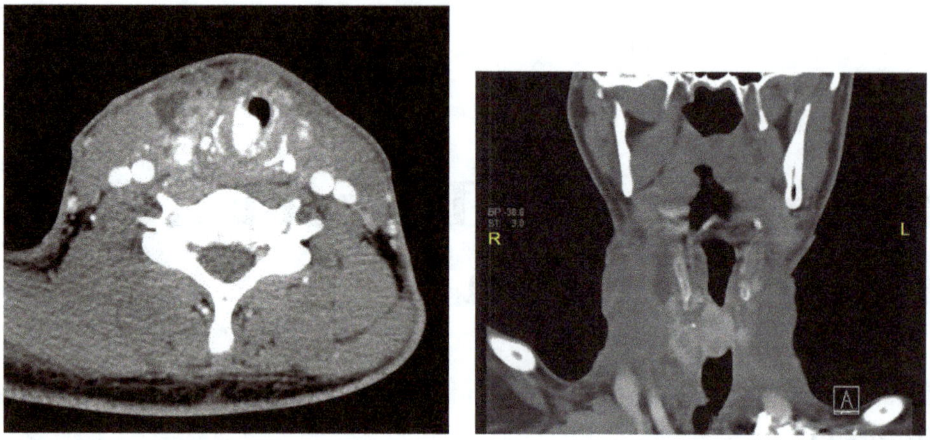

(a) (b)

FIGURE 1: Contrast-enhanced CT showing subglottic soft tissue mass extending at the level of C4, C5, C6, C7 vertebrae, causing marked narrowing of the airways. (a) is axial view and (b) is coronal view.

3. Discussion

Being a rare phenomenon, the number of cases reported with ETT so far is less than 500 [1, 2]. It is most commonly found in the lingual, sublingual, thyroglossal, laryngotracheal, and lateral areas. Very rarely, it has been described at the esophagus, mediastinum, heart, pancreas, adrenals, small intestine, and cutaneous area [3–12].

The percentage of ETT in trachea contributes 6–7% of all primary endotracheal tumors [13]. The first case was described in 1875 by Ziemssen [14–16]. The majority of the cases were reported from endemic goiter regions of the world [17]. Though EITT has been found anywhere from glottis to tracheal bifurcation, its most common appearance is as a submucosal mass on the lateral subglottic and upper tracheal wall [17–19].

The origin of EITT is explained by two theories. "The malformation theory" by Ziemssen in 1875 postulates that tracheal cartilage which develops later splits the thyroid gland, creating a small ectopic nest in the tracheal cavity [15, 16]. "The ingrowth theory" by Paltauf in 1892 states that the improper development of the mesenchymal tissue between the thyroid and trachea results in adherence of the former to the latter thus permitting the ingrowth [20].

Usually, patients are symptomless until a change in their hormonal status happen. Stimulatory factors including TSH, epidermal growth factor, and human chorionic gonadotropin could stimulate thyroid growth [21]. Symptomatic EITT causes difficulty in breathing, cough, stridor, and dysphagia. On physical examination, differentiating stridor of EITT from wheezing of asthma is not easy.

The findings suggestive of malignancy of EITT include multiple nodules, ulceration, and bleeding. 11% of EITT has been reported to undergo malignant transformation [16]. The most common malignancy found is papillary thyroid carcinoma [22, 23].

In a symptomatic patient, complete ENT examination should be carried out. Laboratory studies including thyroid assessment should also be conducted. Indirect laryngoscopy, flexible laryngoscopy, and CT and MR studies must be included. Radionuclide studies are highly sensitive and specific in detecting functional EITT [24]. Tc-99m pertechnetate scans high value in assessing the size, distribution, and activity of EITT. Fusion imaging techniques like single photon emission tomography-computed tomography (SPECT-CT) is valuable in diagnosis of EITT.

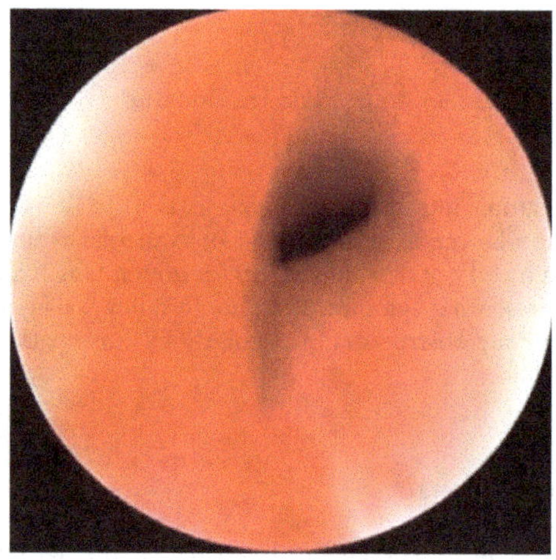

FIGURE 2: Tracheo-laryngoscopic examination showing subglottic mass obstructing the airway.

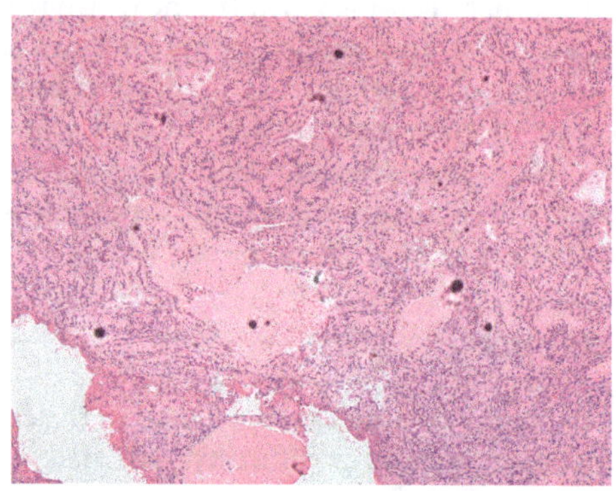

FIGURE 3: Histopathology showing thyroid follicles filled with colloid.

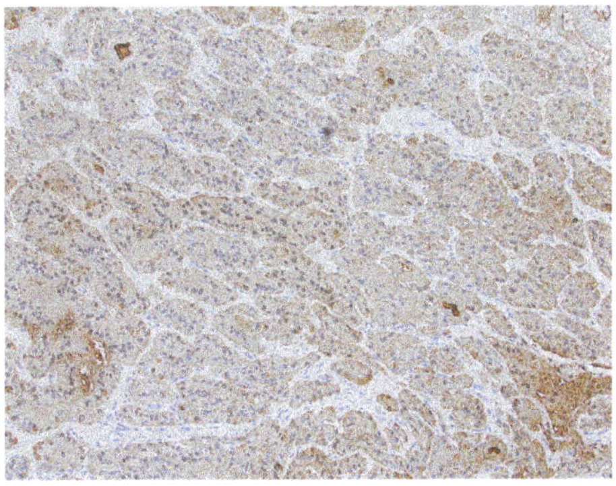

FIGURE 4: Positive cytoplasmic staining with thyroglobulin immunostain confirming the thyroid origin.

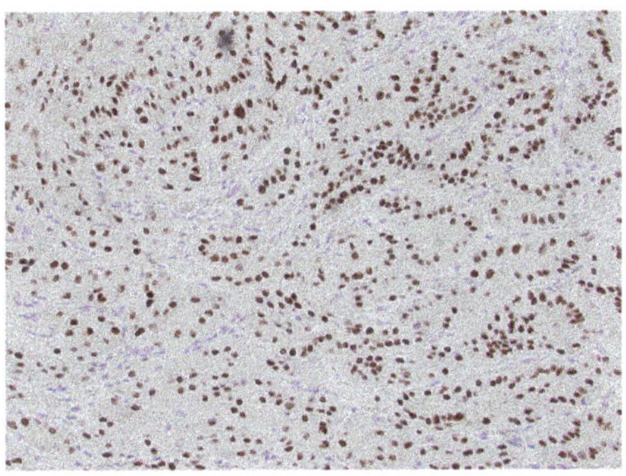

FIGURE 5: Positive nuclear staining with TTF-1 immunostain confirming the thyroid origin.

If associated with multinodular goiter, FNAC can be done. Direct laryngobronchoscopy will help in proper visualization of mass and performing biopsy. Since there is a chance of severe hemorrhage, a biopsy should be carried carefully [16].

The factors determining management of EITT include the size of lesion, the patient's age, the presence of local symptoms, the status of thyroid function, and histological findings. Surgical excision, radioiodine ablation, and thyroid suppression therapy are the main treatment options adapted. The complete surgical excision is indicated in symptomatic cases and in cases of histological malignancy. The two common surgical methods are removal via an endoscopic laser-assisted approach as in the present case and removal of the tumor via an open cricoid procedure [25]. Postoperative thyroid suppression therapy is performed to prevent hypertrophy of residual tissue. Radioiodine ablation with hormonal suppression has only limited success [25]. The risks associated with ablation therapy include radiation thyroiditis and tracheitis. It can be useful in patients who refuse or are unfit for surgery. While considering all the management options, surgical removal should be counted as the best option for the long-term outcomes [26–28].

4. Conclusion

Even though EITT is a rare abnormality with few case reported in the literature, it must be included in the differentials in patients presenting with airway obstruction, particularly in those who have goiters or previous thyroid surgeries.

Conflicts of Interest

The authors declare that there are no conflicts of interest.

References

[1] A. Kalan and M. Tariq, "Lingual thyroid gland: clinical evaluation and comprehensive management," *Ear, Nose, & Throat Journal*, vol. 78, no. 5, p. 340, 1999.

[2] J. S. Yoon, K. C. Won, I. H. Cho, J. T. Lee, and H. W. Lee, "Clinical characteristics of ectopic thyroid in Korea," *Thyroid*, vol. 17, no. 11, pp. 1117–1121, 2007.

[3] M. A. Salam, "Ectopic thyroid mass adherent to the oesophagus," *Journal of Laryngology & Otology*, vol. 106, no. 8, pp. 746-747, 1992.

[4] T. C. Gamblin, G. R. Jennings, D. B. Christie III, W. M. Thompson, and M. L. Dalton, "Ectopic thyroid," *Annals of Thoracic Surgery*, vol. 75, no. 6, pp. 1952-1953, 2003.

[5] G. D. Rieser, K. P. Ober, R. J. Cowan, and A. R. Cordell, "Radioiodide imaging of struma cordis," *Clinical Nuclear Medicine*, vol. 13, no. 6, pp. 421-422, 1988.

[6] R. J. Williams, G. Lindop, and J. Butler, "Ectopic thyroid tissue on the ascending aorta: an operative finding," *Annals of Thoracic Surgery*, vol. 73, no. 5, pp. 1642-1643, 2002.

[7] T. Shiraishi, H. Imai, K. Fukutome, M. Watanabe, and R. Yatani, "Ectopic thyroid in the adrenal gland," *Human Pathology*, vol. 30, no. 1, pp. 105–108, 1999.

[8] E. Eyuboglu, M. Kapan, T. Ipek, Y. Ersan, and F. Öz, "Ectopic thyroid in the abdomen: report of a case," *Surgery Today*, vol. 29, no. 5, pp. 472–474, 1999.

[9] K. Maino, H. Skelton, J. Yeager, and K. J. Smith, "Benign ectopic thyroid tissue in a cutaneous location: a case report and review," *Journal of Cutaneous Pathology*, vol. 31, no. 2, pp. 195–198, 2004.

[10] T. Takahashi, H. Ishikura, H. Kato, T. Tanabe, and T. Yoshiki, "Ectopic thyroid follicles in the submucosa of the duodenum," *Virchows Archiv A Pathological Anatomy and Histopathology*, vol. 418, no. 6, pp. 547–550, 1991.

[11] E. Ihtiyar, S. Isiksoy, C. Algin, A. Sahin, S. Erkasap, and B. Yasar, "Ectopic thyroid in the gallbladder: report of a case," *Surgery Today*, vol. 33, no. 10, pp. 777–780, 2003.

[12] B. Gungor, T. Kebat, C. Ozaslan, and S. Akıllı, "Intra-abdominal ectopic thyroid presenting with hyperthyroidism: report of a case," *Surgery Today*, vol. 32, no. 2, pp. 148–150, 2002.

[13] J. Fish and R. M. Moore, "Ectepic thyroid tissue and ectopic thyroid carcinoma: a review of the literature and report of a case," *Annals of Surgery*, vol. 157, no. 2, pp. 212–222, 1963.

[14] L. Thoren, "Intratracheal goitre," *Acta Chirurgica Scandinavica*, vol. 95, pp. 455–512, 1947.

[15] Ziemssen, "Uber Kopfgeschwuelste im Innern des Kehlkopfs und der Luftrohre und ihre Entfernung," *Beitr Kim Chir*, vol. 41, pp. 1903-1904, 1875.

[16] E. A. Dowling, I. M. Johnson, F. C. Collier, and R. A. Dillard, "Intratracheal goiter: a clinico-pathologic review," *Annals of Surgery*, vol. 156, no. 2, pp. 258-267, 1962.

[17] E. N. Myers and I. P. Pantangco, "Intratracheal thyroid," *Laryngoscope*, vol. 85, no. 11, pp. 1833-1840, 1975.

[18] A. M. Noyer and J. Friedberg, "Thyroglossal duct and ectopic thyroid disorders," *Otolaryngologic Clinics of North America*, vol. 14, no. 1, pp. 187–201, 1981.

[19] R. C. Bone, H. F. Biller, and T. M. Irwin, "Intralaryngotraheal thyroid," *Annals of Otology, Rhinology & Laryngology*, vol. 81, no. 3, pp. 424–428, 1972.

[20] R. Paltauf, "Zur enntniss der Schilddrusentumoren im Innern des Kehlkopfs und der Luftrohre," *Beitrage Zur Pathologischen Anatomie Und Zur Allgemeinen Pathologie*, vol. 11, pp. 71–89, 1892.

[21] H. Dossing, K. E. Jorgensen, E. Oster-Jorgensen, A. Krogdahl, and L. Hegedüs, "Recurrent pregnancy- related upper airway obstruction caused by intratracheal ectopic thyroid tissue," *Thyroid*, vol. 9, pp. 955–958, 1999.

[22] C. K. Hari, M. J. Brown, and I. Thompson, "Tall cell variant of papillary carcinoma arising from ectopic thyroid tissue in the trachea," *Journal of Laryngology & Otology*, vol. 113, no. 2, pp. 183–185, 1999.

[23] A. C. See, S. G. Patel, P. Q. Montgomery, P. H. Rhys Evans, and C. Fisher, "Intralaryngotracheal thyroid-ectopic thyroid or invasive carcinoma?," *Journal of Laryngology & Otology*, vol. 112, no. 7, pp. 673–676, 1998.

[24] A. Sood and R. Kumar, "The ectopic thyroid gland and the role of nuclear medicine techniques in its diagnosis and management," *Hellenic Journal of Nuclear Medicine*, vol. 11, no. 3, pp. 168–171, 2008.

[25] L. Soylu, F. Kiroglu, C. Ersoz, C. Özcan, and B. Aydoğan, "Intralaryngotracheal thyroid," *American Journal of Otolaryngology*, vol. 14, no. 3, pp. 145–147, 1993.

[26] M. Khan, P. G. Michaelson, and M. L. Hinni, "Intratracheal ectopic thyroid tissue presenting with protracted airway obstruction: a case report," *Ear, Nose, & Throat Journal*, vol. 87, no. 8, pp. 476-477, 2008.

[27] B. Karakullukcu, M. G. Guvenc, H. Cansiz, F. Oktem, and B. Oz, "Intratracheal ectopic thyroid: case report and review," *Ear, Nose, & Throat Journal*, vol. 86, no. 7, pp. 406–408, 2007.

[28] H. E. Bowen-Wright and J. Jonklaas, "Ectopic intratracheal thyroid: an illustrative case report & literature review," *Thyroid*, vol. 15, pp. 478–484, 2005.

7

Multifocal Warthin's Tumor: An Uncommon Presentation of Bilateral Cervical Lymphadenopathy

Ryan A. Rimmer and Elizabeth E. Cottrill

Thomas Jefferson University Hospital, Department of Otolaryngology—Head & Neck Surgery, Philadelphia, PA, USA

Correspondence should be addressed to Ryan A. Rimmer; ryan.rimmer@jefferson.edu

Academic Editor: Abrão Rapoport

Warthin's tumor is the second most common benign lesion of the parotid gland. It is most commonly encountered in male smokers in the fifth to seventh decades of life. Uniquely, among benign lesions of the parotid gland, it can be seen bilaterally in 7–10% of cases. Very rarely, Warthin's tumor can also mimic malignant or metastatic disease by presenting within cervical lymph nodes. We present a rare case of a 71-year old male smoker with bilateral parotid lesions in addition to progressively enlarging cervical and mediastinal lymphadenopathy. Excisional biopsy of a cervical lymph node ultimately revealed Warthin's tumor.

1. Introduction

Warthin's tumor (WT), also known as papillary cystadenoma lymphomatomsum, is the second most common benign salivary gland neoplasm representing between 6 and 10% of cases [1, 2]. While it was originally described by Hildebrand in 1895, Dr. Aldred Scott Warthin described additional cases in 1929 and the disease was ultimately renamed after him [3, 4]. It has a predominance for males with a mean age between the fifth and seventh decades. There is a strong association with smoking, but other proposed risk factors include ionizing radiation, viruses, and autoimmune disease [5].

While most commonly occurring within the parotid gland, WT can also be found more rarely in "extra-parotid" locations such as cervical lymph nodes or other salivary tissue [6]. Furthermore, these lesions can be unilateral, bilateral, or multifocal and may occur synchronously or metachronously with greater frequency than other benign salivary lesions [5]. Malignant transformation is exceedingly rare, but can take the form of either lymphomas or carcinomas [7]. We present a rare case of synchronous multifocal Warthin's tumor presenting as bilateral parotid lesions and cervical lymphadenopathy.

2. Case Report

A 71-year-old male presented to an outside institution in 2015 for evaluation of slowly enlarging bilateral cervical lymphadenopathy, parotid swelling, and night sweats. Medical history was significant for melanoma removed from the bridge of his nose in 2015, and active smoking for over 40 years.

During his initial workup at the OSH, computed tomography (CT) imaging showed multiple enlarged bilateral parotid lesions, scattered enlarged level I and II nodes, and upper mediastinal lymph nodes. He underwent ultrasound-guided fine needle aspiration (FNA) and core needle biopsy of a large left neck lymph node measuring 4.0×1.9 cm. Cytology was consistent with WT. Additionally, a level IA neck dissection was performed. Pathology revealed WT and no evidence of malignancy or lymphoma. Six-month follow-up imaging showed stable appearance of the bilateral parotid masses and cervical lymph nodes; however, there was interval enlargement of right upper mediastinal paratracheal lymph nodes.

He relocated in September 2016 and transitioned care to our institution. Thoracic surgery performed endoscopic bronchial ultrasound and transbronchial biopsies of the

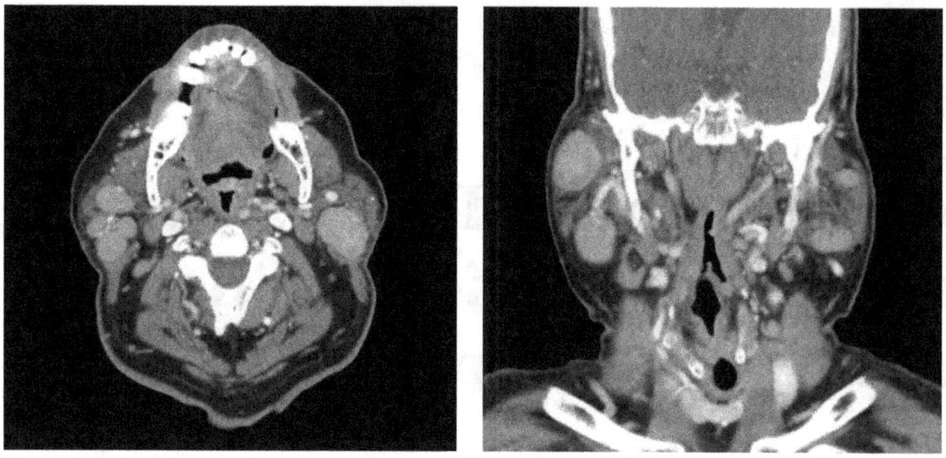

(a) (b)

Figure 1: Computed tomography (CT) with contrast in axial and coronal planes showing bilateral parotid lesions and cervical lymphadenopathy.

right paratracheal node. Cytopathology revealed absence of malignant cells. Flow cytometry was negative for lymphoma. He elected for close surveillance with serial imaging in lieu of mediastinoscopy. Six-month follow up imaging showed stable size of the mediastinal lymph nodes and slight enlargement of a left neck lymph node (Figure 1) and he was subsequently referred to the Department of Otolaryngology.

Physical examination revealed bilateral enlarged parotid glands and bulky cervical lymphadenopathy slightly larger on the right. Facial nerve function was intact bilaterally. The patient was counseled on smoking cessation. He was discussed at our multidisciplinary tumor board. Given the progression of cervical disease, he underwent level II lymph node dissection with removal of a large nodal conglomerate and culture of cystic contents. Histopathology once again confirmed WT (Figure 2). Culture and lymphoma workup were negative. In follow-up, he had quit smoking and elected to continue close observation.

3. Discussion

Unlike other benign salivary masses, WT has unique behavior in that it may occur bilaterally and outside of the major salivary glands. The pathogenesis of "extra-parotid" WT remains controversial. One hypothesis proposes that the tumor originates from heterotopic salivary parenchyma or ductal inclusions in the intra- and peri-glandular lymph nodes during the embryonic development of the parotid gland [5]. Late encapsulation of the parotid in the embryo allows the intermingling of undifferentiated lymphoid stroma with branching salivary ducts. After encapsulation, salivary ducts and acini may be trapped heterotopically within lymph nodes [8]. Heterotopic salivary gland tissue in the neck may arise sporadically via failed closure of the precervical sinus of His within the branchial apparatus [9]. Genetic and environmental factors may then impact these inclusions giving rise to Warthin's tumor.

Other theories using immunohistochemistry propose that WT results from inflammation directed at an unknown antigen. The antigen may be epithelial cells infected by a virus or mutated by tobacco smoke leading to immune response. Alternatively, the inflammation may be an autoimmune response to its own duct cells [10]. Some propose that the tumor is an adenoma with concomitant lymphocytic infiltration; however, this theory has less support given that many classify WT as a "tumor-like lesion" since the epithelial and lymphoid components have been shown to be polyclonal in origin [11, 12].

Tobacco smoking is closely associated with WT. Smoking may trigger ductal hyperplasia and oncocytic metaplasia in preexisting lymph nodes [13]. This transformation occurs with advanced age, which may help to explain the observed age range. Mitochondria-rich oncocytic cells may show structural abnormalities and reduced metabolic function. Smoking may potentiate this damage due to development of reactive oxygen species. Studies have detected high rates of deleted mitochondrial DNA in oncocytic cells of WT [14].

Histologically, WT tissue displays epithelial and lymphoid components. Glandular and cystic structures feature a bilayered epithelial lining composed of inner columnar eosinophilic or oncocytic cells surrounded by smaller basal cells. The lymphoid stroma may display varying degrees of reactivity. A sharply demarcated thin capsule surrounds Warthin's tumor and there may be extensive fibrosis at the periphery [10].

On CT imaging, WT displays oval or round lesions with uniform or heterogeneous density, a clear edge, and no calcifications [15]. These characteristics are consistent with the findings in our case. On magnetic resonance imaging (MRI), T1 shows low to intermediate signal, variable intensity on T2, and lack of enhancement with contrast [16]. Using MR diffusion weighted imaging (DWI), WT has a lower apparent diffusion coefficient (ADC) than pleomorphic adenoma and a comparable ADC to malignant

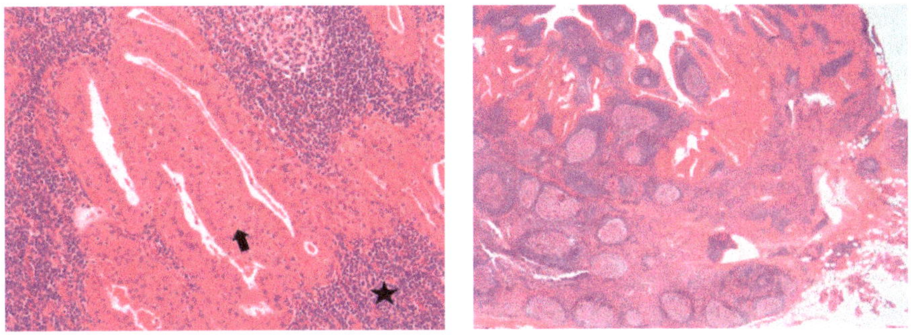

(a) (b)

FIGURE 2: Hematoxylin and eosin stains of pathologic specimen (higher magnification on left). Note dense lymphoid stroma (star) with double layer of epithelial cells (arrow) and cystic spaces.

salivary tumors [17]. A low ADC indicates decreased diffusion of water molecules in tissue, suggesting more cellular tissue. Generally, malignant tumors tend to have lower ADC than benign tumors [18]. WT may be differentiated from malignant lesions based on "hot" uptake with ^{99m}Tc pertechnetate scintography, which is due to the epithelial component's ability to concentrate ^{99m}Tc pertechnetate but not secrete it [18, 19]. WT also exhibits intense uptake on FDG-PET/CT [20].

Patients are typically asymptomatic until identifying a mass. Lesions are most commonly slow growing and firm or fluctuant to palpation. The slow growing nature has been attributed to low levels of MMP-1/Ki-67 expression, which has been associated with reduced cell proliferation [10]. WT typically occurs in the lower pole of the superficial lobe of the parotid gland and rarely in the deep lobe (10%). It can be multicentric in 12–20% and/or bilateral in 5–14% [10]. Multifocal extra-parotid Warthin's tumor has been reported to occur in only 2% of cases [11]. Our patient suffered from bilateral superficial parotid lesions and multifocal cervical lesions. Uniquely, our patient also had mediastinal lymphadenopathy although the EBUS cytology was not diagnostic of WT. Mediastinoscopy could provide additional diagnostic tissue, but was deferred at this time.

Given the low risk of malignancy, conservative management with close observation is often a reasonable consideration. For cases in which surgical resection is sought for cosmesis, superficial parotidectomy is most commonly recommended since WT occurs predominantly in the superficial parotid lobe. Benefits of resection must be weighed against the risk of iatrogenic facial nerve injury and overall risks of anesthesia especially in the case of bilateral tumors. The multifocal nature of WT has made extracapsular dissection more prone to recurrence as residual disease may be left behind [11].

4. Conclusions

Warthin's tumor (papillary cystadenoma lymphomatosum) is the second most common benign lesion of the salivary glands. While most commonly occurring in the parotid gland, unlike other benign salivary masses, it has a propensity for bilaterality and may occur in various extra-parotid locations including cervical lymph nodes. There is a strong association with tobacco smoking, although the exact pathogenesis of Warthin's tumor remains a controversial topic. The risk of malignant transformation is extremely low. In smokers with cervical lymphadenopathy, the suspicion for malignancy is high, however, Warthin's tumor should remain on the differential.

Acknowledgments

Stacey Mardekian, MD for supplying images and descriptions of histologic specimens.

References

[1] J. S. Chapnik, "The controversy of Warthin's tumor," *Laryngoscope*, vol. 93, no. 6, pp. 695–716, 1983.

[2] F. A. Ito, K. Ito, P. A. Vargas, O. P. de Almeida, and M. A. Lopes, "Salivary gland tumors in a Brazilian population: a retrospective study of 496 cases," *International Journal of Oral and Maxillofacial Surgery*, vol. 34, pp. 533–536, 2005.

[3] O. Hildebrand, "Uber angeborene epitheliale cysten und fisteln des halses," *Archiv fur Klinische Chirurgie*, vol. 49, pp. 167–206, 1895.

[4] A. S. Warthin, "Papillary cystadenoma lymphomatosum. A rare teratoid of the parotid region," *Journal of Cancer Research*, vol. 13, pp. 116–125, 1929.

[5] G. D. Orabona, V. Abbate, P. Piombino et al., "Warthin's tumor: aetiopathogenesis dilemma, ten years of our experience," *Journal of Cranio-Maxillofacial Surgery*, vol. 43, no. 4, pp. 427–431, 2015.

[6] G. H. Yoo, D. W. Eisele, F. B. Askin, J. S. Driben, and M. E. Johns, "Warthin's tumor: a 40-year experience at The Johns Hopkins Hospital," *Laryngoscope*, vol. 104, no. 7, pp. 799–803, 1994.

[7] F. O. Moore, R. Z. Abdel-Misih, J. D. Berne, A. W. Zieske, N. R. Rana, and J. G. Ryckman, "Poorly differentiated carcinoma arising in a Warthin's tumor of the parotid gland: pathogenesis, histopathology, and surgical management of malignant warthin's tumors," *American Surgeon*, vol. 73, no. 4, pp. 397–399, 2007.

[8] F. C. Astor, K. L. Hanft, P. Rooney, C. A. Benson, C. T. Flores, and P. Lavertu, "Extraparotid Warthin's tumor: clinical manifestations, challenges, and controversies," *Otolaryngology-Head and Neck Surgery*, vol. 114, no. 6, pp. 732–735, 1996.

[9] A. Haemel, D. R. Gnepp, J. Carlsten, and L. Robinson-Bostom, "Heterotopic salivary gland tissue in the neck," *Journal of the American Academy of Dermatology*, vol. 58, no. 2, pp. 251–256, 2008.
[10] Y. V. Kuzenko, A. M. Romanuk, O. O. Dyachenko, and O. Hudymenko, "Pathogenesis of Warthin's tumors," *Interventional Medicine and Applied Science*, vol. 8, no. 2, pp. 41–48, 2016.
[11] C. Naujoks, C. Sproll, D. S. Daman et al., "Bilateral multifocal Warthin's tumors in upper neck lymph nodes-report of a case and brief review of literature," *Head and Face Medicine*, vol. 8, no. 1, p. 11, 2012.
[12] K. Honda, K. Kashima, T. Daa, S. Yokoyama, and I. Nakayama, "Clonal analysis of the epithelial component of Warthin's tumor," *Human Pathology*, vol. 31, no. 11, pp. 1377–1380, 2000.
[13] W. Cope, C. Naugler, S. M. Taylor, J. Trites, R. D. Hart, and M. J. Bullock, "The association of warthin tumor with salivary ductal inclusions in intra and periparotid lymph nodes," *Head and Neck Pathology*, vol. 8, no. 1, pp. 73–76, 2014.
[14] A. Teymoortash and J. A. Werner, "Tissue that has lost its track: Warthin's tumour," *Virchows Archiv*, vol. 446, no. 6, pp. 585–588, 2005.
[15] C. H. Liang, W. Y. Di, J. P. Ren et al., "Imaging, clinical and pathological features of salivary gland adenolymphoma," *European Review for Medical and Pharmacological Sciences*, vol. 18, no. 23, pp. 3638–3644, 2014.
[16] V. Q. Joe and P. L. Westesson, "Tumors of the parotid gland: MR imaging characteristics of various histologic types," *American Journal of Roentgenology*, vol. 163, no. 2, pp. 433–438, 1994.
[17] Y. Karaman, A. Özgür, D. Apaydın, C. Özcan, R. Arpacı, and M. N. Duce, "Role of diffusion-weighted magentic resonance imaging in the differentiation of parotid gland tumors," *Oral Radiology*, vol. 32, no. 1, pp. 22–32, 2016.
[18] M. Kikuchi, S. Koyasu, S. Shinohara, Y. Imai, M. Hino, and Y. Naito, "Preoperative diagnostic strategy for parotid gland tumors using diffusion-weighted MRI and technetium-99m pertechnetate scintigraphy: a prospective study," *PLoS One*, vol. 11, no. 2, Article ID e0148973, 2016.
[19] G. S. Weinstein, R. T. Harvey, W. Zimmer, S. Ter, and A. Alavi, "Techentium-99m pertechnetate salivary gland imaging: its role in diagnosis of Warthin's tumor," *Journal of Nuclear Medicine*, vol. 35, no. 1, pp. 179–183, 1994.
[20] E. Schwarz, S. Hürlimann, J. D. Soyka, L. Bortoluzzi, and K. Strobel, "FDG-positive Warthin's tumors in cervical lymph nodes mimicking metastases in tongue cancer staging with PET/CT," *Otolaryngology-Head and Neck Surgery*, vol. 140, no. 1, pp. 134-135, 2009.

8

Soft Palate Pleomorphic Adenoma of a Minor Salivary Gland

C. T. Forde, R. Millard, and S. Ali

Department of Otolaryngology, The Royal London Hospital, Whitechapel Road, Whitechapel, London E1 1BB, UK

Correspondence should be addressed to C. T. Forde; cillianforde@gmail.com

Academic Editor: Fernando L. Dias

Approximately 10% of pleomorphic adenomas occur in the minor salivary glands with the palate being the most common site. Pleomorphic adenomas account for the majority of palatal tumours; however, minor salivary gland tumours have a higher risk of malignancy compared to tumours of the major salivary glands, so appropriate diagnostic evaluation should be prompt. We present a case of a 52-year-old man with a longstanding history of a soft palate pleomorphic adenoma which required excision under general anaesthetic via a mandibular swing approach. As well as the surgical approach to access this tumour; this case is unique as it is the largest soft palate pleomorphic adenoma reported in the literature. We discuss the appropriate preoperative investigations and airway considerations for this patient, as well as the factors to consider when planning operative management of palatal tumours.

1. Introduction

Pleomorphic adenomas (PAs) are the commonest tumour of both the major and minor salivary glands, with approximately 10% of PAs occurring in the minor salivary glands. The palate is the most common site of minor salivary gland PA, but other sites may also be affected, including the lips, cheek, floor of mouth, and nasal cavity [1].

To the best of our knowledge, this case is the largest pleomorphic adenoma of the soft palate which has been excised via a mandibular swing procedure. This case required careful preoperative planning with regards to surgical approach and airway management.

2. Case Presentation

A 53-year-old man presented to our department complaining of longstanding progressive dysphagia and a "hot potato" voice. He had only been managing a soft or liquid diet, and he slept with two pillows due to dyspnoea when lying flat and on exertion. He also complained of significant weight loss.

He reported that he had a lump in his mouth for thirty years and had previously presented to ENT services both in England and abroad, but he did not attend follow-up.

Clinical examination revealed a large left-sided oropharyngeal mass originating from the soft palate and extending inferiorly. The overlying mucosa was normal in appearance.

Magnetic resonance imaging (MRI) demonstrated a large tumour which originated from the soft palate and extended to the larynx, measuring 9.96 cm in craniocaudal dimensions (Figure 1). Computed tomography (CT) angiography demonstrated moderate vascularity of the tumour with a hypertrophied left ascending pharyngeal artery.

Radiological assessment was consistent with either a myoepithelioma, a pleomorphic adenoma, or a low-grade mucoepidermoid tumour. Fine-needle aspiration cytology (FNAC) was consistent with an epithelial neoplasm, possibly of salivary gland origin (Figure 2). The multidisciplinary team decision was for surgical management.

Due to the impossibility of oropharyngeal or nasopharyngeal intubation, he underwent a local anaesthetic tracheostomy with transnasal humidified rapid-insufflation ventilatory exchange (THRIVE). Access to the tumour was gained via a lip-split mandibulotomy and mandibular swing procedure. The whole encapsulated mass was excised from the soft palate and left parapharyngeal space via a submucosal dissection (Figures 3 and 4). The wound was then closed primarily using the abundant redundant mucosa which was sutured to the left

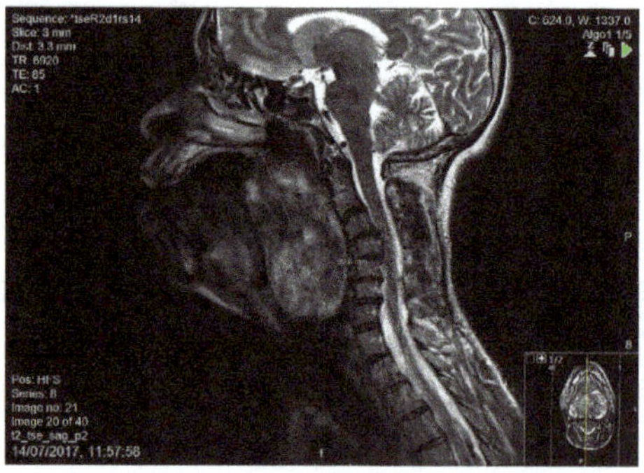

Figure 1: Sagittal T2-weighted MRI image demonstrating the size of the tumour in craniocaudal dimension.

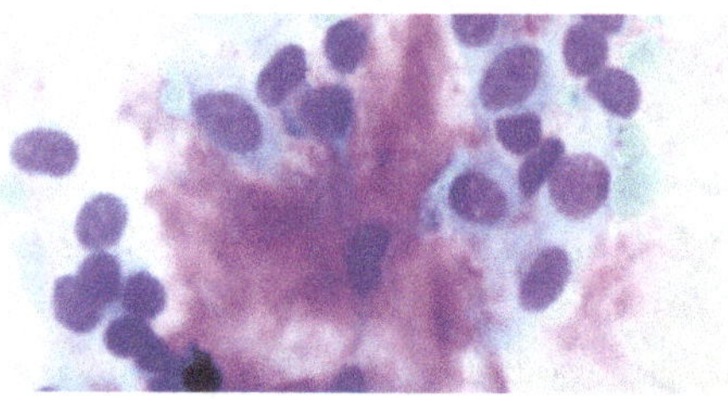

Figure 2: Fine-needle aspiration cytology demonstrating epithelial cells and a metachromatically staining stroma (×400 magnification).

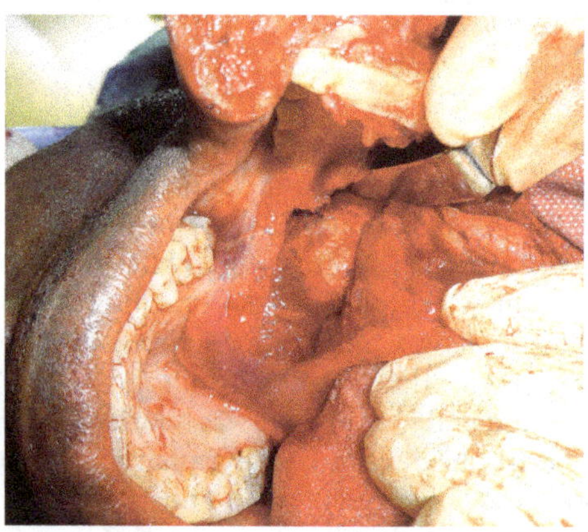

Figure 3: Intraoperative image demonstrating the tumour location.

lateral pharyngeal wall. He had an uneventful postoperative course and, following decannulation, his voice returned to normal, and he was deemed 100% intelligible scoring 0 on the GRBAS scale [2].

Video fluoroscopy demonstrated significant dysphagia due to reduction in pharyngeal bulk and failure of approximation of tongue base. Having been fed via a nasogastric tube for 6 weeks, he is currently tolerating a premashed diet with supraglottic swallowing manoeuvres. He is undergoing further swallow rehabilitation and remains under clinical surveillance.

Histopathological examination of the excised mass demonstrated a benign encapsulated neoplasm composed of epithelium in a variety of architectural patterns consistent with a pleomorphic adenoma (Figures 5 and 6).

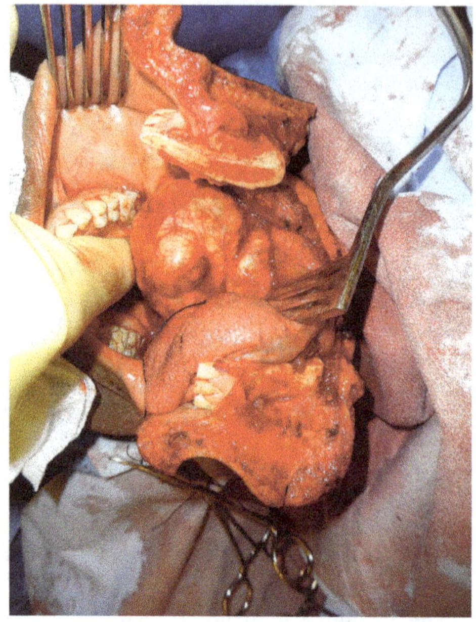

Figure 4: Intraoperative image demonstrating the excision of the tumour.

3. Discussion

Pleomorphic adenomas (PAs) are the commonest tumour of both major and minor salivary glands with about 80–90% of PA occurring in the parotid gland [3]. PA makes up approximately 40% of intraoral minor salivary gland tumours (IMSGT), and about 54% of these occur in the palate [4]. The highest incidence of palatal PA occurs between the fourth and sixth decade with a slight female preponderance [4, 5]. Previous case series have demonstrated that IMSGT are malignant in approximately 41–44% of cases [1, 4].

At $9 \times 7.5 \times 3.9$ cm, the PA in our case represents the largest soft palate PA reported in the literature. The previous largest soft palate PA was 7×6 cm [6], with multiple various midsized tumours also being reported [7].

PAs demonstrate a wide variety of histological features and growth patterns. Three main histologic subgroups of pleomorphic adenoma have been identified: myxoid, cellular, and mixed (classic) type [8], almost all of which have a fibrous pseudocapsule [9].

Due to the higher risk of malignancy with IMSGTs, appropriate preoperative diagnostic investigations are appropriate. von Stempel et al. [10] suggest that MRI is useful for imaging submucosal palatal lesions like a pleomorphic adenoma as they characteristically return low T1-weighted signal and high T2-weighted signal, often with a low-signal fibrous capsule. MRI can evaluate perineural spread and provides excellent soft tissue definition. They also recommend CT scanning to assess for bony erosion, which could indicate a more aggressive lesion. In our case, a CT angiogram was also performed preoperatively due to the size of the neoplasm and the need to identify any large feeding vessels when planning the operative approach.

Intraoral ultrasound is also suggested as an adjunct [10], particularly with regard to obtaining tissue for FNAC.

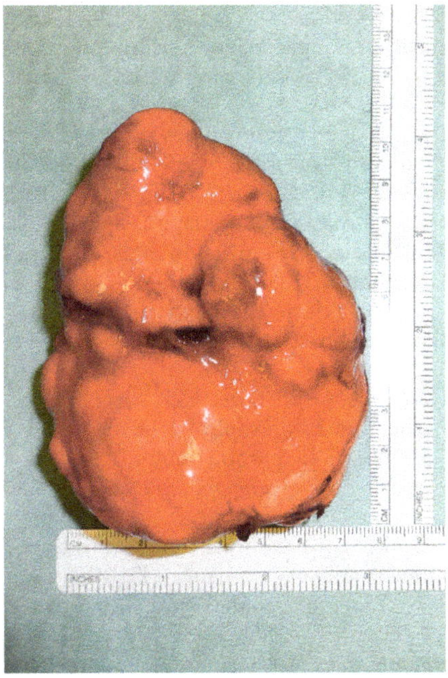

FIGURE 5: Macroscopic picture of the tumour.

Fine-needle aspiration cytology aims to differentiate benign from malignant disease, allowing more accurate counselling of the patient and aiding with surgical planning. FNAC has an accuracy of 82–97% for the preoperative diagnosis of pleomorphic adenoma [11–16]. When aspirated, PA shows combinations of three elements: ductal cells, chondromyxoid matrix, and myoepithelial cells. The diagnosis of PA is reasonably apparent when these three components are present [17]. Other studies [14, 18] have demonstrated that FNAC is reasonably accurate at excluding malignant disease in order to allow more accurate surgical planning.

Anaesthetic considerations when managing IMSGT of the palate are important, particularly given the size of the tumour we report. Due to the extent of the tumour, neither endotracheal nor fibreoptic nasal intubation was an option; therefore, the decision to proceed to tracheostomy was made. In conjunction with our anaesthetic colleagues, transnasal humidified rapid-insufflation ventilatory exchange (THRIVE) was used during the tracheostomy. THRIVE consists of high-flow humidified nasal oxygen therapy, delivered at up to 70 L/min, using OptiFlow (Fisher and Paykel Healthcare Limited, New Zealand). It has been shown to maintain oxygen saturations and extend apnoea time in patients with difficult airways [19]. THRIVE has proved to be an important adjunct during the awake tracheostomy in a previous local anaesthetic tracheostomy [20], and it proved similarly effective in this case.

The best approach for management of palatal pleomorphic adenomas is a wide excision with negative margins [21], especially as malignant transformation has been described at a rate of 1.9–23.3% [22]. Recurrence of minor salivary gland tumours is uncommon [23] but increased by intraoperative tumour spillage and inadequate surgical excision [24]. Radiotherapy is reserved for inoperable or recurrent tumours.

There are many surgical approaches possible for tumours of the soft palate, including intraoral, transcervical, and mandibulotomy and mandibular swing. The surgical approach taken depends on the size and location of the tumour, and as this tumour extended from the soft palate to the parapharyngeal space, a transmandibular approach was deemed necessary to allow adequate exposure in order to ensure complete tumour excision and control of any feeding vessels in order to prevent haemorrhage. Five considerations have been suggested by Papadogeorgakis et al. [25] when deciding the optimal surgical approach for excision of tumour of the soft palate and parapharyngeal space. They are as follows:

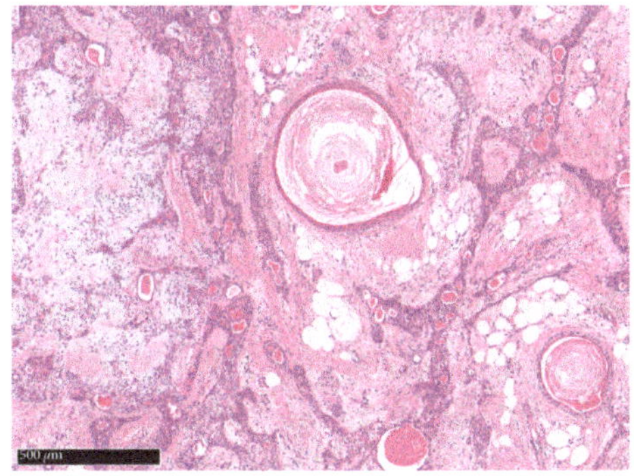

FIGURE 6: H&E stained microscopic image of the tumour (×5 magnification) demonstrating single cells in a myxochondroid stroma, keratin cysts, and tubules with adipocytic stromal change.

(1) Size of the tumour
(2) Suspicion of malignancy
(3) Proximity and the projection of the tumour to the oropharyngeal wall or the neck
(4) Vascularity
(5) Relation of the tumour to the neck neurovascular bundle

Our tumour was mainly oropharyngeal, with extension to the infratemporal fossa. The inferior component was also suprahyoid. Therefore, it was felt that a lip-split mandibulotomy would give good access and delivery of the tumour. We were prepared, however, to extend the neck incision should a combined cervical approach have been necessary.

Our approach gave excellent tumour exposure. From the outset, we were able to fully mobilise and separate the tumour laterally and ensure no major feeding vessels. This approach allowed adequate excision and reduced the chance of capsule rupture and recurrence. The disadvantages of a mandibulotomy include malunion, malocclusion, injury to the mental nerve, and the cosmetic and functional consequences of the lip-split.

4. Conclusion

Soft palate pleomorphic adenomas of this size are rare. Appropriate diagnostic evaluation with FNAC and radiological investigations should be prompt due to the higher risk of malignancy in minor salivary glands compared to tumours of the major salivary glands.

Excisional biopsy is necessary to provide an accurate histopathological diagnosis, and careful preoperative planning should be undertaken in order assess the best surgical approach to ensure complete excision.

A comprehensive airway strategy should be planned before excision of any palatal lesion, including the use of adjuncts, such as THRIVE, if deemed appropriate.

Conflicts of Interest

The authors declare that there are no conflicts of interest regarding the publication of this paper.

References

[1] F. R. Pires, G. A. Pringle, O. P. de Almeida, and S. Y. Chen, "Intra-oral minor salivary gland tumors: a clinicopathological study of 546 cases," *Oral Oncology*, vol. 43, no. 5, pp. 463–470, 2007.

[2] J. M. Wood, T. Athanasiadis, and J. Allen, "Laryngitis," *BMJ*, vol. 349, p. g5827, 2014.

[3] J. W. Eveson and R. A. Cawson, "Salivary gland tumours. A review of 2410 cases with particular reference to histological types, site, age and sex distribution," *Journal of Pathology*, vol. 146, no. 1, pp. 51–58, 1985.

[4] A. Buchner, P. W. Merrell, and W. M. Carpenter, "Relative frequency of intra-oral minor salivary gland tumors: a study of 380 cases from northern California and comparison to reports from other parts of the world," *Journal of Oral Pathology & Medicine*, vol. 36, no. 4, pp. 207–214, 2007.

[5] C. A. Waldron, S. K. El-Mofty, and D. R. Gnepp, "Tumors of the intraoral minor salivary glands: a demographic and histologic study of 426 cases," *Oral Surgery, Oral Medicine, Oral Pathology*, vol. 66, no. 3, pp. 323–333, 1988.

[6] N. K. Sahoo, M. N. Rangan, and R. D. Gadad, "Pleomorphic adenoma palate: major tumor in a minor gland," *Annals of Maxillofacial Surgery*, vol. 3, no. 2, pp. 195–197, 2013.

[7] D. Passi, H. Ram, S. R. Dutta, and L. R. Malkunje, "Pleomorphic adenoma of soft palate: unusual occurrence of the major tumor in minor salivary gland—a case report and literature review," *Journal of Maxillofacial and Oral Surgery*, vol. 16, no. 4, pp. 500–505, 2017.

[8] G. Seifert and K. Donath, "Multiple tumours of the salivary glands–terminology and nomenclature," *European Journal of Cancer Part B: Oral Oncology*, vol. 32, no. 1, pp. 3–7, 1996.

[9] E. Stennert, O. Guntinas-Lichius, J. P. Klussmann, and G. Arnold, "Histopathology of pleomorphic adenoma in the parotid gland: a prospective unselected series of 100 cases," *Laryngoscope*, vol. 111, no. 12, pp. 2195–2200, 2001.

[10] C. von Stempel, S. Morley, T. Beale, and S. Otero, "Imaging of palatal lumps," *Clinical Radiology*, vol. 72, no. 2, pp. 97–107, 2017.

[11] C. M. Heaton, J. L. Chazen, A. van Zante, C. M. Glastonbury, E. J. Kezirian, and D. W. Eisele, "Pleomorphic adenoma of the major salivary glands: diagnostic utility of FNAB and MRI," *Laryngoscope*, vol. 123, no. 12, pp. 3056–3060, 2013.

[12] H. Wang, C. Fundakowski, J. S. Khurana, and N. Jhala, "Fine-needle aspiration biopsy of salivary gland lesions," *Archives of Pathology & Laboratory Medicine*, vol. 139, no. 12, pp. 1491–1497, 2015.

[13] J. K. Gudmundsson, A. Ajan, and J. Abtahi, "The accuracy of fine-needle aspiration cytology for diagnosis of parotid gland masses: a clinicopathological study of 114 patients," *Journal of Applied Oral Science*, vol. 24, no. 6, pp. 561–567, 2016.

[14] N. S. Ali, S. Akhtar, M. Junaid, S. Awan, and K. Aftab, "Diagnostic accuracy of fine needle aspiration cytology in parotid lesions," *ISRN Surgery*, vol. 2011, Article ID 721525, 5 pages, 2011.

[15] S. R. Orell, "Diagnostic difficulties in the interpretation of fine needle aspirates of salivary gland lesions: the problem revisited," *Cytopathology*, vol. 6, no. 5, pp. 285–300, 1995.

[16] S. Zurrida, L. Alasio, N. Tradati, C. Bartoli, F. Chiesa, and S. Pilotti, "Fine-needle aspiration of parotid masses," *Cancer*, vol. 72, no. 8, pp. 2306–2311, 1993.

[17] M. W. Stanley, "Selected problems in fine needle aspiration of head and neck masses," *Modern Pathology*, vol. 15, no. 3, pp. 342–350, 2002.

[18] D. H. Mallon, M. Kostalas, F. J. MacPherson, A. Parmar, A. Drysdale, and E. Chisholm, "The diagnostic value of fine needle aspiration in parotid lumps," *Annals of The Royal College of Surgeons of England*, vol. 95, no. 4, pp. 258–262, 2013.

[19] A. Patel and S. A. R. Nouraei, "Transnasal humidified rapid-insufflation ventilatory exchange (THRIVE): a physiological method of increasing apnoea time in patients with difficult airways," *Anaesthesia*, vol. 70, no. 3, pp. 323–329, 2015.

[20] L. Abeysundara, H. Parker, A. Fowler, and A. Patel, "The use of transnasal humidified rapid-insufflation ventilatory exchange (THRIVE) to facilitate tracheostomy under sedation," *Anaesthesia Cases*, vol. 2016, 2016.

[21] W. M. Mendenhall, C. M. Mendenhall, J. W. Werning, R. S. Malyapa, and N. P. Mendenhall, "Salivary gland pleomorphic adenoma," *American Journal of Clinical Oncology*, vol. 31, no. 1, pp. 95–99, 2008.

[22] M. Ethunandan, R. Witton, G. Hoffman, A. Spedding, and P. A. Brennan, "Atypical features in pleomorphic adenoma—a clinicopathologic study and implications for management," *International Journal of Oral and Maxillofacial Surgery*, vol. 35, no. 7, pp. 608–612, 2006.

[23] R. E. Hickman, R. A. Cawson, and S. W. Duffy, "The prognosis of specific types of salivary gland tumors," *Cancer*, vol. 54, no. 8, pp. 1620–1624, 1984.

[24] Y.-L. Kuo, T.-Y. Tu, C.-Y. Chang et al., "Extra-major salivary gland pleomorphic adenoma of the head and neck: a 10-year experience and review of the literature," *European Archives of Oto-Rhino-Laryngology*, vol. 268, no. 7, pp. 1035–1040, 2011.

[25] N. Papadogeorgakis, V. Petsinis, L. Goutzanis, G. Kostakis, and C. Alexandridis, "Parapharyngeal space tumors: surgical approaches in a series of 13 cases," *International Journal of Oral and Maxillofacial Surgery*, vol. 39, no. 3, pp. 243–250, 2010.

9

Head and Neck Schwannomas: A Surgical Challenge

Ishtyaque Ansari,[1] Ashfaque Ansari,[2] Arjun Antony Graison,[2] Anuradha J. Patil,[3] and Hitendra Joshi[2]

[1]*Department of Neurosurgery, MGM Medical College & Hospital, Aurangabad, India*
[2]*Department of ENT, MGM Medical College & Hospital, Aurangabad, India*
[3]*Department of Plastic Surgery, MGM Medical College & Hospital, Aurangabad, India*

Correspondence should be addressed to Arjun Antony Graison; drarjunantony@yahoo.com

Academic Editor: Abrão Rapoport

Background. Schwannomas, also known as neurilemmomas, are benign peripheral nerve sheath tumors. They originate from any nerve covered with schwann cell sheath. Schwannomas constitute 25–45% of tumors of the head and neck. About 4% of head and neck schwannomas present as a sinonasal schwannoma. Brachial plexus schwannoma constitute only about 5% of schwannomas. Cervical vagal schwannomas constitute about 2–5% of neurogenic tumors. *Methods.* We present a case series of 5 patients of schwannomas, one arising from the maxillary branch of trigeminal nerve in the maxillary sinus, second arising from the brachial plexus, third arising from the cervical vagus, and two arising from cervical spinal nerves. *Result.* Complete extracapsular excision of the tumors was achieved by microneurosurgical technique with preservation of nerve of origin in all except one. *Conclusion.* Head and neck schwannoma though rare should be considered as a differential diagnosis of a unilateral slow growing mass in the head and neck region, particularly in an adult. Schwannomas are always a diagnostic dilemma as they are asymptomatic for long time, and histopathology is the gold standard for diagnosis. As a rule, treatment is surgical and dictated by the location of the tumor and nerve of origin. Due to its rarity, complex anatomical location and morbidity risk postexcision, they can pose a formidable challenge to surgeons. This study aims to describe the presentation, workup, surgical technique, and outcome.

1. Introduction

Neurilemmoma also known as schwannoma is a benign tumor of nerve sheath origin, arising from any nerve covered with a schwann cell sheath, which includes the cranial nerves (except for optic and olfactory), the spinal nerves, and autonomic nervous system [1, 2].

Schwannomas occurring in the head and neck region are frequent, with 25–45% of all reported schwannomas being found in this region [1].

We present our surgical experience with five such tumors, one arising from the maxillary branch of the trigeminal nerve in the maxillary sinus, second arising from the brachial plexus, third arising from the cervical vagus, and two arising from cervical spinal nerves. The clinical presentation, surgical treatment, and outcomes of patients with this pathology are described.

2. Materials and Methods

A retrospective analysis was done at MGM Medical College and Hospital, Aurangabad, from January 2015 to December 2016. Of the five patients, two were female and three were males, with a mean age of 33 years (ranging from 23 to 40 years). Complete excision of the tumors was achieved by extracapsular excision using microneurosurgical technique with operating microscope. Preservation of nerve of origin was achieved in all except one where conventional extracapsular excision technique was applied. Surgical observation, histopathology, and immunochemistry confirmed the tumors to be benign schwannomas in all five cases. There was no recurrence in any of the five patients (on clinical examination) at one year follow-up.

2.1. Case 1. We describe a rare case of schwannoma arising primarily from the maxillary sinus extending into the orbit and intracranially. A 40-year-old female presented with headache since 2 years, left nostril discharge since 1 year, and left eye progressive vision loss since 1 year.

Diagnostic nasal endoscopy (DNE) revealed left-sided nasal mass, pale, firm, pinkish in colour, not bleeding on touch. Clinical examination revealed reduced vision in the left eye with finger counting less than five feet, with mild proptosis of the left eye. There was no motor or sensory loss with no other cranial nerve dysfunction.

Contrast-enhanced CT (CECT) scan with cisternography revealed a large lobulated mass of size 81 × 53 × 82 mm in the left zygomatic and masseteric region with intracranial extension (Figure 1(a)). The lesion was causing thinning and pressure erosion of the posterior wall of maxillary sinus, pterygoid plate, posterior wall of orbit, medial wall of sphenoid on the left side, left lesser wing of sphenoid, and was causing thinning of left anterior clinoid process.

Superiorly, mass was extending to middle cranial fossa and displacing left middle temporal lobe. Medially, it was extending to left nasal cavity causing complete blockage. Posteriorly, it was extending to the posterior nasopharyngeal region. Laterally, it was involving and abutting the masseter and pterygoid muscles and intraorbital muscles. Superiorly, it was extending to the infraorbital region and displacing and compressing the left optic nerve. Lamina papyracea and cribriform plate were intact.

Clinical features and CECT were suggestive of malignant tumor. This divisive situation steered us to keep a possibility of a malignant component in the tumor.

The tumor was approached through Weber Furguson incision with subciliary extension. Left suprastructure maxillotomy was done. Tumor was firm, necrotic, moderately vascular, and grayish white (Figure 2(a)) and found arising from the maxillary nerve. Tumour was found to be arising from the left maxilla, breaching it's posterior wall and floor of orbit, extending into the retroorbital portion of orbit through the superior orbital fissure into the left temporal lobe. Total excision of the tumor was carried out. Left temporal bone base was reached, and temporal lobe was identified. Total excision of intracranial portion of tumor was achieved. Bleeding from the left cavernous sinus was controlled with Abgel® and Surgicel®. Orbital floor reconstruction was done with titanium mesh. Maxilla reconstruction was done with titanium mesh and plate (Figure 2(b)). Postoperatively, patient had an uneventful recovery, with minimal left eye vision improvement (Figure 1(b)).

2.2. Case 2. We describe a 35-year-old female who presented with right-sided supraclavicular swelling since 3 years (Figure 3) and complained of paraesthesia over the right upper limb. There was no history of trauma, fever, and systemic illness. The patient had evidence of right C5, C6 radicular pain, and hypoesthesia. The patient had no complains of weakness, loss of function of upper limb. On local examination, a single spherical swelling was present in the right supraclavicular area measuring 5 × 5 cms. Muscle power in all muscles was 5/5, sensations were intact, and there were no signs of wasting. Tinel sign was positive with the patient, and she reported tingling sensation "pins and needles" along the shoulder tip. Spurling's test was negative in this patient.

Pre- and postcontrast MRI neck screening revealed a well-defined, rounded space occupying lesion in the right side of the neck, that was found to be lateral to the neck vessels and superficial to the subclavian vessels. The lesion was hyperintense on T2-weighted images and STIR (short T1 inversion recovery) images and was found to be isointense on T1-weighted images with heterogeneous contrast enhancement in the lesion (Figure 4). These features were suggestive of a neurogenic tumor.

Under general anaesthesia, the tumor was approached using a V-shaped incision. The brachial plexus was explored. The tumor was found arising from the upper trunk of the brachial plexus and was found to be adherent to the middle and lower trunk of the brachial plexus (Figure 5(a)). The tumor appeared to be greyish white, firm, and globular (Figure 5(b)). The tumor was carefully excised in toto after debulking by microneurosurgical technique. Intra-op nerve stimulator was used for localising the nerve fascicles around the tumor and during excision. After excision, the nerve fascicles were found to be intact. Postoperatively, the patient complained of paraesthesia of the right upper limb which recovered in two weeks.

2.3. Case 3. We describe a 23-year-old male patient who presented with right-sided painless neck swelling since one month. There was no history of trauma, fever, and systemic illness. The patient had no complains of weakness, dysphagia, and hoarseness of voice. On local examination, a single ovoid swelling was present in the right carotid triangle, anterior to the sternocleidomastoid, measuring 3 × 2 cms. Swelling did not move on deglutition or tongue protrusion. There was no loss of muscle power in all muscles, no signs of wasting, or neurological deficits.

USG neck showed a hypoechoic lesion seen at bifurcation of the carotid artery. Moderate central and peripheral vascularity was seen within the lesion. Findings were suggestive of a carotid body tumor/nerve sheath tumor.

CECT neck revealed a well-defined, well-encapsulated, peripherally enhancing soft tissue mass lesion of size 3.4 × 1.8 cm (Figure 6). The mass lesion was noted in the right carotid sheath between the right common carotid artery and internal jugular vein, posterolateral to the right lobe of thyroid. The lesion was seen below the carotid bifurcation. Features were suggestive of a vagal schwannoma.

The tumor was approached by an anterior approach along the medial border of sternocleidomastoid. Platysma and fascia were dissected to reach the tumor. There was a medium-sized globular smooth mass, well-encapsulated seen engulfing the vagus nerve (Figures 7(a)–7(c)). Extracapsular tumor excision was done in toto by conventional technique. Vagus was severed in the process. Vagus was reanastomosed, using the sural nerve graft (Figure 7(d)).

Postoperatively, the patient had mild dysphagia which resolved in two days. The patient reported a minimal change in voice. There were no signs of aspiration. Postoperative videolaryngoscopic assessment revealed right vocal cord palsy. The patient's voice improved with speech therapy.

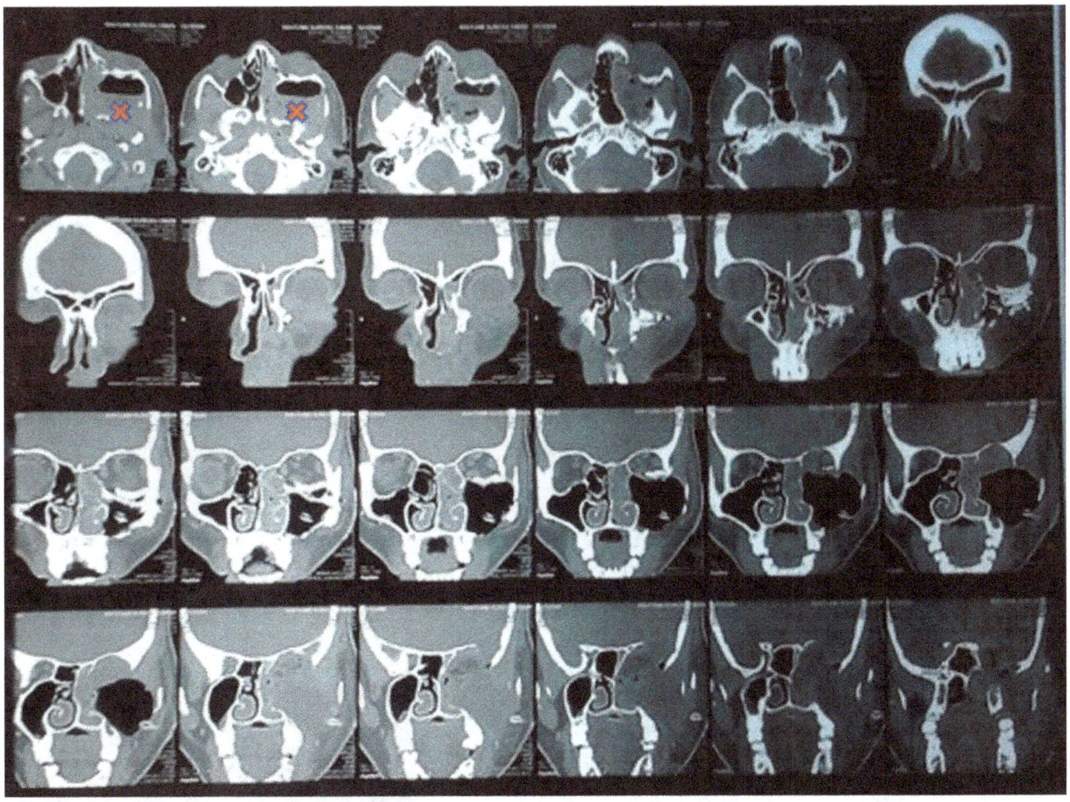

(a)

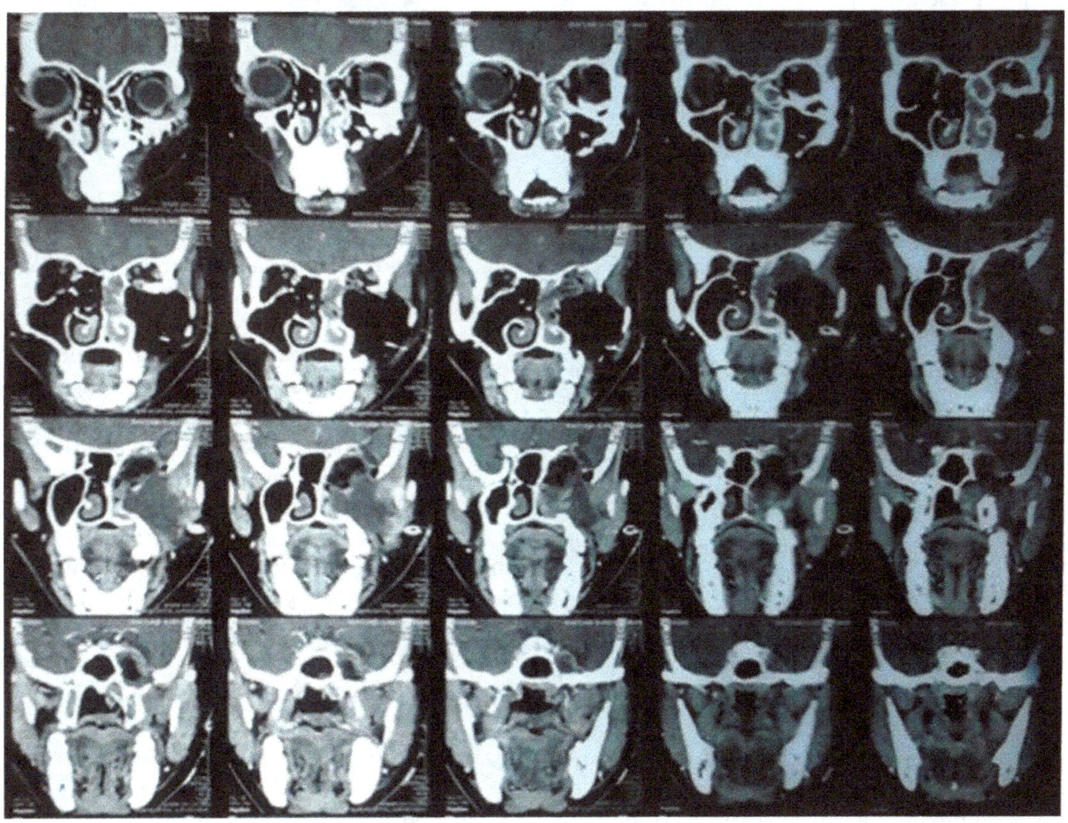

(b)

FIGURE 1: (a) Preoperative CT showing the tumor (*) present in the posterior part of the left maxillary sinus and the left nostril. (b) Postoperative CT.

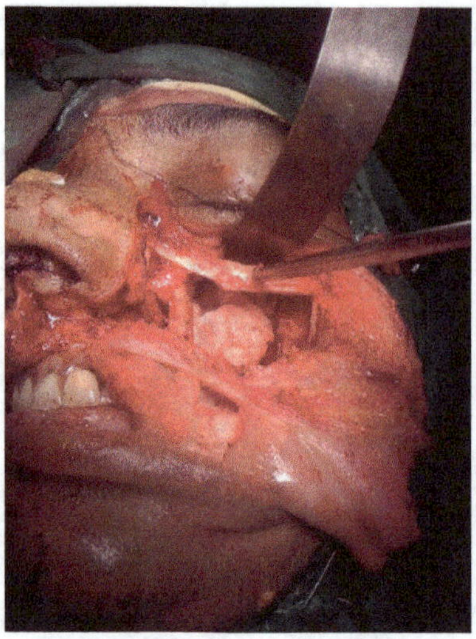

(a)

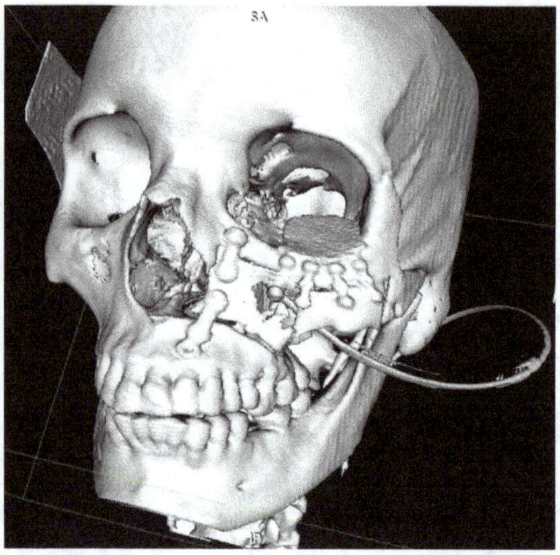

(b)

Figure 2: (a) Intraoperative picture. (b) Postoperative 3DCT reconstruction: orbital floor and maxilla reconstruction done with titanium mesh and plate.

2.4. Case 4. We present a 30-year-old male patient who presented with left-sided painless neck swelling since two years. It was insidious in onset and gradually progressed in size. The patient had no complains of weakness, dysphagia, and hoarseness of voice. On local examination, a single ovoid swelling was present in the left carotid triangle, anterior to the sternocleidomastoid, measuring 5 × 3 cms. Swelling did not move on deglutition or tongue protrusion. There was no loss of muscle power in all muscles, no signs of wasting, or neurological deficits.

MRI neck with angiography and CECT neck revealed a moderately enhancing lesion of size 63 × 45 × 34 mm in left carotid space causing splaying of internal and external carotid artery, anteriorly abutting the submandibular gland with no evidence of encasement of the vessels (Figure 8).

The tumor was approached by an lateral approach along the lateral border of sternocleidomastoid, 3.5 cms below the auricle. External jugular vein ligated. Tumor was found attached to the C1 spinal nerve. Extracapsular tumor excision was done in toto by microneurosurgical technique (Figure 9). Minivac® drain was placed.

Postoperatively, the patient had mild ptosis of the left eye lid with marginal mandibular nerve paresis and features suggestive of first bite syndrome, all of which improved with physiotherapy. There was no vocal cord paralysis. The patient is currently free of all symptoms at one year follow-up.

2.5. Case 5. We present a 35-year-old male patient who presented with right-sided neck swelling since six months. The patient had complaints of right-sided mild ear pain and no complains of weakness, dysphagia, and hoarseness of voice. On local examination, a single ovoid swelling was present in the left carotid triangle, anterior to the sternocleidomastoid, measuring 4 × 4 cms. There was no loss of muscle power in all muscles, no signs of wasting, or neurological deficits.

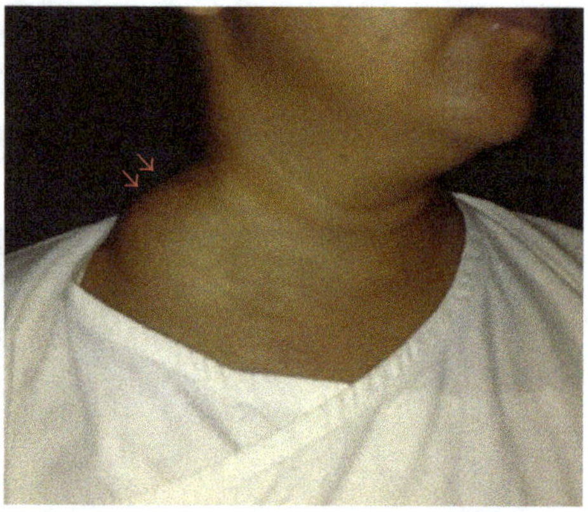

Figure 3: Pre-op image (arrows indicating tumor).

MRI neck revealed an oval solid lesion of size 42 × 41 × 28 mm in the right carotid triangle, laterally abutting sternocleidomastoid and posteriorly the paraspinal muscle. The lesion was hyperintense on T2W and FLAIR (Fluid Attenuated Inversion Recovery) images and hypointense on T1W images (Figure 10).

The tumor was approached by anterior approach along the medial border of sternocleidomastoid. The tumor was seen involving the cervical spinal nerve. Extracapsular tumor excision was done in toto by microneurosurgical technique, preserving the involved nerve. Post-op recovery was uneventful and devoid of any complications or deficits.

3. Discussion

Schwannomas can arise from any nerve which has schwann cells except optic and olfactory nerve as they lack those cells [1].

These tumors are generally encapsulated except from the sinonasal tract and nasopharynx [3].

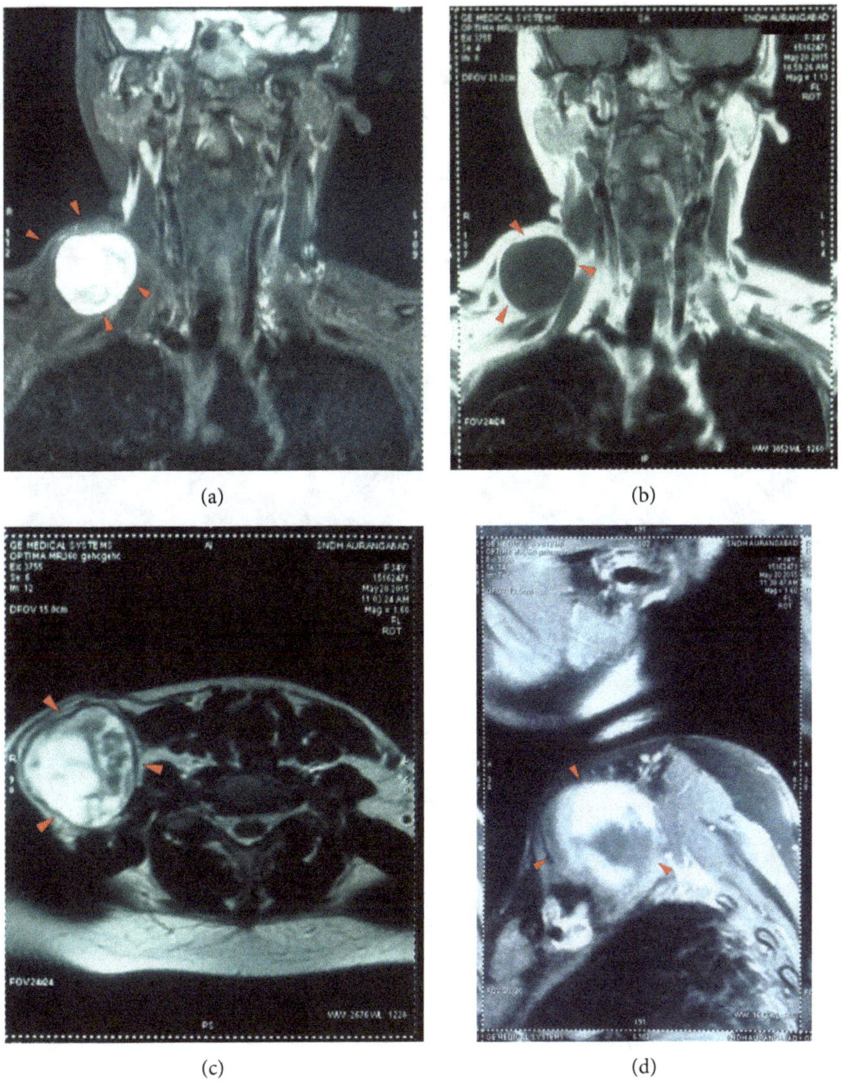

(a) (b) (c) (d)

FIGURE 4: (a) T2-weighted coronal cut. (b) T1-weighted coronal cut. (c) T2-weighted axial cut. (d) Postcontrast T1 sagittal cut.

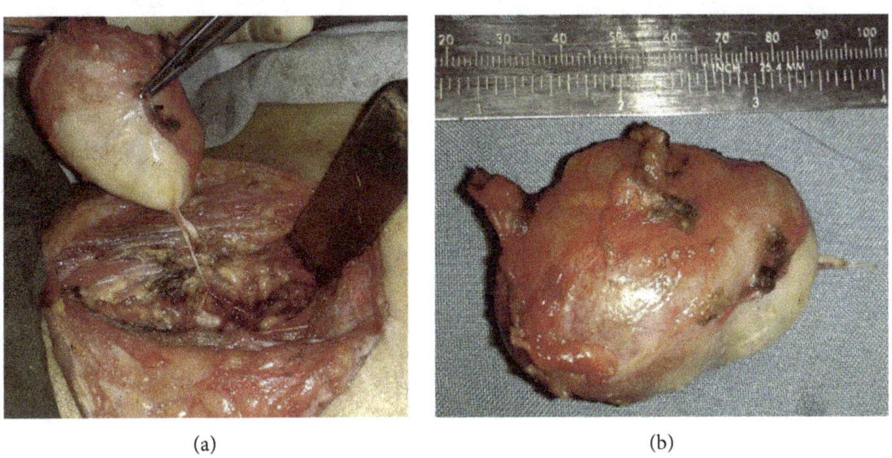

(a) (b)

FIGURE 5: (a) Tumor with nerve attachment. (b) Enucleated tumor with intact capsule.

Most often these tumors are solitary but can occur in multiple areas also. Multiple occurrences are usually associated not only with neurofibromatosis II but also schwannomatosis [4, 5]. Head and neck are the most commonly affected regions (25–45%) with the lateral neck being the frequently involved site [6, 7]. Cytogenetic abnormality of chromosome 22 is

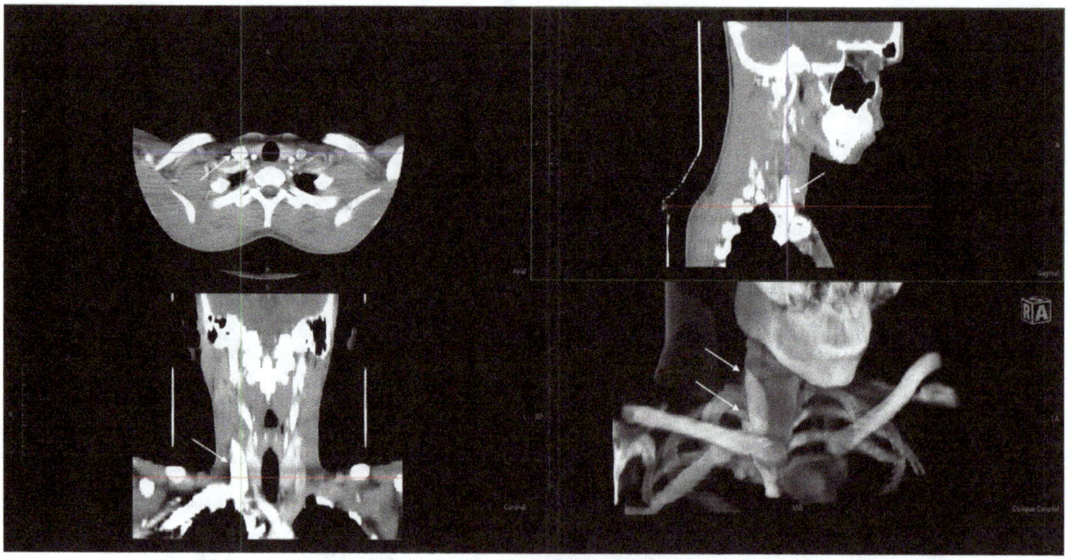

FIGURE 6: Neck mass (arrows).

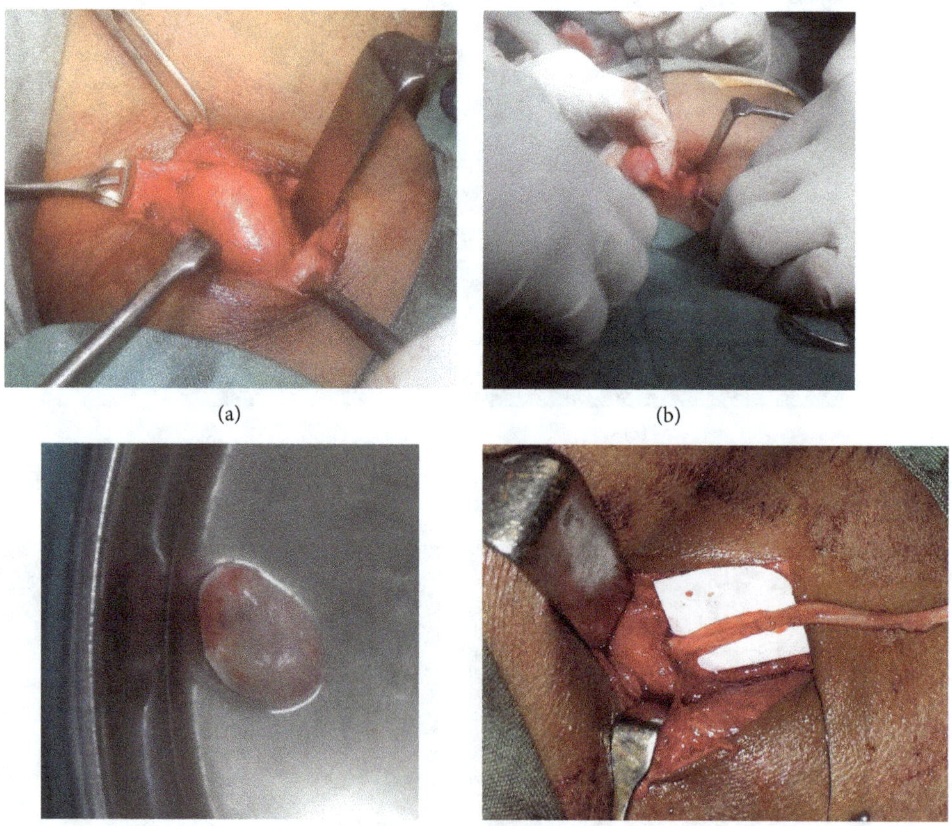

(a) (b) (c) (d)

FIGURE 7: (a) Intra-op tumor excision. (b) Showing the tumor nerve attachment. (c) Enucleated tumor with intact innermost layer of capsule. (d) Vagus reanastomosis using sural nerve graft.

seen in 50% cases, and those are associated with neurofibromatosis II [3, 6].

Sinonasal schwannoma contributes about 4% of head and neck schwannomas [8].

It remains asymptomatic for a quite long period because of slow growth. Nasal obstruction is the main symptom of this tumor. Pain, bony dehiscence including skull base and neural symptoms develop later as the tumor enlarges. It can also simulate rhinosinusitis as clinical features are similar [8].

Brachial plexus tumors are rare comprising of only 5% of all tumors of upper limb [9]. The most frequent site is in the

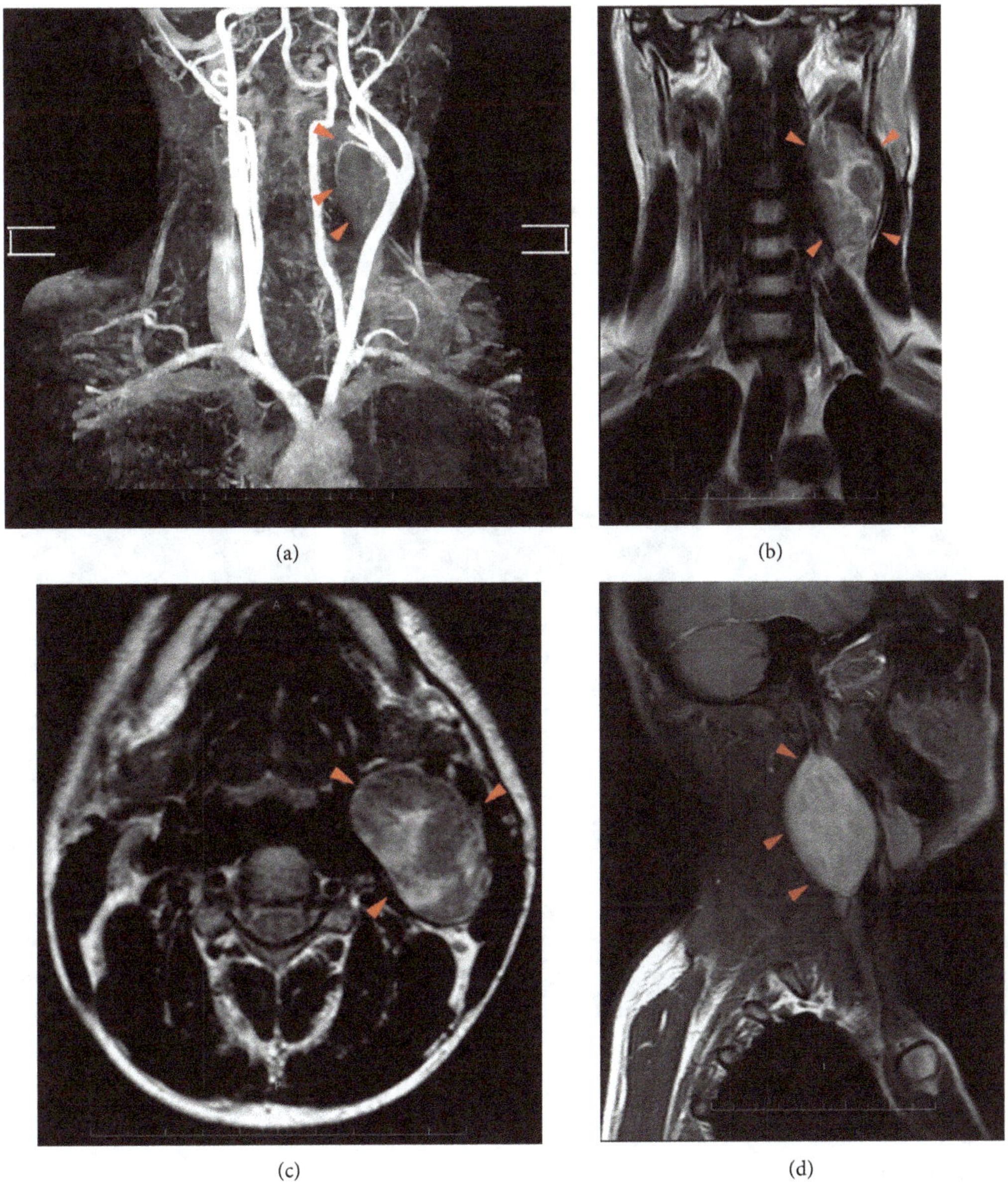

FIGURE 8: (a) MRI angiography showing splaying of the carotids by the tumor. (b) T2-weighted coronal cut. (c) T2-weighted axial cut. (d) Postcontrast T1 sagittal cut.

head and neck, which comprises 25% of all schwannomas and only about 5% of schwannomas present as brachial plexus tumors [10, 11].

The two most common brachial plexus region tumors are the schwannomas and neurofibromas, both of which are benign and arise from the nerve sheath [12].

Most often, early in the course, minimal neurological deficit will be present, or there will be none at all. Manipulation of the mass can produce paraesthesias or "shocks" in the distribution of the affected nerve, and this can be an important aid to diagnosis. Side-to-side mobility greater than longitudinal mobility of the mass from the nerve is more common in cases of benign lesions, whereas malignancy is associated with firmness and immobility [12, 13]. In cases of brachial plexus lesions, MR imaging is the study of choice to delineate the margins of the tumor from surrounding tissues with greatest contrast [13]. Importantly, however, MR imaging is currently unable to differentiate between schwannoma and neurofibroma [13].

Computerized tomography scanning is optimal at revealing osseous erosion around the spine or changes in neural foramina. A newer modality, MR neurography (MR-magnetic resonance), has the potential to demonstrate the entire course of visualized peripheral nerves [13]. Schwannomas of the vagus nerve grow between the common carotid artery and the internal jugular vein. This growth pattern often leads to a divergence of both structures, which is visible in CT scan or MRI [14].

Cervical vagal schwannomas constitute about 2–5% of neurogenic tumors [3]. These tumors usually present as asymptomatic masses as in our case, if symptomatic patients will present with hoarseness as the main symptom. The sign

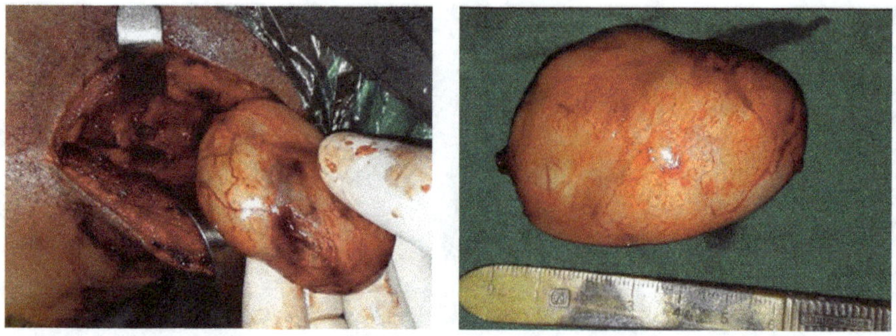

(a) (b)

FIGURE 9: (a) Intraoperative tumor excision. (b) Enucleated tumor with intact innermost layer of capsule.

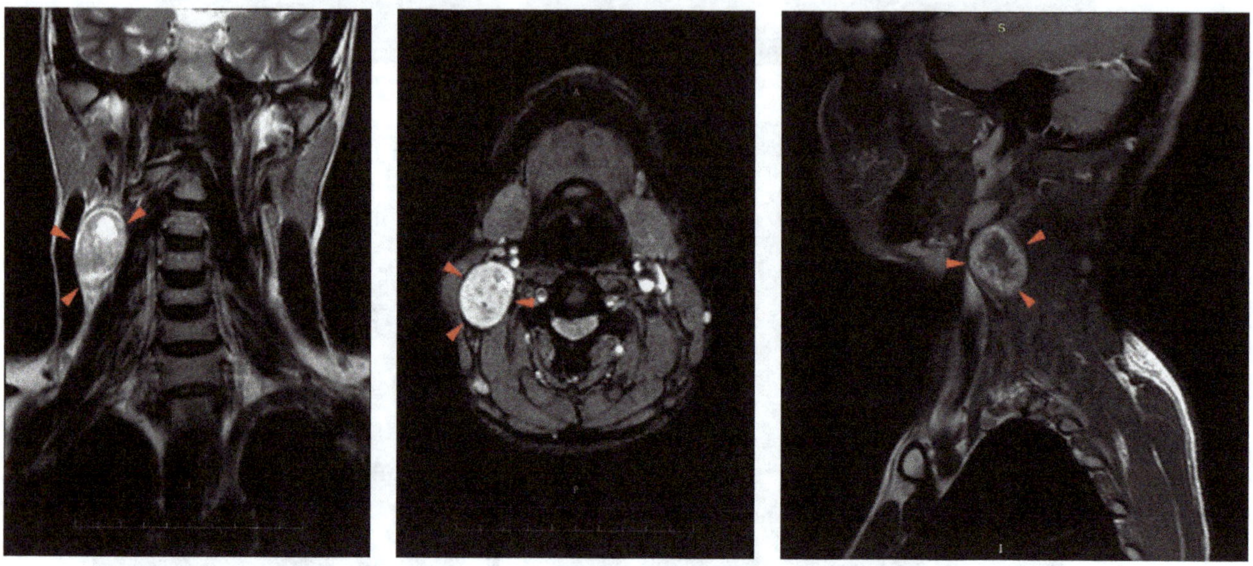

(a) (b) (c)

FIGURE 10: (a) T2-weighted coronal cut. (b) T2-weighted axial cut. (c) Postcontrast T1-weighted sagittal cut.

usually seen in these cases is unilateral vocal cord paralysis. The reported incidence of preoperative vocal cord paralysis is about 12%. Clinical sign elicited in case of vagal schwannoma is a paradoxical cough on palpating the mass due to vagal stimulation. The presence of this sign together with palpation of mass medial to the sternocleidomastoid should arouse the suspicion of a neurogenic tumor [3, 6].

Microscopically (Figure 11), spindle-shaped cells in Antoni-A and Antoni-B arrangement interspersed with Verocay bodies are the characteristic features [2]. These tumor cells typically show a diffuse positive immunoreactivity for S-100 protein [2] and are negative for neurofilament protein. S-100 protein demonstrates a neuroectodermal origin of the tumor [15].

Neurilemmomas are resistant to radiotherapy [2], and as they are well encapsulated, the treatment of choice is conservative surgical enucleation with periodic follow-up. The choice of operation is mainly determined by the relationship between the tumor and the nerve of origin.

Conventional extracapsular excision can damage the normal fascicles during dissection of the capsule. Intracapsular excision with gentle dissection between the tumor capsule and normal fascicles minimizes the risk of nerve damage. The epineurial layer covering the tumor capsule should be dissected in a manner similar to peeling an onion to allow for safe removal of the tumor, which should be approached by its proximal and distal poles (Figure 12). The fascicles located in the tumor are usually nonfunctional; therefore, excision of these fascicles does not lead to neurologic deficits [9]. The use of operating microscope and microneurosurgical technique has modified the outcome of conventional extracapsular excision as was seen in our case series, with minimal postoperative morbidity. This technique facilitates extracapsular tumor excision by microscopic technique along with the nerve fibre coursing through it (if it cannot be separated), thus sparing the other nerve fibres, and maintaining minimum morbidity.

Complete extracapsular excision preserving the nerve of origin should be attempted when feasible [16], but for extensive schwannomas, nerve sacrifice with reconstruction and rehabilitation are important considerations.

The choice of surgical approach is dictated by the size of the tumor, its location, its relationship to the great vessels, and the suspicion of malignancy.

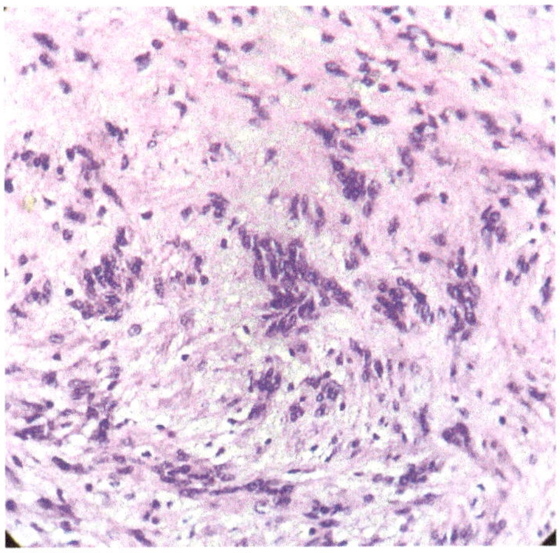

(a)

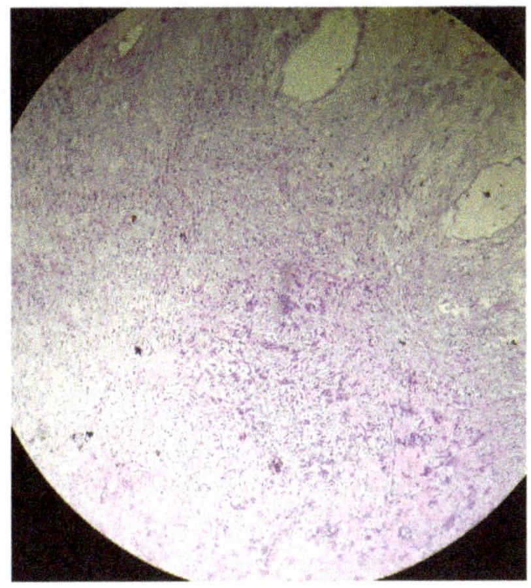

(b)

FIGURE 11: (a) Schwannoma under high power resolution (H&E stain 40x). (b) Schwannoma under low power resolution (H&E stain 10x).

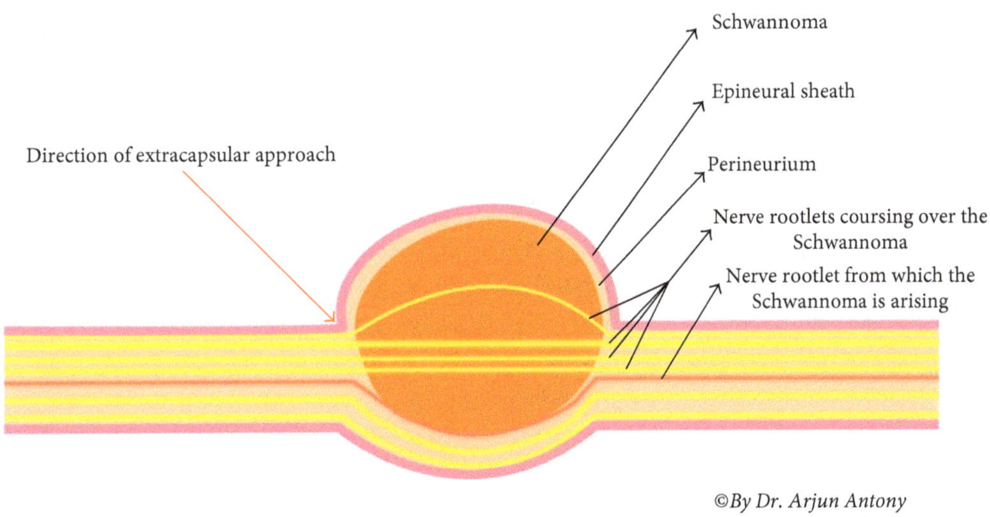

FIGURE 12: Technique of extracapsular excision.

4. Conclusion

This case report emphasises the rarity of schwannomas in maxillary sinus involving the trigeminal, arising from the brachial plexus, vagus nerve, and cervical spinal nerves, respectively. Among surgical techniques, complete extracapsular excision using microneurosurgical technique with operating microscope is the preferred technique advocated. A schwannoma though rare should be considered as a differential diagnosis of a unilateral slow growing mass in the head and neck region particularly in an adult. They are difficult to diagnose preoperatively. Radiologic findings are usually nondiagnostic. Diagnosis relies on clinical suspicion, and confirmation is often obtained by means of surgical pathology. Thorough preoperative counselling of patients to inform them of the potential occurrence of neurological deficit is important. Long-term surveillance is not recommended, even though these tumors are benign and mostly asymptomatic. Recurrence is rare.

Consent

Written informed consents were obtained from the patients for publication of these cases and accompanying images.

Authors' Contributions

Ishtyaque Ansari is the primary author and was the main operating surgeon, involved in design, project supervision, data analysis, editing, and final approval. Ashfaque Ansari was the operating surgeon and involved in project supervision, data analysis, and editing. Arjun Antony Graison is the corresponding author and was the assisting surgeon, responsible for data collection, data analysis, manuscript drafting and editing. Hitendra Joshi and Anuradha J. Patil were the operating surgeons and responsible for editing.

References

[1] J. G. Batsakis, *Tumours of the Peripheral Nervous System*, Williams and Wilkins, Baltimore, MD, USA, 2nd edition, 1979.

[2] A. Verma, K. Banerjee, A. Verma, S. Singh, J. Rao, and P. Om, "Maxillary neurilemmoma-rarest of the rare tumour: report of 2 cases," *International Journal of Surgery Case Reports*, vol. 4, no. 11, pp. 1044–1047, 2013.

[3] S. Vijendra, R. Rao, V. Prasad, S. Haseena, and M. Niprupama, "A giant vagal schwannoma with unusual extension from skull base to the mediastinum," *Journal of Cancer Research and Therapeutics*, vol. 11, no. 4, p. 970, 2015.

[4] J. Gosk, O. Gutkowska, S. Kulinski, M. Urban, and A. Halon, "Multiple schwannomas of the digital nerves and superficial radial nerve: two unusual cases of segmental schwannomatosis," *Folia Neuropathologica*, vol. 53, no. 2, pp. 158–167, 2015.

[5] A. Gonzalvo, A. Fowler, R. J. Cook et al., "Schwannomatosis, sporadic schwannomatosis, and familial schwannomatosis: a surgical series with long-term follow-up," *Journal of Neurosurgery*, vol. 114, no. 3, pp. 756–762, 2010.

[6] S. C. Chang and Y. M. Schi, "Neurilemmoma of the vagus nerve. A case report and brief literature review," *Laryngoscope*, vol. 94, no. 7, pp. 946–949, 1984.

[7] M. P. Colreavy, P. D. Lacy, J. Hughes et al., "Head and neck schwannomas–a 10 year review," *Journal of Laryngology & Otology*, vol. 114, no. 2, pp. 119–124, 2000.

[8] R. S. Minhas, J. S. Thakur, and D. R. Sharma, "Primary schwannoma of maxillary sinus masquerading as malignant tumour," *BMJ Case Reports*, vol. 2013, pp. 10–12, 2013.

[9] T. R. Donner, R. M. Voorhies, and D. G. Kline, "Neural sheath tumors of major nerves," *Journal of Neurosurgery*, vol. 81, no. 3, pp. 362–373, 1994.

[10] J. H. Huang, U. Samadani, and E. L. Zager, "Brachial plexus region tumors: a review of their history, classification, surgical management, and outcomes," *Neurosurgery Quarterly*, vol. 13, no. 3, pp. 151–161, 2003.

[11] K. M. Ahn, H. K. Lee, K. D. Lee, and T. H. Yu, "A case of neurilemmoma of the brachial plexus," *Korean Journal of Otolaryngology*, vol. 8, pp. 733–735, 2002.

[12] A. Ganju, N. Roosen, D. G. Kline, and R. L. Tiel, "Outcomes in a consecutive series of 111 surgically treated plexal tumors: a review of the experience at the Louisiana State University Health Sciences Center," *Journal of Neurosurgery*, vol. 95, no. 1, pp. 51–60, 2001.

[13] D. K. Binder, J. S. Smith, and N. M. Barbaro, "Primary brachial plexus tumors: imaging, surgical, and pathological findings in 25 patients," *Neurosurgical Focus*, vol. 16, no. 5, p. E11, 2004.

[14] S. Jain, K. Houseknecht, A. M. Rojiani, M. Setzer, and F. D. Vrionis, "Management of nerve sheath tumors arising in the sympathetic chain," *Cancer Control: Journal of the Moffitt Cancer Center*, vol. 15, no. 4, pp. 352–357, 2008.

[15] V. A. Budu, I. A. Bulescu, C. G. Popp, B. C. Mocanu, and C. A. Mogoanta, "Vagus nerve schwannoma in the parapharyngeal space: surgical, histological and immunohistochemical aspects. A case report," *Romanian Journal of Morphology and Embryology*, vol. 56, no. 1, pp. 273–276, 2015.

[16] A. Krishnamurthy, V. Ramshankar, and U. Majhi, "A large extra cranial cystic trigeminal schwannoma of the parapharyngeal space-exploring the right approach," *Indian Journal of Surgical Oncology*, vol. 5, no. 3, pp. 196–198, 2014.

10

Hunter Syndrome Diagnosed by Otorhinolaryngologist

Ayako Hashimoto,[1] Tadayuki Kumagai,[2] and Hiroyuki Mineta[3]

[1]*Department of Otorhinolaryngology, Shizuoka Children's Hospital, Shizuoka, Japan*
[2]*Department of Pediatrics, Fujieda City General Hospital, Fujieda, Japan*
[3]*Department of Otorhinolaryngology, Head and Neck Surgery, Hamamatsu University School of Medicine, Hamamatsu, Japan*

Correspondence should be addressed to Ayako Hashimoto; takadaayako@hotmail.com

Academic Editor: Nicolás Pérez Fernández

Hunter syndrome is a lysosomal disease characterized by deficiency of the lysosomal enzyme iduronate-2-sulfatase (I2S). It has an estimated incidence of approximately 1 in 1,62,000 live male births. We report a case of Hunter syndrome diagnosed by an otorhinolaryngologist. To our knowledge, this is the first study diagnosed by an otorhinolaryngologist despite the fact that otorhinolaryngological symptoms manifest at a young age in this disease. The patient was a 4-year-old boy. He underwent adenotonsillectomy. Intubation was difficult, and he had some symptoms which are reasonable as a mucopolysaccharidosis. The otorhinolaryngologist should play an integral role in the multidisciplinary approach to the diagnosis and management of many children with MPS (mucopolysaccharidoses) disorders.

1. Introduction

Hunter syndrome (mucopolysaccharidosis type II (MPS II)) is a lysosomal disease characterized by deficiency of the lysosomal enzyme iduronate-2-sulfatase (I2S). It has an estimated incidence of approximately 1 in 1,62,000 live male births [1] and represents the major type of MPS disorder in East Asian countries. Patients with Hunter syndrome usually appear normal at birth, with clinical signs and symptoms manifesting between 2 and 4 years of age [2]. Clinical manifestations include severe airway obstruction, skeletal deformities, cardiomyopathy, mixed hearing loss, and, in most patients, neurological decline. Most patients exhibit ear, throat, and airway problems and, accordingly, visit ear, nose, and throat (ENT) clinics at a young age [3]. We report a case of Hunter syndrome, which, to our knowledge, is the first to be diagnosed by an otorhinolaryngologist despite the fact that otorhinolaryngological symptoms manifest at a young age in this disease.

2. Case Presentation

The patient was a 4-year-old boy, born at 38 weeks and 3 days of gestation, with a birth weight of 2110 g. He was examined by a neurologist for an arachnoid cyst and intellectual disability. He had a medical history of hospitalization for Kawasaki disease at 2 years of age and underwent operations for inguinal hernia at 10 months and 3 years of age. The patient was referred by an ENT physician from another general hospital, for airway obstruction and hearing loss. An informed consent from parents was obtained.

The patient exhibited a coarse face, stiff joints, and claw hand deformity (Figure 1). The result of conditioned orientation response audiometry was 65 dB. Examination of the oropharynx revealed marked hypertrophy of the tonsils, adenoids, and tongue. A lateral neck X-ray revealed obstruction of the nasopharyngeal airway due to adenoid hypertrophy (Figure 2), and the arytenoid was swollen (Figure 3). A sleep study revealed an apnea-hypopnea index of 19.5 events/h, and obstructive sleep apnea was 98.5%. He also exhibited an ectopic Mongolian spot (Figure 4).

The patient underwent adenotonsillectomy. During the operation, intubation was difficult and was performed using a video laryngo scope. The anesthesiologist suggested the possibility of Hunter syndrome. It was difficult to insert the mouth opener and visualize the lower edge of the tonsils during the operation because of tongue hypertrophy. The patient remained intubated in the pediatric intensive care

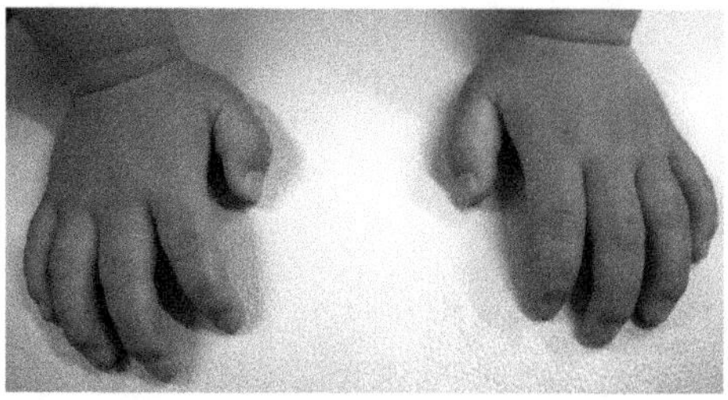

Figure 1: Hand X-ray imaging the clawhand deformity.

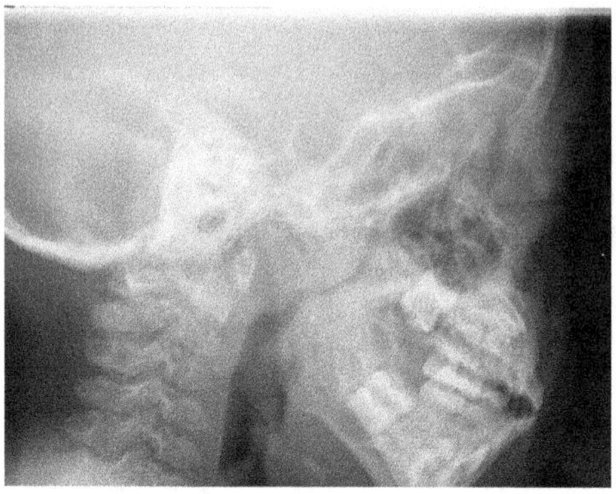

Figure 2: Lateral neck X-ray. Obstruction of the nasopharyngeal airway due to adenoid hypertrophy is apparent.

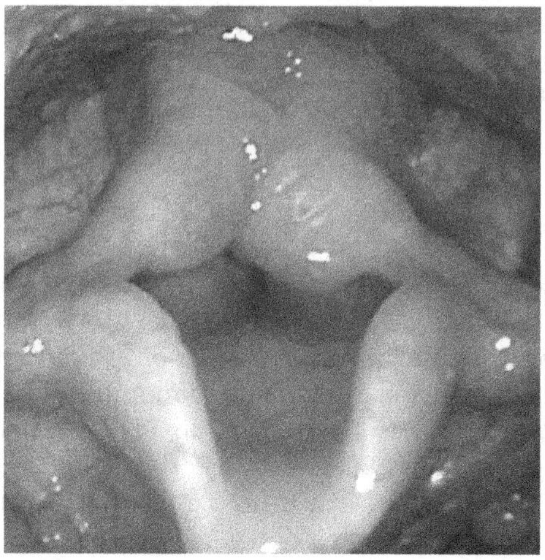

Figure 3: Laryngeal endoscopy revealing swelling in the arytenoid.

unit for two days after operation because of oropharyngeal swelling, especially the uvula. After two days, he was extubated without problem, and the orthopedics department consulted. Chest radiography revealed oar-like ribs (Figure 5) and an egg-shaped chest vertebra (Figure 6). Sharp metacarpal bones in the fingers (Figure 7) and genu valgum (Figure 8) were also revealed by radiography. Furthermore, head magnetic resonance imaging revealed an enlarged Virchow-Robin space (Figure 9). These findings were reasonably consistent with the characteristics of MPS. Uronic acid testing suggested MPS I or MPS II, and an enzyme activity test for I2S yielded a value of <0.7 nmol/mg protein/4 h. He was diagnosed with Hunter syndrome (MPS II).

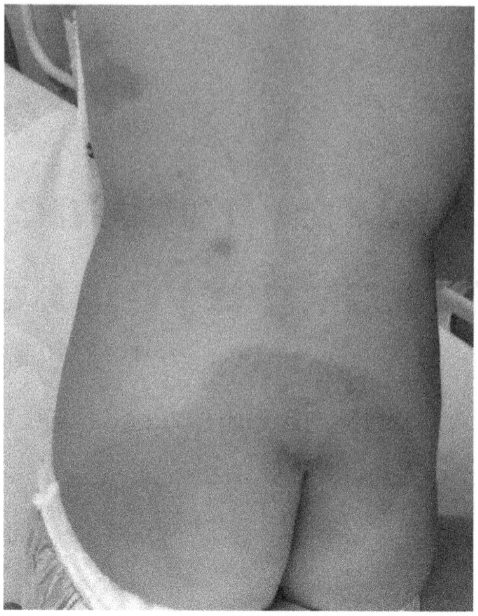

Figure 4: Mongolian spot.

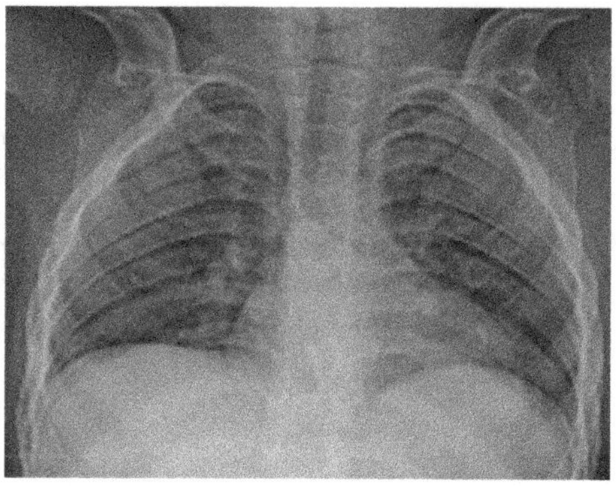

Figure 5: Chest X-ray image revealing oar-like ribs.

Enzyme replacement therapy (ERT) was initiated, which led to improved joint stiffness.

3. Discussion

Treatments for MPS include bone marrow transplantation, umbilical cord blood transplantation, ERT, and symptomatic treatment. ERT is not highly effective for the bone and the brain [4]; moreover, once symptoms progress, they are not improved with any therapy [5]. Therefore, early diagnosis and early initiation of treatment is crucial [6]. Important symptoms for early diagnosis are hernia and otitis media [6, 7]. However, these symptoms are common childhood complaints; consequently, it is difficult to definitively associate these symptoms with MPS disorder [3].

We experienced difficult intubation in a case with a medical history of inguinal hernia operation; the patient exhibited an ectopic Mongolian spot, coarse face, stiff joints, and claw hand deformity, some of which are clearly characteristic symptoms of MPS. Cohn et al. reported that these symptoms are a mnemonic screening tool for the diagnosis

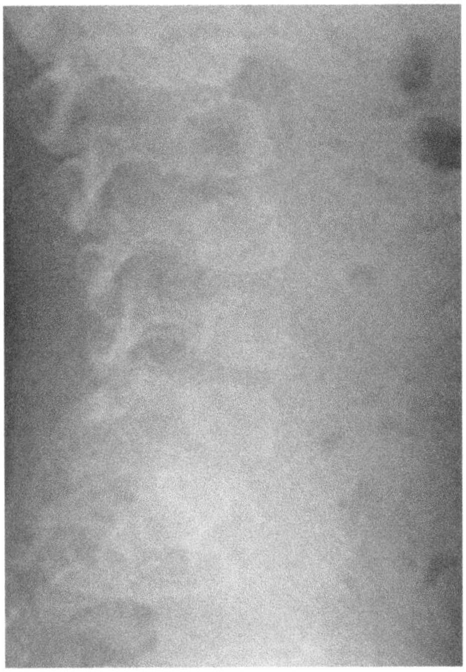

FIGURE 6: Chest X-ray image revealing egg-shaped vertebra.

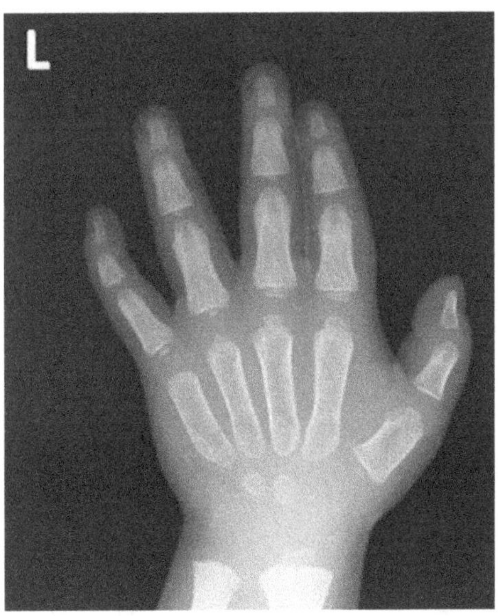

FIGURE 7: X-ray image of the fingers revealing sharp metacarpals.

of Hunter syndrome and, according to that report, our case suggested a likelihood of Hunter syndrome >95% [7]. If otorhinolaryngologists can verify ectopic Mongolian spot (s) and hernia, including hernia operation history, when the refractory otitis media is treated, it may be possible to diagnose MPS earlier, given that many patients with MPS II exhibit some otorhinolaryngological symptoms from younger age [8–10].

Otorhinolaryngologists and pediatricians can suspect MPS, and it is important that both cooperate to diagnose and treat MPS as early as possible.

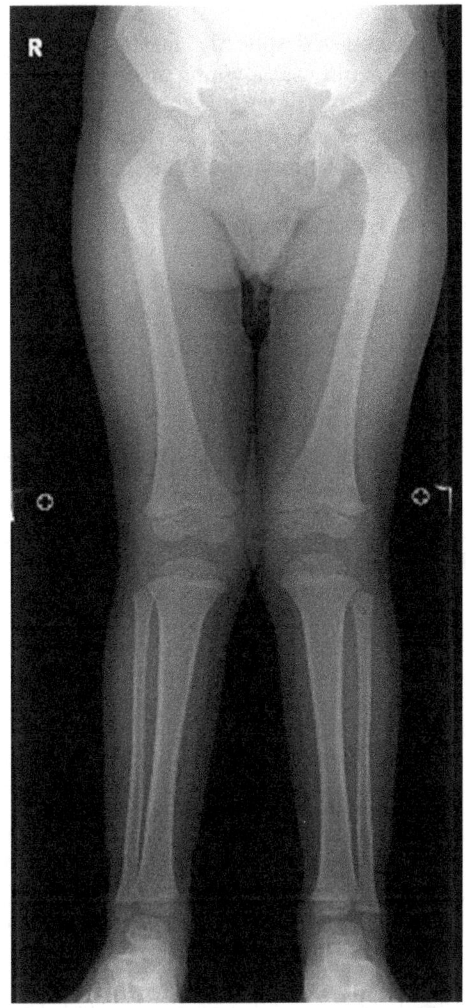

FIGURE 8: Genu valgum.

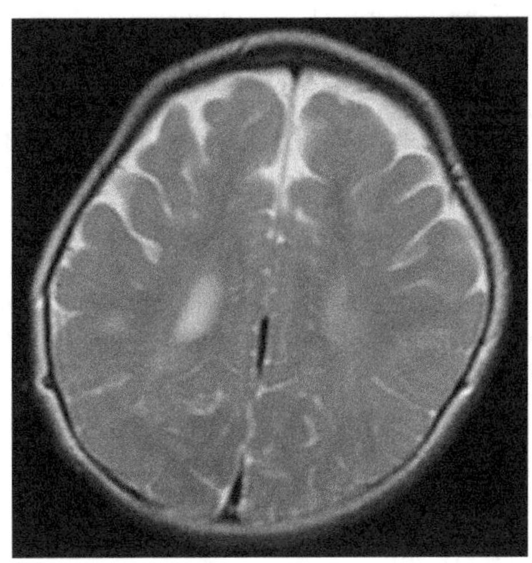

FIGURE 9: Head magnetic resonance image revealing an enlarged Virchow-Robin space.

4. Conclusions

Hunter syndrome is a lysosomal disease. We report a case of Hunter syndrome diagnosed by an otorhinolaryngologist.

To our knowledge, this is the first reported diagnosis by an otorhinolaryngologist despite the fact otorhinolaryngological symptoms manifest at a young age in this disease. This case report illustrates the significant role of otorhinolaryngologists and the importance of cooperation with pediatricians for early diagnosis and treatment of MPS.

Conflicts of Interest

The authors declare that there are no conflicts of interest regarding the publication of this article.

References

[1] P. J. Meikle, J. J. Hopwood, A. E. Clague, and W. F. Carey, "Prevalence of lysosomal storage disorders," *JAMA*, vol. 281, no. 3, pp. 249–254, 1999.

[2] H. S. Jeong, D. Y. Cho, K. M. Ahn, and D. K. Jin, "Complications of tracheotomy in patients with mucopolysaccharidoses type II (Hunter syndrome)," *International Journal of Pediatric Otorhinolaryngology*, vol. 70, no. 10, pp. 1765–1769, 2006.

[3] B. K. Burton and R. Giugliani, "Diagnosing Hunter syndrome in pediatric practice: practical considerations and common pitfalls," *European Journal of Pediatrics*, vol. 171, no. 4, pp. 631–639, 2012.

[4] C. Lampe, A. K. Bosserhoff, B. K. Burton et al., "Long-term experience with enzyme replacement therapy (ERT) in MPS II patients with a severe phenotype: an international case series," *Journal of Inherited Metabolic Disease*, vol. 37, pp. 823–829, 2014.

[5] Ç. Gökdoğan, Ş. Altinyay, O. Gökdoğan et al., "Audiologic evaluations of children with mucopolysaccharidosis," *Brazilian Journal of Otorhinolaryngology*, vol. 81, no. 3, pp. 281–284, 2015.

[6] J. E. Wraith, M. Beck, R. Giugliani et al., "Initial report from the Hunter Outcome Survey," *Genetics in Medicine*, vol. 10, no. 7, pp. 508–516, 2008.

[7] G. M. Cohn, I. Morin, D. A. Whiteman, and Hunter Outcome Survey Investigators, "Development of a mnemonic screening tool for identifying subjects with Hunter syndrome," *European Journal of Pediatrics*, vol. 172, pp. 965–970, 2013.

[8] B. Gönüldaş, T. Yılmaz, H. S. Sivri et al., "Mucopolysaccharidosis: otolaryngologic findings, obstructive sleep apnea and accumulation of glucosaminoglycans in lymphatic tissue of the upper airway," *International Journal of Pediatric Otorhinolaryngology*, vol. 78, no. 6, pp. 944–949, 2014.

[9] R. Parini, M. Rigoldi, L. Tedesco et al., "Enzymatic replacement therapy for Hunter disease: up to 9 years experience with 17 patients," *Molecular Genetics and Metabolism Reports*, vol. 3, pp. 65–74, 2015.

[10] A. Keilmann, T. Nakarat, I. A. Bruce, D. Molter, G. Malm, and HOS Investigators, "Hearing loss in patients with mucopolysaccharidosis II: data from HOS-the Hunter Outcome Survey," *Journal of Inherited Metabolic Disease*, vol. 35, no. 2, pp. 343–353, 2012.

11

Type 3 Thyroplasty for a Patient with Female-to-Male Gender Identity Disorder

Yu Saito ,[1] Kazuhiro Nakamura,[2] Shigeto Itani,[1] and Kiyoaki Tsukahara[1]

[1]*Department of Otolaryngology, Head and Neck Surgery, Tokyo Medical University, 6-7-1 Nisisinnjuku, Shinjuku-ku, Tokyo 160-0023, Japan*
[2]*Department of Otolaryngology, Todachuo General Hospital, 1-19-3 Honthou, Toda-shi, Saitama 335-0023, Japan*

Correspondence should be addressed to Yu Saito; sysesy20121111117@yahoo.co.jp

Academic Editor: Marco Berlucchi

Objective. In most cases, about the voice of the patient with female-to-male/gender identity disorder (FTM/GID), hormone therapy makes the voice low-pitched. In success cases, there is no need for phonosurgery. However, hormone therapy is not effective in some cases. We perform type 3 thyroplasty in these cases. *Method.* Hormone therapy was started in 2008 but did not lower the speaking fundamental frequencies (SFFs). We therefore performed TP3 under local anesthesia. *Results.* In our case, the SFF at the first visit was 146 Hz. The postoperative SFF was 110 Hz. *Conclusions.* TP3 was performed under local anesthesia in a patient with FTM/GID in whom hormone therapy proved ineffective. With successful conversion to a lower-pitched voice, the patient could begin to live daily life as a male. QOL improved significantly with TP3. If hormone therapy proves ineffective, TP3 may be selected as an optional treatment and appears to show few surgical complications and was, in this case, a very effective treatment.

1. Introduction

Gender identity disorder is a state in which self-consciousness of sex and biological sex is different. Treatments for female-to-male/gender identity disorder (FTM/GID) include hormone therapy, plastic surgery, sex reassignment surgery, voice therapy, and phonosurgery. In most cases, hormone therapy results in the voice of patients with FTM/GID becoming low-pitched. In successful cases, no phonosurgery is needed. However, hormone therapy is ineffective in some cases, and we perform type 3 thyroplasty (TP3) for such cases. TP3 is a surgical technique used to reduce the anteroposterior diameter of the thyroid cartilage. This causes the vocal folds to shorten and relax. With the decrease in tension of the vocal fold, speaking fundamental frequencies (SFFs) decrease and the voice becomes lower-pitched. The surgery is also effective for improving laryngeal efficiency. TP3 is effective for diseases such as vocal fold atrophy, sulcus vocalis, mutation voice disorder, and scarring.

2. Patient and Methods

The patient was a 46-year-old individual with FTM/GID, before sex reassignment surgery (SRS). The chief complaint was a high-pitched voice. In terms of past history, she had a history of appendicitis and panic disorder. The subject became aware of GID around 4 years old. FTM/GID was diagnosed at the age of 42 years. Hormone therapy was started in 2008 but did not lower the SFF, and Kayser-Gutzmann voice therapy was ineffective. She came to our hospital for phonosurgery in August 2015. Figures 1 and 2 showed preoperative endoscopic findings in aspiration and phonation. SFF at the first visit was 146 Hz, and no abnormalities of the vocal folds were identified. To measure the F0, the patient was instructed to phonate the sustained vowel /e/ with a comfortable tone and loudness. Hormone therapy and speech therapy failed to sufficiently lower the pitch of the voice. We therefore selected TP3 under local anesthesia for this case.

3. Operation Methods and Results

The surgery was performed under local anesthesia to allow the voice to be monitored. A horizontal skin incision was made in the neck. A vertical incision was made to separate and retract the strap muscles laterally and expose the thyroid ala on one side. An incision about 7 mm long is then made with a number 11 scalpel on the lateral side of the thyroid

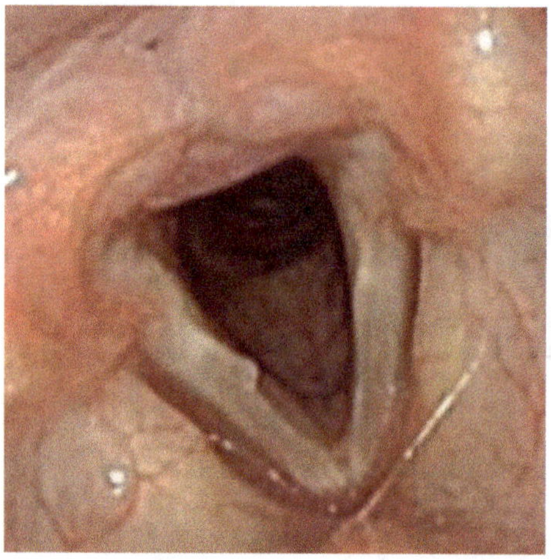

FIGURE 1: Preoperative endoscopic findings in aspiration.

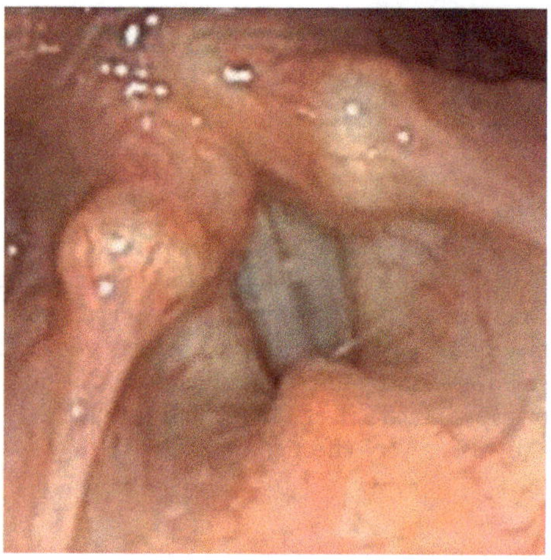

FIGURE 2: Preoperative endoscopic findings in phonation.

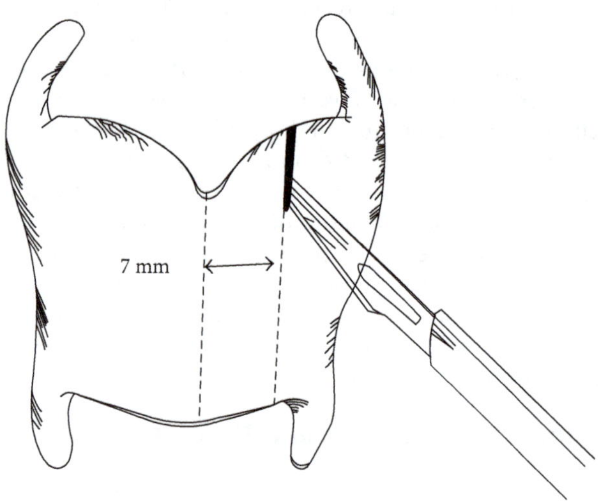

FIGURE 3: Cartilage incision. An incision with a number 11 scalpel is made on the lateral side of the thyroid cartilage.

cartilage (Figure 3). TP3 was started from one side according to the original Isshiki method. After splitting the thyroid cartilage on the right side, the cartilage was overlapped. The voice then became markedly lower-pitched. Next, the thyroid cartilage was split on the left side and overlapped. At this time, the voice turned rough and spasmodic. Finally, overlapping up to a width of 3 mm was carried out on the right side, while the left side was returned and fixed face-to-face (FTF). Fixation is important. The thyroid cartilage was fixed by a 3-0 nylon suture and a 17 mm curved conventional cutting needle. Further monitoring showed the voice was not spasmodic and remained low-pitched. We confirmed that the patient was satisfied with her voice and the operation was finished (Figure 4). The operation lasted 1 h 35 min. Postoperative SFF was 110 Hz, and quality of life (QOL) improved significantly with TP3 (Table 1). The Jitter and Shimmer score was not changed from preoperation to postoperation (Table 1). Figures 5 and 6 showed postoperative endoscopic findings in aspiration and phonation.

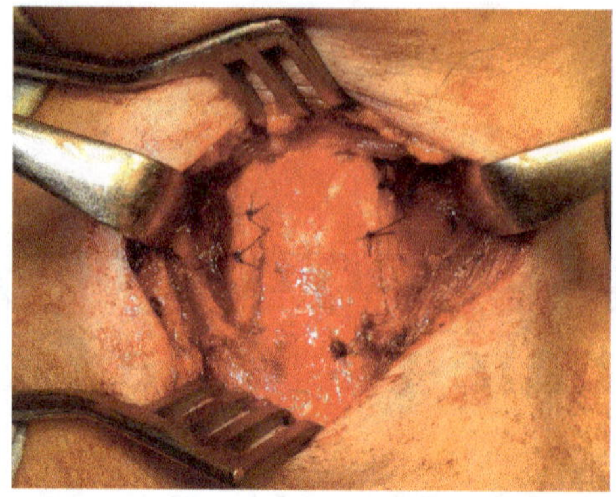

FIGURE 4: Findings of thyroid cartilage at the end of surgery. The right was overlapped, and the left side was returned and fixed FTF.

TABLE 1: Pitch range, acoustic analyzed data and VHI of pre- and post-operative voice.

	Lowest (Hz)	SFF (Hz)	Highest (Hz)	Jitter (%)	Shimmer (%)	VHI-30
Preope	136	146	493	0.54	1.01	9/120
Post-ope	92	110	402	0.91	1.82	4/120

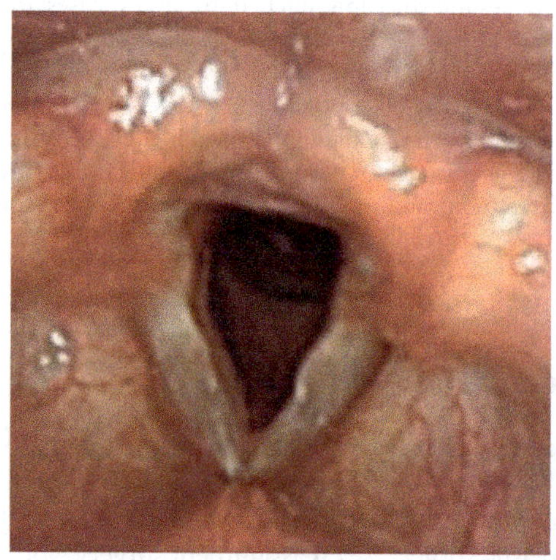

FIGURE 5: Postoperative endoscopic findings in aspiration.

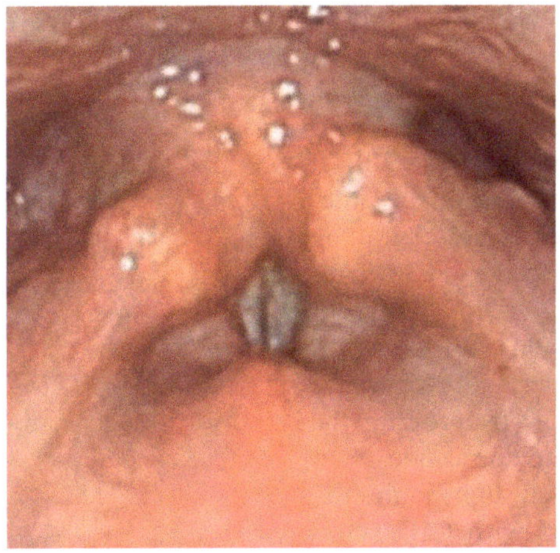

FIGURE 6: Postoperative endoscopic findings in phonation.

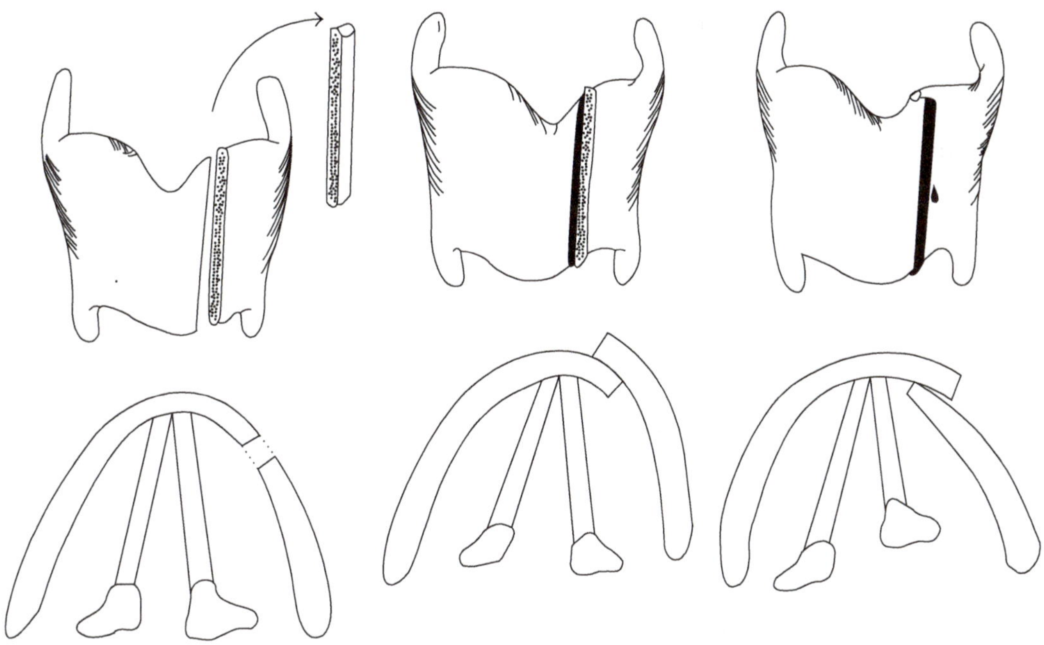

FIGURE 7: Three fixation patterns (a) FTF fixation. (b) OL fixation: lateralization. (c) OL fixation: medialization.

4. Discussion

In the treatment of FTM/GID, hormone therapy makes the voice low-pitched in most cases. As a result, phonosurgery is not needed. In hormone therapy, an androgen or anabolic steroid is administered, and there are few side effects [1]. SFF becomes low-pitched within 1-2 months, stabilizing at 6 months. However, predicting how much vocal degradation will be seen is difficult, given the individual differences [2]. In voice therapy, the Kayser-Gutzmann method is often performed and usually effective in mutation voice disorders. In this case, hormone therapy and voice therapy failed to sufficiently lower the pitch of the voice. TP3 under local anesthesia was selected for this Case [3–6]. TP3 was first reported by Isshiki et al. in 1974 [7], with further descriptions by the same group in 1983 [3]. TP3 surgery involves relaxation of the vocal folds. Partial resection of the thyroid cartilage causes the vocal folds to shorten and relax, and with decreased tension of the vocal folds, the SFF decreases and the voice becomes lower-pitched [4–6]. During TP3, monitoring the voice is very important. TP3 should therefore be performed under local anesthesia, not general anesthesia, and we continued surgery while confirming the patient's voice. In this manner, it is possible to choose the voice the patient wants, and the patient can also be satisfied [8].

Under voice monitoring, the edges may also be overlapped, if necessary. There are two kinds of OL: medialization and lateralization (Figure 7). Medialization or lateralization and the OL width are determined under voice monitoring. In this case, firstly, the voice turned good with lateralization OL, the right side was fixed in a lateralization OL manner. Secondly, the thyroid cartilage was split on the left side and overlapped, the voice was did not turn out to be good. Whereas the left side was returned and fixed in a face-to-face (FTF) manner as before. The major indications include patients with a high SFF associated with vocal fold atrophy, mutational voice disorder, FTM/GID, or laryngeal trauma, and patients with sulcus vocalis, who show unsatisfactory responses to voice therapy [4, 5, 9, 10]. In either case, tension decreases due to shortening of the anteroposterior diameter of the vocal fold and SFF decreases, leading to vocal improvement. Unlike other thyroplasties, TP3 is irreversible surgery because it involves cartilage resection in cases of fixed FTF. Appropriate preoperative evaluation of the patient is thus important. The AP test is the most important preoperative exam. We confirm whether the SFF is low by pressing the thyroid cartilage from the ventral side to the dorsal side.

In our case, the VHI score was decreased slightly, and the QOL improved. In Japan, many patients with GID stand miserable situations. Many Japanese have prejudice and discrimination against GID. His preoperative voice is almost normal as shown in Table 1, but he has been taking a lot of prejudices and discriminations against the high-pitched SFF. He looked real man, but his voice was high-pitched, he has been worried about his voice long time. So, he came to us to take TP3. TP3 could change his voice low-pitched; he was reborn as real man. His QOL improved by TP3.

5. Conclusion

TP3 was performed in a patient with FTM/GID in whom hormone therapy proved ineffective. With successful conversion to a lower-pitched voice, the patient could begin to live daily life as a male. QOL improved significantly with TP3, which was performed under local anesthesia. Voice characteristics can be adjusted to some extent and patient feedback improves satisfaction with the operation. If hormone therapy proves ineffective, TP3 may be selected as optional treatment.

References

[1] W. Futterweit, "Endocrine therapy of transsexualism and potential complications of long-term treatment," *Archives of Sexual Behavior*, vol. 27, no. 2, pp. 209–226, 1998.

[2] G. Van Borsel, R. De Cuypere, B. Rubens, and J. Destaerke, "Voice problems in female-to-male transsexuals," *International Journal of Language & Communication Disorders*, vol. 35, no. 3, pp. 427–442, 2000.

[3] N. Isshiki, T. Taira, and M. Tanabe, "Surgical alteration of the vocal pitch," *Journal of Otolaryngology*, vol. 12, no. 5, pp. 335–340, 1983.

[4] D. H. Slavit, N. E. Maragos, and R. J. Lipton, "Physiologic assessment of Isshiki type III thyroplasty," *Laryngoscope*, vol. 100, no. 8, pp. 844–848, 1990.

[5] G. D. Li, L. Mu, and S. Yang, "Acoustic evaluation of Isshiki type 3 thyroplasty for treatment of mutational voice disorders," *Journal of Laryngology & Otology*, vol. 113, no. 1, pp. 31–34, 1999.

[6] M. Remacle, N. Matar, I. Verduyckt, and G. Lawson, "Relaxation thyroplasty for mutational falsetto treatment," *Annals of Otology, Rhinology & Laryngology*, vol. 119, no. 2, pp. 105–109, 2010.

[7] N. Isshiki, H. Morita, H. Okamura, and M. Hiramoto, "Thyroplasty as a new phonosurgical technique," *Acta Oto-Laryngologica*, vol. 78, no. 1-6, pp. 451–457, 1974.

[8] K. Nakamura, T. Muto, T. Yoshida, H. Hiramatsu, Y. Watanabe, and M. Suzuki, "Efficacy of total intravenous anesthesia without intubation for laryngeal framework surgery," *Acta Oto-Laryngologica*, vol. 128, no. 9, pp. 1037–1042, 2008.

[9] K. Nakamura, K. Tsukahara, Y. Watanabe, D. Komazawa, and M. Suzuki, "Type 3 thyroplasty for patients with mutational dysphonia," *Journal of Voice*, vol. 27, no. 5, pp. 650–654, 2013.

[10] N. Isshiki, K. Shoji, H. Kojima, and S. Hirano, "Vocal fold atrophy and its surgical treatment," *Annals of Otology, Rhinology & Laryngology*, vol. 105, no. 3, pp. 182–188, 1996.

12

Squamous Cell Carcinoma Originating from Adult Laryngeal Papillomatosis

Vivian Narana Ribeiro El-Achkar,[1] **Andressa Duarte**,[2] **Fabiano Pinto Saggioro**,[3] **Francisco Veríssimo De Mello Filho**,[4] **Jorge Esquiche León**,[5] **Alfredo Ribeiro-Silva**,[6] **and Estela Kaminagakura**[7]

[1]*DDS, PhD Student at Department of Bioscience and Oral Diagnosis, Science and Technology Institute, Universidade Estadual Paulista (UNESP), Sao Jose dos Campos, Brazil*
[2]*PhD Student at Department of Pathology and Legal Medicine, Ribeirão Preto Medical School, University of São Paulo, Ribeirao Preto, Brazil*
[3]*PhD, Assistant Physician at Pathology Service of Department of Pathology and Legal Medicine, Ribeirão Preto Medical School, University of São Paulo, Ribeirao Preto, Brazil*
[4]*MD, PhD, Associated Professor at Department of Ophthalmology, Otorhinolaryngology and Head and Neck Surgery, Ribeirão Preto Medical School, University of São Paulo, Ribeirão Preto, Brazil*
[5]*PhD, Professor at Department of Stomatology, Collective Health and Legal Dentistry, Ribeirão Preto Medical School, University of São Paulo, Ribeirao Preto, Brazil*
[6]*MD, PhD, Associated Professor at Department of Pathology and Legal Medicine, Ribeirão Preto Medical School, University of São Paulo, Ribeirao Preto, Brazil*
[7]*DDs, PhD, Associated Professor at the Department of Bioscience and Oral Diagnosis, Science and Technology Institute, Universidade Estadual Paulista (UNESP), Sao José dos Campos, Brazil*

Correspondence should be addressed to Estela Kaminagakura; estela.tango@unesp.br

Academic Editor: Abrão Rapoport

Background. The malignant transformation of laryngeal papillomatosis (LP) into squamous cell carcinoma (SCC) can occur in up to 4% of LP cases. The low-risk HPV types 6 and 11 are those that are most commonly related to LP; however, high-risk HPV types may be present. The present study reviews the literature on cases of malignant transformation of LP in adults and reports a clinical case. *Case Report.* A 47-year-old male patient exhibiting hoarseness for 4 months presented an exophytic lesion in the right palatine tonsil and a digitiform-like lesion in the right vocal fold. The biopsy revealed a well-differentiated SCC in the vocal cord, which showed a transition zone with a squamous papillomatous lesion. By using the chromogenic *in situ* hybridization (CISH) test, both lesions showed a positive result for high-risk HPV types 16 and 18 and negative for low-risk HPV types 6 and 11. The final diagnosis was SCC arising from LP. The patient underwent surgical treatment. After 36 months of follow-up, no signs of recurrence were observed. *Results.* The literature review revealed 25 cases of malignant transformation into SCC of LP with adult onset. Of these, only 9 cases were assessed by CISH and/or PCR for HPV identification, of which 7 were positive. The current study focuses on the eighth case, suggesting the involvement of the high-risk HPV types in its pathogenesis. *Conclusions.* LP is considered a benign lesion with the potential for malignant transformation, which reinforces the need for its early diagnosis and the constant monitoring of patients with LP.

1. Introduction

Papilloma is the most common benign tumor affecting the larynx, which may present as a single event or as recurring and/or affecting more than one topography, as occurs in laryngeal papillomatosis (LP) [1]. LP is distributed bimodally, affecting juvenile patients (JLP), with onset of disease before 5 years of age and adult patients, aged 20–40 years (ALP) [1]. ALP is prevalent in male patients [1] and tends to be less aggressive than JLP [2].

ALP is considered to be the most important clinical manifestation of human papillomavirus (HPV) larynx infection and is correlated mainly with low-risk HPV's of malignancy types 6 and 11 [3]. The disease may be progressive, with a high relapse rate and requiring more than 100 surgical procedures, but spontaneous remission may also occur [4, 5].

Malignant transformation of LP is rare, having been described in about 1–4% of cases [1]. The following is a case of malignant transformation of LP in an adult patient with no history of recurrence, a rare case that shows that even nonrecurrent lesions have a potential for malignancy. We also performed a brief review of the literature, looking for cases of malignancy in patients who had suffered their first manifestation of the disease in adulthood.

2. Materials and Methods

A search for English language articles was carried out in the PubMed, Scopus, and Web of Science databases using the following keywords: malignancies in ALP and epidermoid carcinoma/squamous cell carcinoma from ALP. The search period extended from 1988 to the present, and only the reports in which the onset of the disease occurred in the adult phase were considered; cases in which malignancy occurred in patients of juvenile onset LP were discarded.

3. Case Report

A 47-year-old male patient noticed a change in his voice (hoarseness) 4 months previously. During the anamnesis, he did not report any addictions or habits, but systemic hypertension had been diagnosed and controlled. During intraoral physical examination, a pediculated exophytic lesion with a rough surface and coloration similar to adjacent mucosa was observed in the right tonsil. Examination by laryngoscopy revealed an exophytic lesion in the right paralyzed vocal fold, occupying its anterior two-thirds, in which the mucosa was covered by fibrinopurulent exudate. An incisional biopsy was performed on the vocal cord and excisional on the palatine tonsil. Microscopically, the vocal cord biopsy revealed a squamous epithelium exhibiting architectural disorganization, covered by a fibrinopurulent membrane. This epithelium exhibited projections towards the connective tissue and was infiltrated into the connective tissue, forming islands and strands of malignant epithelial cells (Figure 1).

The squamous layer showed clear epithelial cells with a vacuolized nuclei, and some cells similar to koilocytes were present in the upper layers of the epithelium. The epithelium was found with digitiform projections and fibrovascular connective tissue centers containing mononuclear inflammatory infiltrate (Figure 1(a)). A transitional zone was found in this biopsy, where the atypical epithelium protrudes exophytically with a digitiform aspect (Figure 1(b)). The malignant component showed atypical cells, with nuclear pleomorphism, sometimes binucleated cells, with a hyperchromatic nucleus and individual keratinization. Atypical mitoses and areas of necrosis were also found (Figure 1(c)). The result of the incisional biopsy was of a well-differentiated squamous cell carcinoma (SCC) present in the right vocal cord. Histological examination suggested that the SCC originated from a papillomatous lesion, and chromogenic in situ hybridization (CISH) was performed. Both lesions showed a positive result in CISH for high-risk HPV types 16 and 18 (Figures 1(d) and 1(e)) and negative for low-risk HPV types 6 and 11.

On the other hand, the histological sections of the right palatine tonsil region revealed a squamous papilloma demonstrated by proliferation of the stratified squamous epithelium, predominantly nonkeratinized, presenting exocytosis and basal layer hyperplasia with typical mitoses.

3.1. Chromogenic in situ Hybridization (CISH). The following procedures were carried out from the biopsy block: dewaxing, peroxidase blockade, and enzymatic digestion, followed by a pretreatment with a 95% EDTA bath for 15 min, followed by several rinses with distilled water and dehydration. After drying, the probe was added onto the material, the slices were covered by a coverslip, and sealing was performed. The material was denatured for 5 min at 75°C, and hybridization was performed at 37°C for 60 min for high-risk HPV. The ZytoFast Plus CISH Implementation Kit-HRP-DAB (ZytoVision, Bremerhaven, Germany, and the ZytoFast HPV-type 6/11 Probe and 16/18 Probe) was used. In the next step, the coverslip was removed, and the slides were washed in TBS buffer at 55°C for 5 min, and then, the primary antibody was incubated at 37°C for 30 min in a humid chamber. For tagging, chromogen diaminobenzidine (DakoCytomation, Carpinteria, CA, USA) was used for 10 min, and Mayer's Hematoxylin was used for the counterstaining. Reactions were performed with negative and positive controls.

3.2. Treatment and Prognosis. Surgery was performed, including tracheostomy, with the final diagnosis of SCC originating from LP, staging T3N0M0. One month after the surgical procedure, the patient returned without complaints. In the other nasofibroscopy and bronchoscopy examinations, no changes were observed. Follow-up by a speech therapist was fundamental for significant voice improvement. The patient has been undergoing maintenance for 36 months and has no complaints and no signs of relapse.

3.3. Literature Review. Fifteen articles were found, totaling 27 cases of malignant transformation of LP with onset in

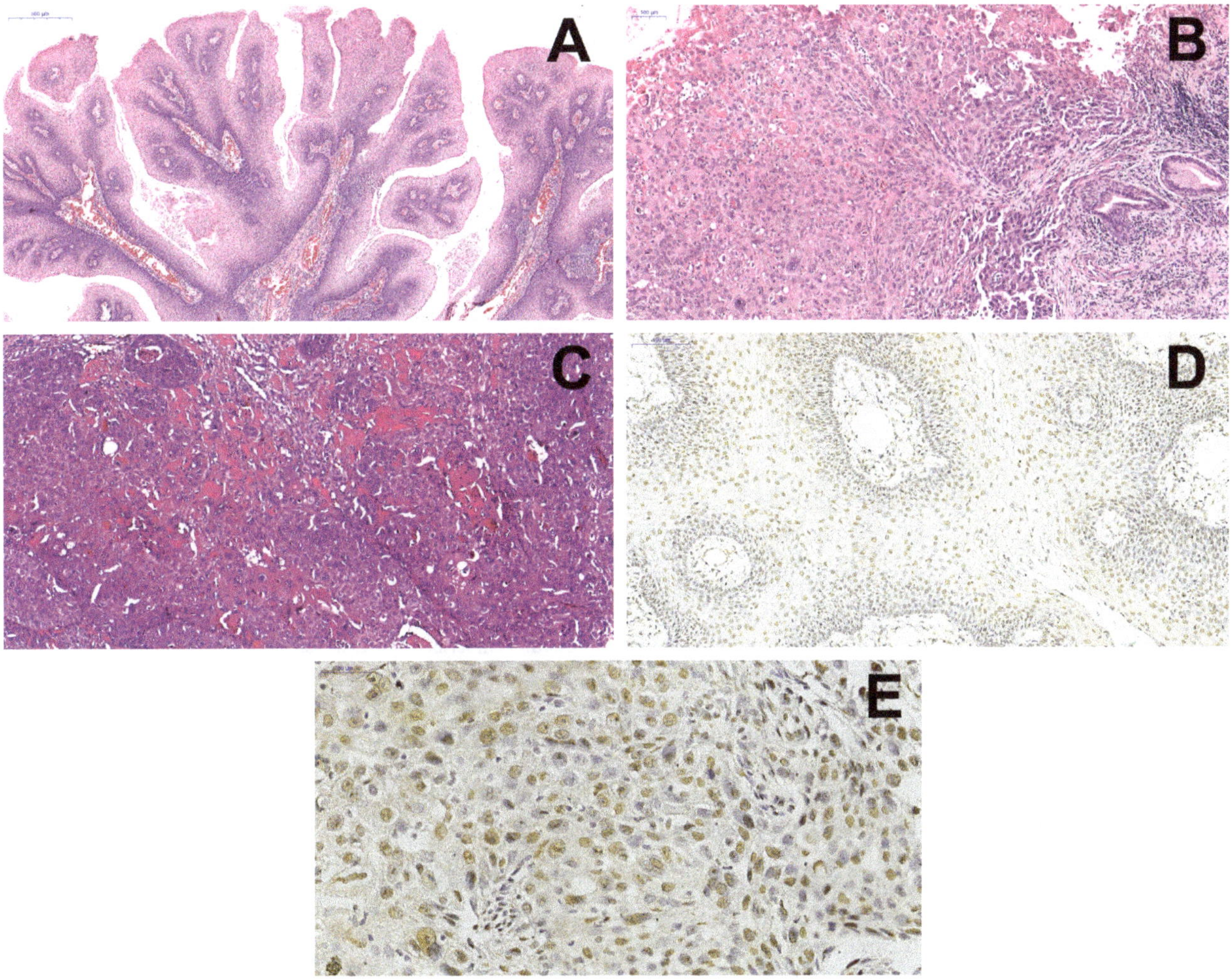

FIGURE 1: Photomicrographs: lesion with papillary appearance showing exophytic projections of epithelial proliferation with benign appearance (a), transition zone of malignant neoplasm in the right vocal fold (b), well-differentiated SCC (c), dotted brown nuclei showing positive CISH result for high-risk HPV (16/18) in LP (d), and in SCC (e).

adult patients. The mean age of the patients was 57.03 years (SD = 13.76). Of these, including the present case, 25 (89.28%) were male patients (Table 1), and in 3 (10.71%) cases, there was no history of recurrent LP. The localization of the carcinoma was cited in 10 cases, of which 3 (30%) were malignant lesions in the lung, due to dissemination. In the remaining 7 (70%), the larynx was affected, mainly in the vocal cords. There were 9 (47.36%) smokers, and HPV was identified in 9 of the reports, 2 negative tests, 4 with low-risk HPV and 4 with high-risk HPV.

4. Discussion

In adults, the exact mode of infection is controversial; transmission during sexual contact and reactivation of a slow-progressing latent infection acquired in childhood has been suggested [1]. The aggressive clinical course of LP can lead to malignant transformation and death by extending through the lower respiratory tract [1]. The rates of LP malignancy are around 1 to 4% [1]; however, there are few studies with an extensive review of these cases [21]. In this present review, only cases in which the disease started in adulthood were considered.

Gastroesophageal reflux and immunosuppression may also be aggravating factors for patients with papillomatosis [15, 16]. In the present case, no signs of reflux or immunosuppression were found. Tobacco use, irradiation [21], and p53 mutation [22] may also favor malignant transformation. However, it may also occur in the absence of these factors [23].

Pou et al. [11] reported that, of 17 patients who underwent a LP aggressive clinical course, the malignant transformation occurred in 3 of them, there being 2 of juvenile onset, with more than 100 relapses, and HPVs 6 and 11 were found. Another case occurred in the adult patient after 12 recurrences, and HPV 16 was identified. Our report highlights the rapid progression to SCC; the patient presented symptoms for only 4 months and the malignant lesion was diagnosed together with papillomatosis; it being able to attribute this to an aggressive progression of high-risk HPV 16. The rarity of cases in which the malignant transformation has a rapid course was observed; in 3 reported

Table 1: Clinical information of adult patient's onset who developed SCC and was reported in the English language literature.

Author(s), year	Age	Gender	RRP	Risk factors	HPV
Byhardt et al, 1988 [6]	61	Male	Yes	Smoker and Rxt	NR
Kashima et al, 1988 [7]	28	Male	Yes	Rxt	6
Zarod et al, 1988 [8]	72	Female	Yes	NR	6
Lindeberg et al, 1989 [9]	62.5	Male	Yes	Smoker	Negative
Lindeberg et al, 1989 [9]	34.4	Male	Yes	NR	Negative
Hasan et al, 1995 [10]	30	Male	Yes	Nonsmoker, without Rxt	NR
Pou et al, 1995 [11]	46	Male	Yes	Nonsmoker	16
Sakakura et al, 1996 [12]	63	Female	Yes	Nonsmoker	18
Klozar et al, 1997 [13]	81	Male	Yes	NR	NR
Klozar et al, 1997 [13]	58	Female	Yes	NR	NR
Klozar et al, 1997 [13]	56	Male	No	NR	NR
Behl et al, 2001 [14]	28	Male	Yes	Nonsmoker	NR
Azadamaki et al, 2013 [15]	77	Male	Yes	Nonsmoker	NR
Hao et al, 2013 [16]	52	Male	No	Passive smoker	16/18
Hasegawa et al, 2013 [17]	75	Male	Yes	NR	11
Jeong et al, 2009 [18]	55	Male	Yes	NR	6, 11
Jeong et al, 2009 [18]	64	Male	Yes	NR	NR
Ilmarinen et al, 2014 [19]*	—	Male	Yes	7 smokers, 2 nonsmokers	NR
Zhang et al, 2015 [20]	43	Male	No	Multiple sex partners, second-hand smoker	NR
Present study	47	Male	No	No	16/18

RRP: recurrent respiratory papillomatosis; Rxt: radiotherapy; NR: not reported. *The authors described 9 cases of malignancy, all were male and the mean age was 62 years (range: 41–79).

cases, the patients did not have recurrent disease, and in 1 case, the carcinoma was detected only 6 months after the diagnosis of LP [20]. Other factors associated with more aggressive LP are the higher number of recurrences and evolution time greater than 10 years [5].

The incidence of high-grade dysplasia for LP is between 10% and 17.6% [24–26]. The progression of LP with dysplasia with multiple recurrences to carcinoma was reported [10]. Hall et al. [27] reported that only one (2%) of the 54 adult patients with recurrent respiratory papillomatosis developed SCC. However, the patient had a history of smoking and had a severe dysplasia. In another study, there were 9 male patients with adult onset LP, which had transformed into SCC. Initially, in 2 cases, there was no dysplasia; 2 cases were diagnosed with a mild condition, 3 were moderate, and 2 exhibited severe dysplasia [19]. In the presented case, there was a papillomatosis lesion with low-grade dysplasia associated with carcinoma. Recently, squamous hyperplasia and mild dysplasia were grouped into low-grade lesions and moderate and severe dysplasia in high-grade lesions, according to the malignancy potential [1].

Pulmonary imaging (RX or CT or PET scan) is recommended, in addition to careful histopathological examination, which should be repeated every time a surgery is performed to remove papillomatosis. There should be routine following-up of patients with LP, since there are reports of pulmonary dissemination, which develops into malignancy in a short period of time and which, if detected early, guarantees a greater survival time for the patient [17]. Within 36 months of follow-up of the patient in the present study, there was no involvement of the lungs.

Although LP is a benign lesion, it can present a severe course with malignant transformation, especially when high-risk HPV is detected. Therefore, the follow-up of these patients is highly recommended.

Conflicts of Interest

The authors declare that they have no conflicts of interest.

Acknowledgments

The authors acknowledge with thanks the financial support received from FAPESP (São Paulo Research Foundation, process number 16/24019-0) and CAPES (Coordination for the Improvement of Higher Education Personnel).

References

[1] M. Richardson, N. Gale, J. Hille, and N. Zidar, *WHO Classification Head and Neck Tumours*, IARC Press, Lyon, France, 2017.

[2] M. Carifi, D. Napolitano, M. Morandi, and D. Dall'Olio, "Recurrent respiratory papillomatosis: current and future perspectives," *Therapeutics and Clinical Risk Management*, vol. 5, no. 11, pp. 731–738, 2015.

[3] V. Gerein, E. Rastorguev, J. Gerein, W. Draf, and J. Schirren, "Incidence, age at onset, and potential reasons of malignant transformation in recurrent respiratory papillomatosis patients: 20 years' experience," *Otolaryngology-Head and Neck Surgery*, vol. 132, no. 3, pp. 392–394, 2005.

[4] T. Kanazawa, N. Fukushima, S. Imayoshi et al., "Rare case of malignant transformation of recurrent respiratory papillomatosis associated with human papillomavirus type 6 infection and p53 overexpression," *SpringerPlus*, vol. 2, no. 1, p. 153, 2013.

[5] T. Omland, H. Akre, K. A. Lie, P. Jebsen, L. Sandvik, and K. Brøndbo, "Risk factors for aggressive recurrent respiratory papillomatosis in adults and juveniles," *PLoS One*, vol. 9, no. 11, Article ID e113584, 2014a.

[6] R. W. Byhardt and U. Almagro, "The role of radiation therapy in the treatment of recurrent adult laryngeal papillomatosis,"

American Journal of Clinical Oncology, vol. 11, no. 2, pp. 131–137, 1988.

[7] H. Kashima, T. C. Wu, P. Mounts, D. Heffner, A. Cachay, and V. Hyams, "Carcinoma ex-papilloma: histologic and virologic studies in whole-organ sections of the larynx," *Laryngoscope*, vol. 98, no. 6, pp. 619–624, 1988.

[8] A. P. Zarod, J. D. Rutherford, and G. Corbitt, "Malignant progression of laryngeal papilloma associated with human papilloma virus type 6 (HPV-6) DNA," *Journal of Clinical Pathology*, vol. 41, no. 3, pp. 280–283, 1988.

[9] H. Lindeberg, S. Syrjänen, J. Kärjä, and K. Syrjänen, "Human papillomavirus type 11 DNA in squamous cell carcinomas and pre-existing multiple laryngeal papillomas," *Acta Oto-Laryngologica*, vol. 107, no. 1-2, pp. 141–149, 1989.

[10] S. Hasan, S. N. Dutt, U. Kini, S. Shariff, K. M. Nalinesha, and D. Prasad, "Laryngeal carcinoma ex-papilloma in a non-irradiated, non-smoking patient: a clinical record and review of the literature," *Journal of Laryngology & Otology*, vol. 109, no. 8, pp. 762–766, 1995.

[11] A. M. Pou, F. L. Rimell, J. A. Jordan et al., "Adult respiratory papillomatosis: human papillomavirus type and viral coinfections as predictors of prognosis," *Annals of Otology, Rhinology & Laryngology*, vol. 104, no. 10, pp. 758–762, 1995.

[12] A. Sakakura, Y. Yamamoto, T. Takasaki, K. Makimoto, M. Nakamura, and H. Takahashi, "Recurrent laryngeal papillomatosis developing into laryngeal carcinoma with human papilloma virus (HPV) type 18: a case report," *Journal of Laryngology & Otology*, vol. 110, no. 1, pp. 75–77, 1996.

[13] J. Klozar, M. Taudy, J. Betka, and R. Kana, "Laryngeal papilloma-precancerous condition?," *Acta Oto-Laryngologica*, vol. 117, no. 527, pp. 100–102, 1997.

[14] A. Behl, E. James, P. Kelkar, and N. Chawla, "Malignant transformation in a young adult with recurrent laryngeal papillomatosis," *Medical Journal Armed Forces India*, vol. 57, no. 2, pp. 154-155, 2001.

[15] R. Azadarmaki and M. N. Lango, "Malignant transformation of respiratory papillomatosis in a solid-organ transplant patient: case report and literature review," *Annals of Otology, Rhinology & Laryngology*, vol. 122, no. 7, pp. 457–460, 2013.

[16] Z. Hao, T. Dillard, P. Biddinger, and V. Patel, "Suppression of respiratory papillomatosis with malignant transformation by erlotinib in a kidney transplant recipient," *BMJ Case Reports*, vol. 2013, article bcr2013008757, 2013.

[17] Y. Hasegawa, N. Sato, H. Niikawa et al., "Lung squamous cell carcinoma arising in a patient with adult-onset recurrent respiratory papillomatosis," *Japanese Journal of Clinical Oncology*, vol. 43, no. 1, pp. 78–82, 2013.

[18] W. J. Jeong, S. W. Park, M. Shin et al., "Presence of HPV type 6 in dysplasia and carcinoma arising from recurrent respiratory papillomatosis," *Head Neck*, vol. 31, no. 8, pp. 1095–1101, 2009.

[19] T. Ilmarinen, J. Hagström, C. Haglund et al., "Low expression of nuclear Toll-like receptor 4 in laryngeal papillomas transforming into squamous cell carcinoma," *Otolaryngology-Head and Neck Surgery*, vol. 151, no. 5, pp. 785–790, 2014.

[20] Z. Zhang, M. Chang, and L. M. Moreta-Sainz, "Case report: pulmonary papillomatosis in a patient presenting with cough and hemoptysis," *Permanente Journal*, vol. 19, no. 3, pp. e125–e127, 2015.

[21] E. S. Lie, V. Engh, M. Boysen et al., "Squamous cell carcinoma of the respiratory tract following laryngeal papillomatosis," *Acta Oto-Laryngologica*, vol. 114, no. 2, pp. 209–212, 1994.

[22] P. L. Rady, V. J. Schnadig, R. L. Weiss et al., "Malignant transformation of recurrent respiratory papillomatosis associated with integrated human papillomavirus type 11 DNA and mutation of p53," *Laryngoscope*, vol. 108, no. 5, pp. 735–740, 1998.

[23] C. Bewtra, R. Krishnan, and S. S. Lee, "Malignant changes in nonirradiated juvenile laryngotracheal papillomatosis," *Archives of Otolaryngology-Head and Neck Surgery*, vol. 108, no. 2, pp. 114–116, 1982.

[24] T. Omland, K. A. Lie, H. Akre, L. E. Sandlie, P. Jebsen et al., "Recurrent respiratory papillomatosis: HPV genotypes and risk of high-grade laryngeal neoplasia," *PLoS ONE*, vol. 9, no. 6, Article ID e99114, 2014b.

[25] G. I. Sanchez, R. Jaramillo, G. Cuello, K. Quintero, A. Baena et al., "Human papillomavirus genotype detection in recurrent respiratory papillomatosis (RRP) in Colombia," *Head Neck*, vol. 35, no. 2, pp. 229–234, 2012.

[26] S. Karatayli-Ozgursoy, J. A. Bishop, A. Hillel, L. Akst, and S. R. Best, "Risk factors for dysplasia in recurrent respiratory papillomatosis in an adult and pediatric population," *Annals of Otology, Rhinology & Laryngology*, vol. 125, no. 3, pp. 235–241, 2016.

[27] J. E. Hall, K. Chen, M. J. Yoo, K. C. Fletcher, R. H. Ossoff, and C. G. Garrett, "Natural progression of dysplasia in adult recurrent respiratory papillomatosis," *Otolaryngology-Head and Neck Surgery*, vol. 144, no. 2, pp. 252–256, 2011.

13

Pneumomediastinum, Pneumopericardium, and Epidural Pneumatosis following Adenotonsillectomy: A Very Rare Complication

Feride Fatma Görgülü ,[1] **Ayşe Selcan Koç** ,[1] **and Orhan Görgülü**[2]

[1]*Radiology Department, Adana City Research and Training Hospital, University of Health Sciences, Adana, Turkey*
[2]*Otorhinolaryngology Department, Adana City Research and Training Hospital, University of Health Sciences, Adana, Turkey*

Correspondence should be addressed to Feride Fatma Görgülü; drferide@yahoo.com

Academic Editor: Kamal Morshed

Adenotonsillectomy is a common surgical otolaryngology procedure that is associated with several complications, including hemorrhage, odynophagia, damage to teeth, taste disorders, atlantoaxial subluxation, lingual edema, infection, and injury of the carotid artery. Pneumomediastinum, pneumopericardium, and epidural pneumatosis are an extremely unusual condition in children with adenotonsillectomy. Treatment should be conservative in the majority of cases and based on benign self-limiting course of these diseases; early recognition can prevent further complications. The combination of pneumomediastinum with epidural pneumatosis, pneumopericardium, retropharyngeal-prevertebral pneumatosis, axillar-perihumeral pneumatosis, and subcutaneous emphysema is also a very rare condition. We present a unique case with the radiological findings of air in all of these areas in a 6-year-old male child with adenotonsillectomy. The case was unusual in that the patient developed this complication 3 hours later after adenotonsillectomy with severe vomitting. The possible mechanism, the algorithm of treatment, and precautions in such cases will be discussed.

1. Case

A 6-year-old male child was admitted to our hospital with his parents for adenotonsillectomy with the history of recurrent tonsillitis and obstructive sleep apnea. Examination revealed grade five enlarged tonsils that were almost meeting at the midline. His adenoids were found to be blocking 90% of his airway in a lateral nasopharyngeal X-ray. Preoperative workup including chest radiography and electrocardiography was normal.

Adenotonsillectomy was performed under general anesthesia with endotracheal intubation. Standard surgical technique was used, and dissection of palatine tonsil was performed meticulously on the subcapsular plane to avoid excessive trauma. Adenoids were removed gently by curettage. Hemostasis was performed by means of careful bipolar electrocoagulation. The surgical procedure proceeded uneventfully with no intraoperative or early postoperative complications. The patient recovered from anesthesia well within 15 minutes.

During the first postoperative hours, there were no episodes of coughing, but the patient had an episode of emesis, one severe vomitting attack. Dyspnea and generalised swelling of his face, neck, and chest wall developed immediately after vomitting at the three-hour postoperative period.

He was conscious and in sitting position because of dyspnea. He did not state an obvious chest pain. But he was uncomfortable and moderately anxious. His vital signs were blood pressure, 110/70 mmHg; pulse rate, 135 beats/minute; respiratory rate, 35 breaths/minute with shallow breathing; temperature, 36.7°C; and oxygen saturation, 98% at room air. A physical examination revealed painless swelling of the face, neck, and chest area with marked crepitus on palpation consistent with cervicofacial subcutaneous emphysema.

Emphysema was palpated on anterior chest wall from sternum to axillary regions. Inspection of the oropharynx and nasopharynx did not evidence any bleeding from the operation sides or the presence of any mucosal tear and muscle dehiscence. He had a normal neurologic examination including intact cranial nerves, sensation, and muscle strength.

Because of suspicion of subcutaneous emphysema and pneumomediastinum on chest X-ray, a computed tomography (CT) of the thorax was obtained simultaneously. The CT showed the subcutaneous emphysema of the neck and the chest wall along with a large volume of air (Figures 1 and 2). The emphysema extended to both axillae, even the perihumeral region and along the precervical and anterolateral cervical soft tissues (Figure 3). The CT also showed extensive pneumomediastinum, the presence of pneumopericardium, large epidural pneumatosis, retropharyngeal-prevertebral pneumatosis, and air in paraesophageal spaces without pneumothorax (Figure 4). No masses, bullae, and blebs were seen.

Since the patient did not present with additional cardiorespiratory compromise and was hemodynamically stable, conservative management was decided. He was transferred to pediatric intensive care unit for close monitorization and conservative treatment. The patient also was instructed to refrain from coughing. The patient was administered analgesics, oxygen, cold-vapor, and broad-spectrum prophylactic antibiotics, and food intake was forbidden. He was followed up by chest radiographs. He was relieved from signs and symptoms around the sixth day, and his thorax CT revealed absence of air at seventh day after adenotonsillectomy. Then he was discharged at the seventh day, and follow-up examinations did not reveal any abnormal findings.

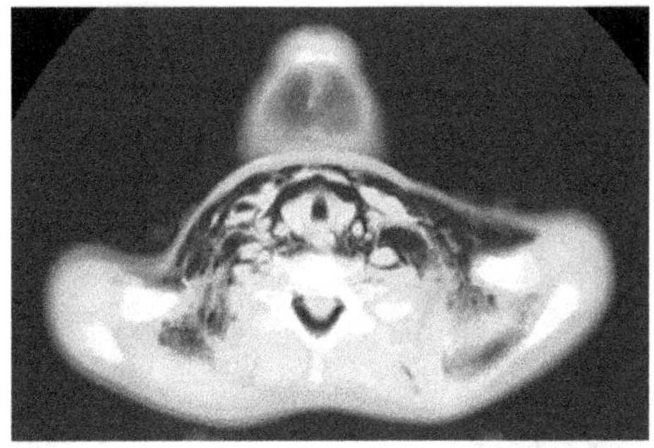

FIGURE 1: A large volume of emphysema in subcutaneous tissue, the neck planes, peritracheal, and periesophageal spaces.

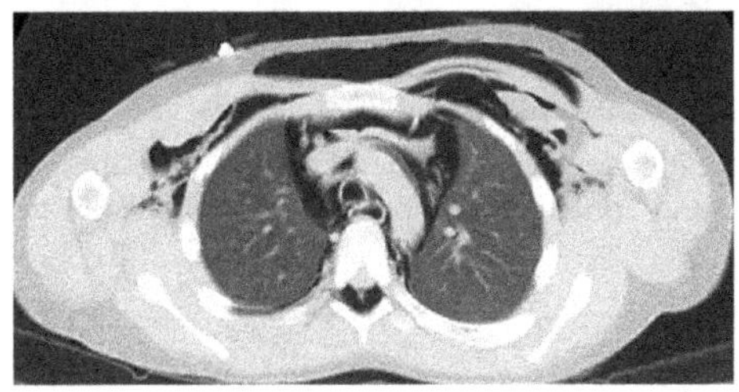

FIGURE 2: The emphysema of chest wall extended to mediastinum and both axillae.

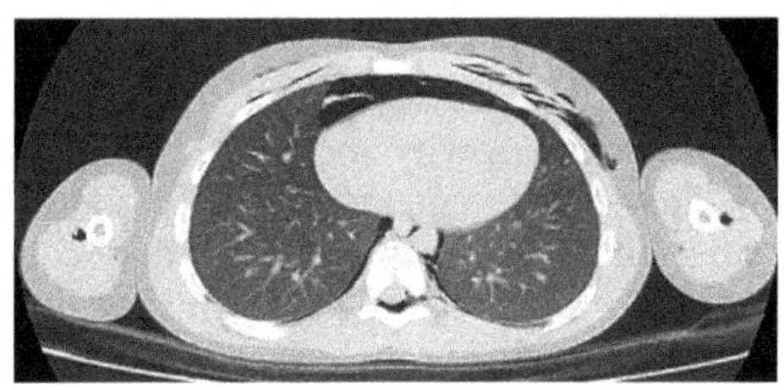

FIGURE 3: The presence of pneumopericardium, large epidural pneumatosis, air in perihumeral region, and prevertebral pneumatosis without pneumothorax.

2. Discussion

Subcutaneous emphysema, pneumomediastinum, pneumopericardium, retropharyngeal-prevertebral pneumatosis, and epidural pneumatosis are a quite rare complication of adenotonsillectomy that tends to develop intraoperatively or during the postoperative period [1]. This case is unusual in that these frightening complications developed extensively with severe vomitting at the third hour of postoperative period when there was no other problem.

Pneumomediastinum is the presence of air or another gas within the mediastinum. This is a rare and generally benign self-limited condition that can be categorized as spontaneous or traumatic [2]. Pneumopericardium can be occasionally accompanied with pneumomediastinum and is defined as a collection of air in the pericardial space. If cardiac tamponade develops, mortality increases up to 58% [3]. Epidural pneumatosis secondary to pneumomediastinum is also a benign situation that does not usually cause a neurological deficit. Most cases recover without treatment. However, close follow-up is suggested because of the risk that intracranial infection or paralysis may occur [4].

The mechanism leading to subcutaneous emphysema, pneumomediastinum, and epidural pneumatosis after adenotonsillectomy have not been conclusively identified. There may be two explanations of this mechanism. Firstly, such pneumatic injuries can be caused by surgical trauma where mucosa and muscle are damaged at the surgical site of adenotonsillectomy. In this situation, this injury provides a route for air to enter the parapharyngeal space by following the cervicofascial plane from entering in through the superior constrictor muscle. Because the paraphayrngeal and retropharyngeal spaces are connected anatomically, the air then travels to the mediastinum. The process is facilitated by events such as coughing, vomitting, respiratory infections, and straining that raise upper airway pressure [1, 2, 5]. In the second mechanism, these complications can also arise from injury during intubation, excessive intra-alveolar pressure, and activities that increase the intrathoracic pressure. These may lead to rupture of tracheal mucosa and perivascular alveoli, and then the free air dissects from the ruptured alveoli along the pulmonary vasculature to reach the mediastinum to produce pneumomediastinum. Accumulated mediastinal air may decompress along cervical fascial planes

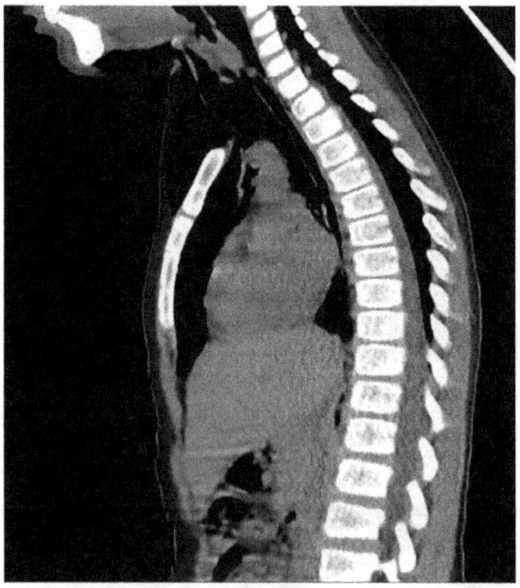

Figure 4: Extensive pneumomediastinum, pneumopericardium, large epidural pneumatosis, and retropharyngeal-prevertebral pneumatosis.

into the subcutaneous tissue to produce subcutaneous emphysema at the chest, head, and neck [6, 7]. Epidural pneumatosis is thought to be due to free air dissecting posteriorly through fascial planes in the nerve roots from the posterior pharynx and mediastinum, axillary arteries, or intervertebral foramina [8]. In our case, there was no obvious mucosal tear and passage of air to the mediastinum in the adenotonsillectomy cavity and upper aerodigestive site. It was more likely that air entered the mediastinum from the lower airways. This event may be a secondary condition to increased intrathoracic pressure with a rupture of the defect in any part of the tracheobronchial tree.

The clinical presentation of subcutaneous emphysema, pneumomediastinum, and pneumopericardium is chest pain, dyspnea, dysphagia, chest and back pain, cyanosis, severe swelling, Hamman's sign (crunching-rasping sound like crepitus synchronous with systole), and crepitus on palpation [9]. Hamman's sign is caused by the heart beating against air-filled tissues, mostly with a decrease in heart sounds, and it is pathognomonic for pneumomediastinum [2]. This sign has also relation with Hamman's syndrome that is a rare condition represented by spontaneous pneumomediastinum and subcutaneous emphysema [10].

Differential diagnosis of neck and chest swollen after adenotonsillectomy includes hematoma, cellulitis, allergic reaction, angioedema, subcutaneous emphysema, and pneumomediastinum [11]. Common predisposing factors for pneumomediastinum were vomiting, coughing, use of cocaine, barotrauma, asthma, excess alcohol consumption, secondary condition to increased intrathoracic pressure, valsalva maneuver, and weight lifting. Uncommon causes of pneumomediastinum include arthroscopy, tooth extraction, vocal training maneuvers, and endotracheal intubation with pyriform sinus, vallecula, or tracheal lacerations [12].

These air containing complications can be detected readily by radiological imaging. If the patient shows the abovementioned clinical conditions, pneumomediastinum should be suspected. A plain neck radiograph will demonstrate the finding of subcutaneous emphysema. Pneumomediastinum should be excluded with an anteroposterior and a lateral chest radiograph [13]. With the increased use of chest CT scan and technologic advancement in the initial evaluation of trauma, the sensitivity of detecting pneumomediastinum has increased, and findings that were not seen on a chest radiograph are increasingly identified. Because the presence of pneumomediastinum posterior to the heart was associated with increased mortality, this location of pneumomediastinum noted on the CT could be immediately assessed on admission. These findings on the CT should alert the clinician that the patient has an increased risk of a mortality of up to 40% and may help guide subsequent management [14]. So the surgeon can consider them for patients as close monitoring in the ICU, aggressive operation, and the possibility of additional diagnostic studies.

In adenotonsil surgery, avoiding harmful maneuvers and using of meticulous bipolar dissection or careful blunt dissection should be performed that delivers less damage, instead of high-voltage electrodissection and aggressive snare technique. This would most probably prevent the development of these frustrating complications. Additionally, as to prevent these complications, intubation should be carefully done to avoid upper airway lesions, and ventilation of high positive oxygen pressure should be avoided in case of significant tissue damage at operative area [2].

Treatment of patients with these complications in children involves intensive cardiorespiratory assessment and monitoring. Any activity that increases upper airway pressure such as coughing, valsalva, or forced expiration should be avoided, and the injured mucosa may be sutured. This provides to prevent further air and microbial tracking within tissue planes. Uncomplicated pneumomediastinum and epidural pneuomatosis are managed conservatively with oxygen, analgesia, sedation, bed rest, restriction of oral intake, the administration of a cough suppressant, and a stool softener. Broad-spectrum antibiotics may also be prescribed to prevent development of life-threatening mediastinitis. In severe cases with airways involvement, orotracheal intubation and tracheotomy are indicated. Surgical approach for decompression is not routinely adopted, if tension pneumothorax, tension pneumomediastinum, air tamponade, and cardiac herniation do not accompany these disorders. Most cases are usually solved after supportive treatment in 7–10 days of observation. The prognosis is excellent with conservative management, and the risk for recurrence is low [15].

3. Conclusions

In conclusion, an association between a skin emphysema, a pneumomediastinum, a pneumopericardium, and epidural pneumatosis is extremely rare in children. They are usually benign self-limited conditions that require early differentiation from more serious causes. The defined complications' successfull treatment depends on immediate and accurate diagnosis. Careful examination of initial chest X-ray is important for avoiding unnecessary investigations. CT scanning has an importance in diagnosing clinically suspected cases when chest X-ray is uncertain. In our case, it was more likely that air entered through the lower airway to the mediastinum with a rupture anywhere along a defect or bullous formation of the tracheobronchial tree. Intubation should be carefully performed to avoid airway lesions. Ultimately, the surgical approach should be the least aggressive.

Conflicts of Interest

The authors declare that they have no conflicts of interest.

References

[1] N. P. Shine, C. Sader, and H. Coates, "Cervicofacial emphysema and pneumomediastinum following pediatric adenotonsillectomy: a rare complication," *International Journal of Pediatric Otorhinolaryngology*, vol. 69, no. 11, pp. 1579–1582, 2005.

[2] J. P. Kim, J. J. Park, H. S. Kang, and M. S. Song, "Subcutaneous emphysema and pneumomediastinum after tonsillectomy," *American Journal of Otolaryngology*, vol. 31, no. 3, pp. 212–215, 2010.

[3] R. G. Cummings, R. L. Wesly, D. H. Adams, and J. E. Lowe, "Pneumopericardium resulting in cardiac tamponade," *Annals of Thoracic Surgery*, vol. 37, no. 6, pp. 511–518, 1984.

[4] P. D. Koelliker and L. A. Brannam, "Epidural pneumatosis associated with spontaneous pneumomediastinum: case report and review of the literature," *Journal of Emergency Medicine*, vol. 17, no. 2, pp. 247–250, 1999.

[5] A. E. Stewart, D. F. Brewster, and P. E. Bernstein, "Subcutaneous emphysema and pneumomediastinum complicating tonsillectomy," *Archives of Otolaryngology-Head & Neck Surgery*, vol. 130, no. 11, pp. 1324–1327, 2004.

[6] C. Gillot, S. Tombu, V. Crestani et al., "Subcutaneous emphysema and mediastinitis: unusual complications of tonsillectomy," *B-ENT*, vol. 1, no. 4, pp. 197–200, 2005.

[7] K. F. Watters, P. D. Lacy, and R. M. Walsh, "Massive subcutaneous emphysema following routine endotracheal intubation," *Journal of Laryngology & Otology*, vol. 117, no. 11, pp. 899–901, 2003.

[8] V. S. Dontu and D. Kramer, "Spontaneous pneumothorax, pneumomediastinum and epidural emphysema presenting as neck pain suspicious for meningitis," *Pediatric Emergency Care*, vol. 23, no. 7, pp. 469–471, 2007.

[9] H. Nishino, M. Kenmochi, S. Kasugai, T. Okada, and T. Ohashi, "Subcutaneous emphysema secondary to tonsillectomy: a case report," *Auris Nasus Larynx*, vol. 30, pp. 135-136, 2003.

[10] D. Khurram, B. Patel, and M. W. Farra, "Hamman's syndrome: a rare cause of chest pain in a postpartum patient," *Case Reports in Pulmonology*, vol. 2015, Article ID 201051, 4 pages, 2015.

[11] N. Patel and G. Brookes, "Surgical emphysema following tonsillectomy," *Ear, Nose and Throat Journal*, vol. 84, no. 10, pp. 660-661, 2005.

[12] D. T. Damore and P. S. Dayan, "Medical causes of pneumomediastinum in children," *Clinical Pediatrics*, vol. 40, no. 2, pp. 87–91, 2001.

[13] P. I. Abbas, A. C. Akinkuotu, M. L. Peterson, and M. V. Mazziotti, "Spontaneous pneumomediastinum in the pediatric patient," *American Journal of Surgery*, vol. 210, no. 6, pp. 1031–1035, 2015.

[14] W. S. Lee, V. E. Chong, and G. P. Victorino, "Computed tomographic findings and mortality in patients with pneumomediastinum from blunt trauma," *JAMA Surgery*, vol. 150, no. 8, pp. 757–762, 2015.

[15] C. J. Allen, L. F. Teisch, and K. D. Stahl, "Spontaneous pneumomediastinum, pneumopericardium and epidural pneumatosis: insights on clinical management," *Acute Cardiac Care*, vol. 17, no. 1, pp. 20–23, 2015.

14

Multimodality Surgical Approach in Management of Laryngotracheal Stenosis

Ashfaque Ansari and Annju Thomas

E. N. T. Department, MGM Medical College and Hospital, Aurangabad, Maharashtra, India

Correspondence should be addressed to Annju Thomas; thannju@gmail.com

Academic Editor: Andrea Gallo

Introduction. Postintubation laryngotracheal stenosis requires a precise diagnosis and an experienced operator in both endoscopic and surgical treatment. This report presents surgically treated cases of laryngotracheal stenosis secondary to long-term intubation/tracheostomy with review of the literature. *Materials and Methods.* In this retrospective study, we present 5 cases (a 23-year-old male, 13-year-old male, 22-year-old male, 19-year-old male, and 33-year-old female) of postintubation/tracheostomy laryngotracheal (glottic/subglottic) stenosis in the years 2016 and 2017. Each patient was managed differently. Intubation characteristics, localization of stenosis, surgical technique and material, postoperative complications, and survival of patients were recorded. *Results.* The site of stenosis was in the subglottis in 4 patients and glottis in 1 patient. The mean length of the stenosis was greater in the postintubation group. Postintubation stenosis had a mean duration of intubation of 6.8 days, compared to 206.25 days of cannulation following tracheostomies. Each patient underwent an average of 2 procedures during their treatment course. One patient underwent open surgical anastomosis because of recurrent subglottic stenosis after multiple treatments. Phonation improved immediately in almost all except in the patient who underwent only endoscopic dilatation. *Discussion.* The reasons for laryngeal stenosis and its delayed diagnosis have been reviewed from the literature. Suture tension should be appropriate, and placement of the suture knot outside the trachea minimizes formation of granulation tissue. The published reports suggest that resection by endoscopy with laser and open technique resection and primary anastomosis are the best treatment modality so far as the long-term results are concerned. *Conclusion.* Resection of stenotic segment by open surgical anastomosis and laser-assisted resection is a safe option for the treatment of subglottic stenosis following intubation without the need for repeated dilation. Endoscopic dilation can be reserved for unfit patients.

1. Introduction

Laryngotracheal stenosis is a congenital or acquired narrowing of the airway that may affect the supraglottis, glottis, and/or subglottis. It has several grades. Incidence of laryngotracheal stenosis following intubation has been reported up to 21% [1]. However, only a few (1-2%) of these patients present with the symptoms. Resection and anastomosis has been established as the definitive treatment of stenosis more than one cm in length [2]. The current study aims to present cases of laryngotracheal stenosis managed by different methods at our hospital.

2. Materials and Methods

2.1. Setting and Patients. The study was conducted by the department of ENT in a teaching hospital in western India. Patients were identified from the prospectively maintained admission and operation theater registers. A total of 5 patients were identified between April 2016 and November 2017. The 5 patients were treated for glottic/subglottic stenosis following tracheostomy and after prolonged endotracheal intubation. Cases with high-grade stenosis (Cotton–Meyer's III and IV) with loss of structural integrity were included in this study. Patients having GERD were excluded.

Demographic data were obtained for each patient: age, sex, comorbid conditions, and corticosteroid therapy received. The following data regarding the stenosis were also obtained: the circumstances leading to the development of stenosis (postintubation/tracheostomy/surgery/trauma), type of stenosis (web-like stenosis, granulation tissue formation, and adhesions), and the procedures performed.

Each patient underwent a standard preoperative assessment, including physical examination, routine laboratory tests, chest radiography, and computed tomography of the chest with virtual bronchoscopy. An initial diagnostic flexible bronchoscopy was performed for each patient to identify the type, location, and severity of the stenosis. The stenosis was characterized severe if it was causing symptoms, primarily dyspnea, and was complex in nature (stenosis combined with cartilage fracture or tracheomalacia), and the obstruction of the tracheal lumen exceeded 50%.

2.2. Case Report 1. A 23-year-old male came to our OPD with complaints of change of voice and noisy breathing. Examination revealed that the young man had inspiratory stridor and hoarseness of voice with portex tracheostomy tube in situ. History revealed that he was admitted previously for organophosphorus poisoning 3 years back, during that time he was intubated for 15 days. After extubation, he was kept in the ward for 5 days after which he was discharged. The patient developed dyspnea 1 month after discharge from primary hospital, and the patient was admitted and taken up for emergency tracheostomy, following which a clinical diagnosis of tracheal stenosis was made.

CT neck revealed tracheal stenosis proximal to tracheostomy stoma involving length of 2 cm and transverse diameter of 6 mm.

After which, the patient underwent 6 check bronchoscopies and 1 dilatation and followed stenting of the stenosis at the previous hospital, which did not relieve him of his complaints. He underwent a check bronchoscopy with dilatation of the tracheal stenosis at our hospital 1 year later.

The patient returned back to our ENT OPD 1 year after the dilatation with complaints of hoarseness of voice and stridor. 3D CT neck (Figures 1 and 2) revealed tracheal stenosis over approximately 11 mm length, noted at the level of cricoid cartilage. Transverse diameter measures 5.5 mm, and AP diameter measures 5.1 mm. There was grade III (90%) stenosis over the third tracheal ring with narrowing extending proximally up to the second ring. CT scan showed a stenotic segment of 2.5 cm. The patient and his relatives were explained about the condition and the procedure to be performed. They agreed for a reconstructive surgery, and a tracheal resection and anastomosis was planned.

The patient underwent surgery, and apron's neck incision was taken. Flaps elevated superiorly till the hyoid bone and inferiorly till the clavicle. Strap muscles were separated, and thyroid gland was dissected. Trachea was visualized, and stenotic portion of the trachea was resected, and end-to-end anastomosis was done with 3/0 Prolene suture material, and a Romo vac drain was kept in situ. A mentosternal suture with neck in flexion to restrict neck movement was placed with 1/0 Prolene. Postoperatively, the patient was kept in ICU with nasal intubation. Nasal intubation and Romo vac drain was removed on the 5th postoperative day. The patient was shifted out of ICU on the 8th postoperative day due to uneventful recovery and was discharged on the 14th postoperative day. At 1-month follow-up, the patient was asymptomatic with normal breathing and voice.

CT neck 6 month postoperatively (Figure 3) suggested of no evidence of stenosis. Tracheal lumen and tracheal bifurcation were normal, and on 70 degree scopy, vocal cord mobility was normal.

2.3. Case Report 2. A 13-year-old male was referred to our OPD with complaints of dyspnea and noisy breathing. Examination revealed that the patient had inspiratory stridor with metallic tracheostomy tube in situ. On indirect laryngoscopy, bilateral vocal cords were mobile. History revealed that the patient was admitted in the Government Medical College in view of neuroparalysis secondary to snake bite. The patient was ventilated through an endotracheal tube for 10 days after which he underwent a tracheostomy. The patient was shifted to the ward on the 23rd day after admission. The patient was discharged with a metallic tube in situ. After discharge, the patient complained of noisy breathing. The patient underwent flexible bronchoscopy which revealed subglottic stenosis, bilateral fixed vocal cords due to thickening, and fibrosis. The patient was referred to our hospital for further management. The patient's relatives were explained about the condition and the procedure to be performed. They agreed for the surgery, and laser-assisted transglottic stenosis excision was planned.

The patient underwent the surgery under general anaesthesia, and flexible bronchoscopy was done. Floppy epiglottis was visualized, and glottis stenosis with interarytenoid adhesion was seen. Subglottic soft stenosis (Cotton–Meyer's grade 4) was visualized. Rigid bronchoscopy was done, and stenotic segment length was assessed. Bogdasarian grade 4 postglottic stenosis was noted and partly released with CO_2 laser. Bougie was used for dilatation of the subglottic stenosis. CO_2 laser was used to release the stenotic bands of the subglottic stenosis. Endotracheal tube number 4 was inserted through the tracheostomy (Figures 4 and 5) site upward in a retrograde fashion through the stenosis to maintain patency.

Postoperatively, the patient was kept in ICU. The patient was shifted out of ICU on the 3rd postoperative day. The patient made uneventful recovery with no complaints of dyspnea and noisy breathing. The patient was discharged on the 20th postoperative day after Montgomery T-tube insertion. Postoperatively, after the 6 month, the Montgomery T-tube was removed. One month after T-tube removal, there was no evidence of stridor and no recurrence of stenosis.

2.4. Case Report 3. A 22-year-old male presented to our OPD with complaints of dyspnea on lying down and hoarseness of voice. Examination revealed that the patient had orthopnea and stridor. On indirect laryngoscopy, bilateral vocal cords were fixed with interarytenoid adhesion and with subglottic stenosis. History revealed that the patient had history of hospitalization in view of OP poisoning. The patient was

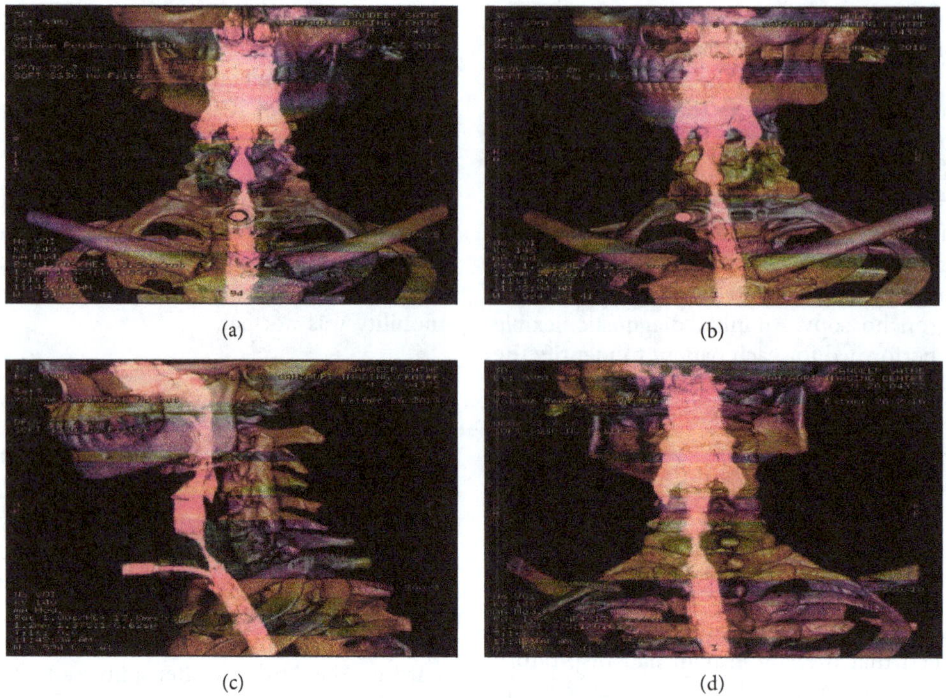

Figure 1: 3D CT neck showing stenotic portion.

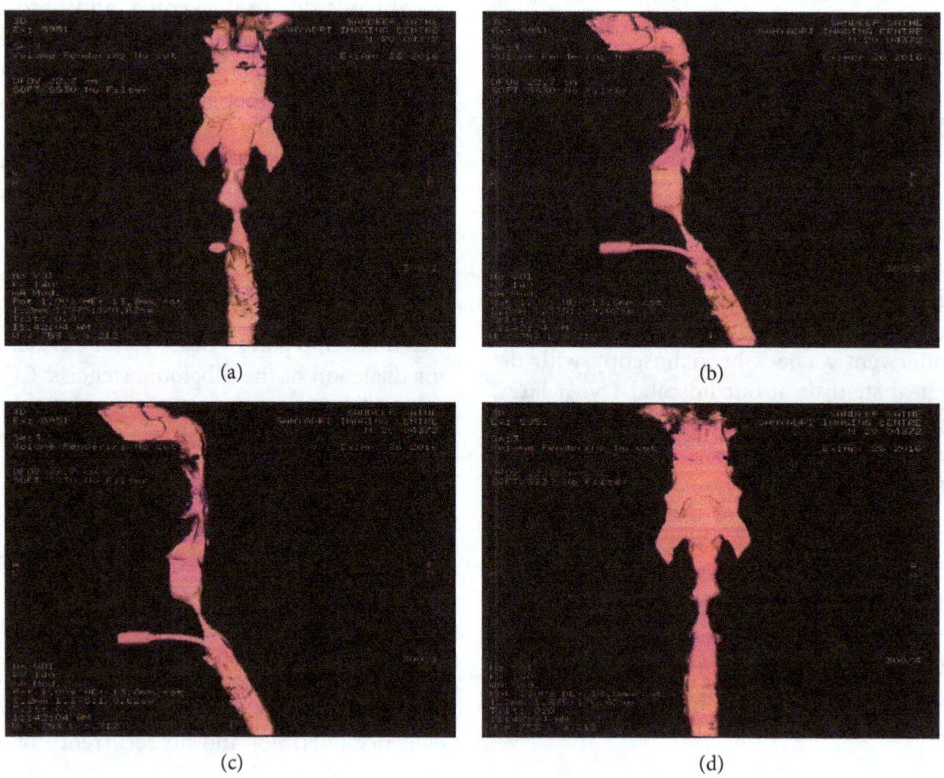

Figure 2: 3D CT neck showing stenotic portion.

intubated for 2 weeks. The patient was shifted to the ward after extubation on the 3rd week after admission. The patient was discharged. After discharge, the patient complained of hoarseness of voice and dyspnea. The patient came to our OPD where on indirect laryngoscopy it was revealed that the patient has bilateral abductor cord palsy with interarytenoid adhesion, and on flexible bronchoscopy, there was a stenosis seen, 4 cm (Figure 6) below the glottis which was grade II soft stenosis. The patient's relatives were explained about the condition of the patient and the procedure to be performed.

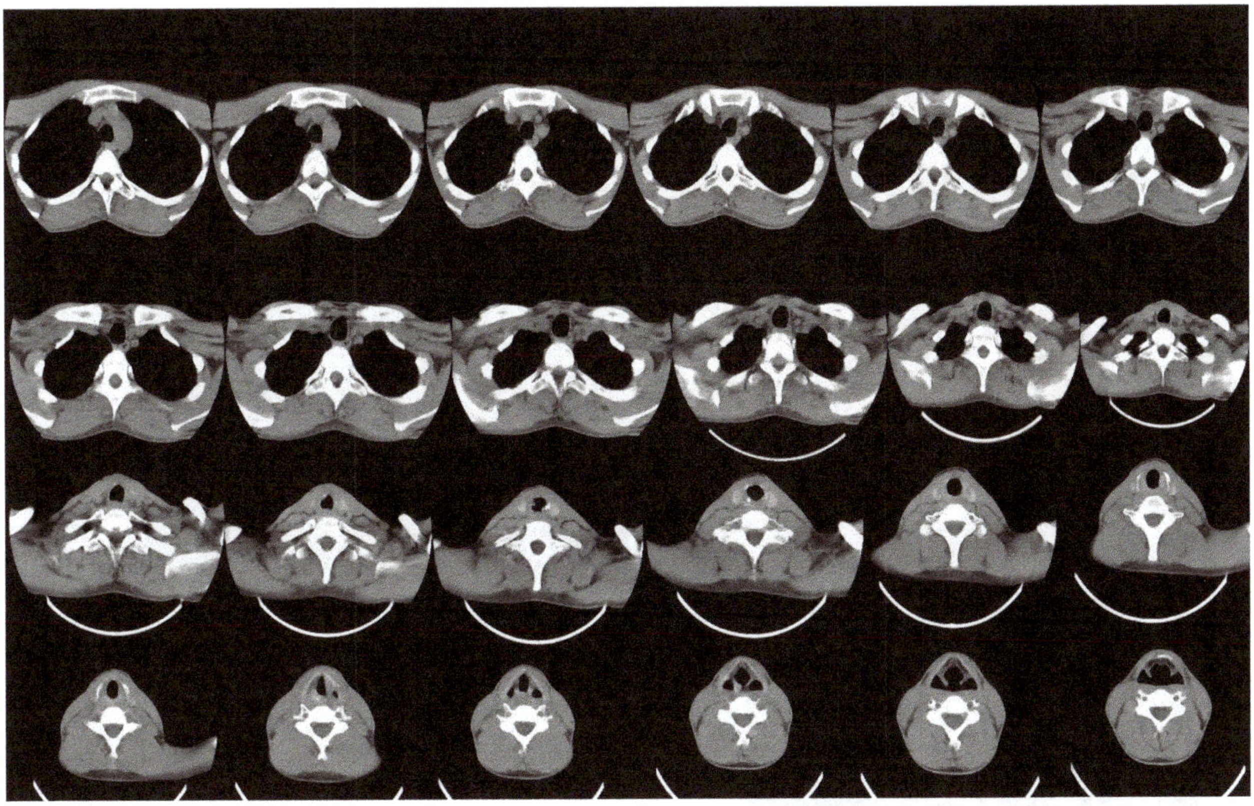

FIGURE 3: CT neck 6 month postoperatively.

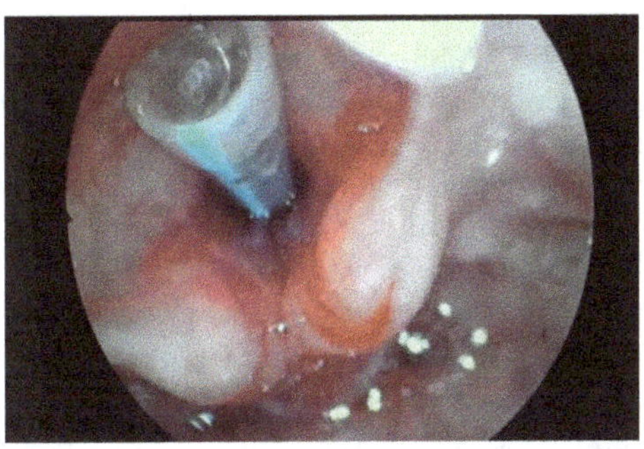

FIGURE 4: Endotracheal tube number 4 inserted after laser-assisted release of stenosis.

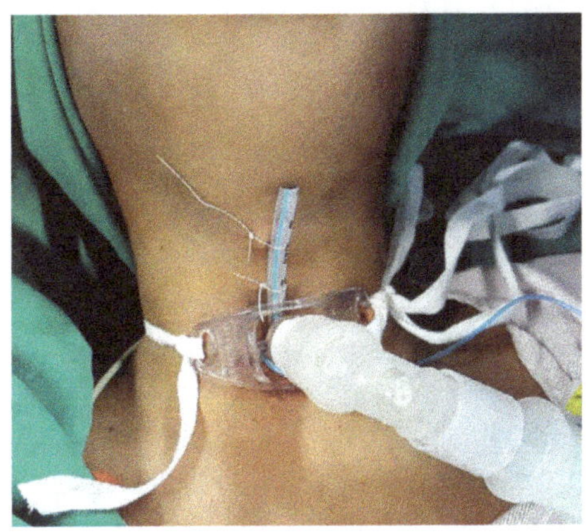

FIGURE 5: Endotracheal tube number 4 inserted after laser-assisted release of stenosis.

They agreed for the surgery, and MLscopic Kashima's cordotomy by laser was planned.

The patient underwent surgery on 18 March 2017. Under general anaesthesia, after intubation, MLscope was introduced. Bilateral vocal cords were visualized, and posterior commissure was visualized. Right side cordotomy was done using CO_2 laser (Figure 7), followed by dilatation of stenotic portion using rigid bronchoscope. The patient was shifted to ICU postoperatively and was shifted out on the 3rd postoperative day. The patient made an uneventful recovery and was discharged from the ENT ward on the 9th postoperative day. Six months postoperatively, on endoscopic examination, there was no evidence of glottic or subglottic stenosis and there was no evidence of stridor.

2.5. Case Report 4. A 19-year-old boy was brought to our OPD with complaints of dyspnea. Examination revealed that the patient had stridor and portex tracheostomy tube in situ. On indirect laryngoscopy, bilateral vocal cords were mobile. History revealed that the patient was admitted in another hospital 1 month prior to visit at our hospital in view of head injury. The patient had undergone craniotomy for the same with tracheostomy. The patient was discharged after an uneventful recovery after decannulating him. The patient started developing dyspnea 15 days after discharge. The patient underwent tracheostomy once again. The patient was discharged

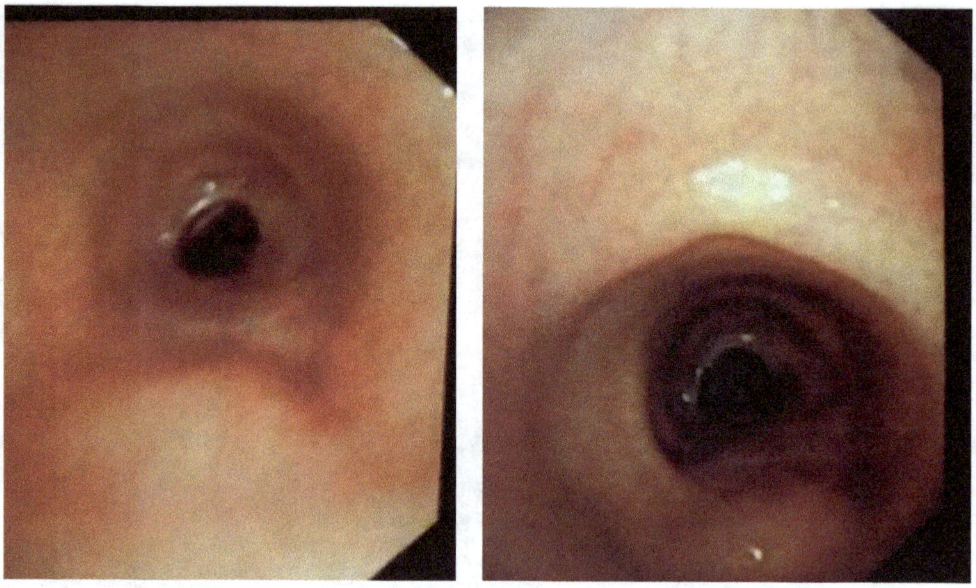

(a) (b)

FIGURE 6: Stenosis seen 4 cm below the glottis.

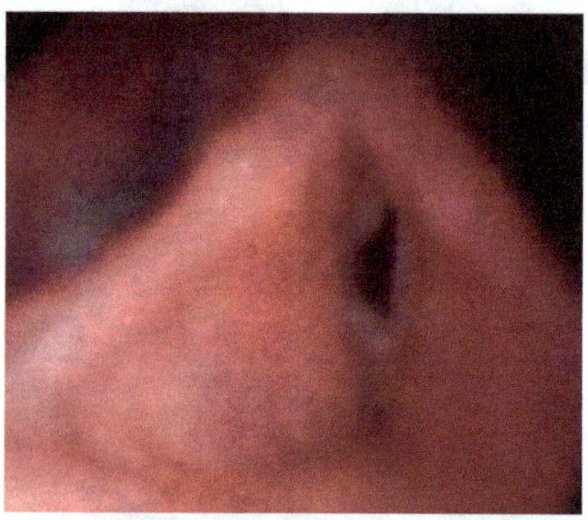

FIGURE 7: Postoperative image of Kashima's cordotomy.

with portex tracheostomy tube number 8. The patient came to our OPD in view of dyspnea after which a CT neck was performed suggestive of tracheostomy in situ 3 cm from the carina with tracheal stenosis at the level of tracheostomy tube. The patient's relatives were explained about the condition of the patient and the procedure to be performed. They agreed for the surgery, and flexible bronchoscopy was planned.

The patient underwent surgery on 20 September 2016. Under local anaesthesia, flexible bronchoscopy was done. Portex tracheostomy tube no. 8 was slightly pulled out for better visualization. Tracheal stenosis was visualized at level of tracheostoma (Figure 8). Tracheal stenosis was mild, and granulation tissue was positive. Dilatation was done using balloon dilator, and tracheostomy tube number 7 was inserted. The patient was shifted to the ward postoperatively and was discharged with metallic tracheostomy tube on the 3rd postoperative day. The patient followed up on the 15th postoperative day, and tracheostomy decannulation was done. After check bronchoscopy and dilatation, the patient was discharged. The patient required one more sitting of dilatation in the 2nd postoperative month. On the 6th postoperative month, check bronchoscopy revealed no evidence of stenosis.

2.6. Case Report 5. A 33-year-old female was referred to our OPD with complaints of hoarseness of voice and dyspnea on exertion. Examination revealed that the patient had stridor. On indirect laryngoscopy, bilateral vocal cords were mobile. History revealed that the patient was admitted in view of clozapine poisoning and was kept intubated for 10 days. After extubation, the patient made an uneventful recovery and was discharged on the 5th day after shifting to the ward. The patient came to our OPD with complaints of hoarseness of voice and dyspnea on exertion. CT scan revealed narrowing of trachea for an approximate length 2 cm from C7-T1 to T1-T2. Since the stenosis involved the distal airway fibreoptic visualization with holmium laser excision was planned. The patient's relatives were explained about the condition of the patient and the procedure to be performed.

They agreed for the surgery and excision of stenosis by holmium laser (Figure 9) with balloon dilatation followed by mitomycin C application was done. The patient was shifted to ICU postoperatively and was shifted out on the 2nd postoperative day. The patient made an uneventful recovery and was discharged from the ENT ward on the 5th postoperative day. There was no evidence of stridor and no evidence of stenosis on check bronchoscopy when the patient followed up in the 4th postoperative month.

3. Results

Five patients were included: 1 female and 4 males (Figure 10). Patients were predominantly male in the case study. Mean

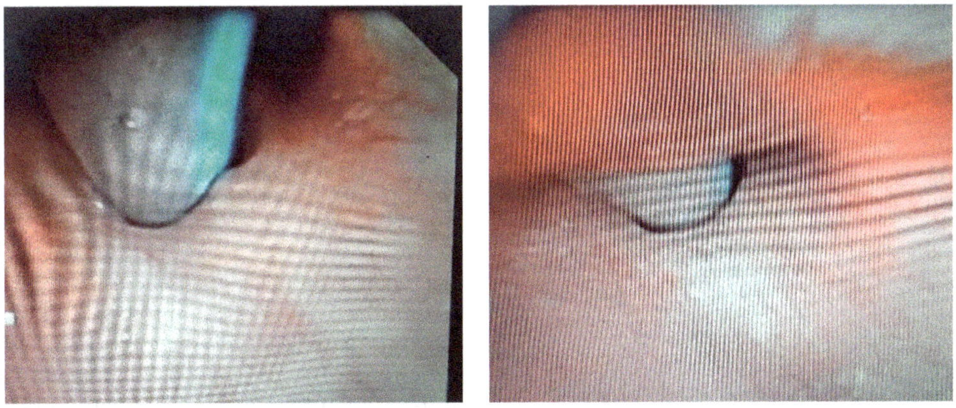

(a) (b)

FIGURE 8: Tracheal stenosis at level of tracheostoma.

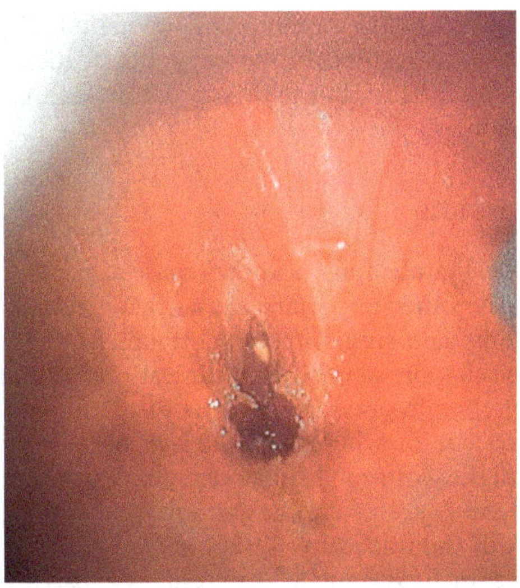

FIGURE 9: Laser excision of stenosis.

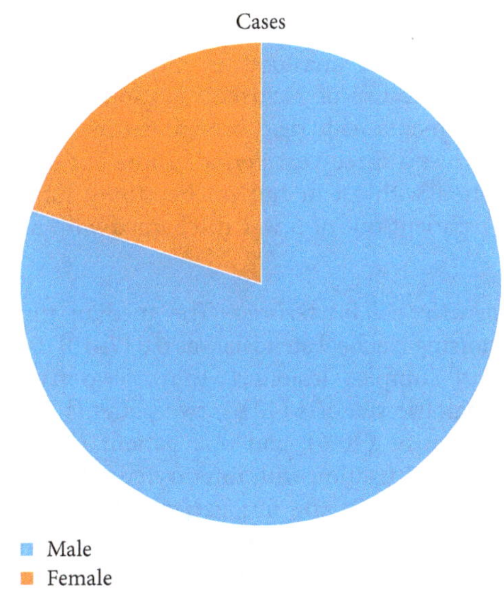

FIGURE 10: Male and female pie graph.

age was 22 ± 10 years (range: 13 to 33 years). Reason for intubation/tracheostomy is noted in Table 1.

The comorbidities found were diabetes mellitus and hypothyroidism (1 patient each). Two each were addicted to smoking and alcohol. Three patients were on corticosteroid therapy.

Patients' characteristics and comorbidities as seen in patient at the time of the first interventional bronchoscopy procedure performed are listed in Table 2 and Figure 11.

The site of stenosis was localized in the subglottis in 4 patients (80%) and glottis with subglottis in 1 patient (20%) (Figure 12).

The characteristics of the laryngotracheal stenosis varied depending on whether the development of stenosis followed postintubation or tracheostomy and are presented in Table 3. The mean length of the stenosis was greater in the post-intubation group due to the formation of a web-like stenosis along the distribution of the endotracheal tube cuff. Patients with postintubation stenosis had a mean duration of intubation of 6.8 days. Patients with tracheal stenosis following tracheostomy had a much longer duration of cannulation, with a mean of 206.25 days.

TABLE 1: Reason for tracheostomy/intubation.

	Cases (n = 5)
Poisoning	4 (80%)
Head injury	1 (20%)

The types of the glottic stenosis developed in the patients are presented in Figure 13. No significant difference was noted between males and females with regards to the predisposing factors or comorbid conditions and the type of glottic stenosis. A variety of modalities and treatments were applied as mentioned in Table 4.

All patients underwent indirect laryngoscopy upon admission. No complications related to the procedure were reported. Four patients underwent flexible bronchoscopy first. HCT3D was performed in 1 patient. Postintubation injury was the most frequent cause of stenosis in 4 patients (80%) and 1 due to posttracheostomy trauma (20%) (Figure 14).

Each patient underwent an average of 2 procedures during their treatment course. One patient was treated with

TABLE 2: Comorbidities.

	Cases (n = 5)
Male/female	4/1
Age (median range)	22 ± 10 years (range: 13 to 33 years)
Diabetes mellitus	1 (20%)
Cardiovascular disease	0
Systemic hypertension	0
Gastroesophageal reflux disease	0
Chronic obstructive pulmonary disease	0
Asthma	0
Obstructive sleep apnea	0
Hypothyroidism	1 (20%)
Alcohol	2 (40%)
Smoking	2 (40%)
Corticosteroid therapy	3 (10%)

5 procedures prior to admission and finally underwent surgical management by anastomosis. This patient underwent open surgery because of recurrent subglottic stenosis after multiple treatments with rigid bronchoscopy and stent implantations over a three-year period. Three out of 5 patients were admitted with an in situ tracheostomy tube. Postoperatively, 1 patient out of 5 was discharged with a stent.

3.1. Preoperative Characteristics. The median time of intubation causing tracheal stenosis was 6.8 [7–10] days All the patients had complex lesions (>1cm). Two patients had grade 3 subglottic stenosis (40%), two patients had grade 2 subglottic stenosis (40%), and one patient (20%) had bilateral vocal cord fixation with interarytenoid adhesion and subglottic stenosis. Of the five patients, two patients had previous endoscopic dilation, and one of the 2 patients who had underwent dilatation in the past had tracheal stents prior to surgery.

3.2. Operative Findings. An endoscopic visualization of the glottis and subglottis was sufficient in 4 patients of which 1 (20%) patient with bilateral vocal cord paralysis underwent endoscopic laser-assisted cordotomy with removal of interarytenoid adhesion and subglottic stenosis, 1 (20%) patient with subglottic stenosis with lax tracheal underwent endoscopic laser-assisted resection with placement of stent, 1 (20%) patient with stenosis at the level of tracheostoma underwent dilation using bougies, and one patient (20%) with subglottic stenosis at the level of C7-T1 and T1-T2 underwent excision of stenosis by holmium laser followed by dilatation of excised stenotic part by balloon followed by mitomycin C application around the excised region. Only one patient of the five (20%) with subglottic stenosis with a history of previous endoscopic dilations and stenting which were unsuccessful underwent open surgical tracheal resection and anastomosis.

3.3. Postoperative Results. Postoperative intubation and ventilator support were required in 1 patient, and remaining 4 patients did not requir any assisted ventilation postoperatively (Figure 15). ICU admission was required for 4 patients out of 5. Median length of ICU stay was 5.5 (range: 4–7 days)

The median length of hospital stay was 9 days (range: 7–21 days). The postoperative success rate was 100%. None of the 5 patients in the study had severe perichondritis and postoperative stridor.

3.4. Follow-Up Review. The median follow-up duration was 6 months (range: 2–12 months). All the 5 patients were asymptomatic and very satisfied with their results after the procedure. The patient who underwent resection and anastomosis by open surgical technique and using holmium laser with balloon dilatation had improvement in phonation immediately after 1-month follow-up. The patient with bilateral vocal cord paralysis had no airway problems, and the patient with laser-assisted resection with stenting and phonation improved over the six-month follow-up period. The patients who underwent flexible bronchoscopy with dilation alone had no airway complaints, but there was not much improvement in phonation.

4. Discussion

Endotracheal intubation is a known cause of glottic/subglottic stenosis. The other important causes being complication of tracheostomy and surgical/external trauma.

Postintubation stenosis is a clinical problem caused by regional ischemic pressure necrosis of the airway [7]. Stenosis can occur anywhere from the level of the endotracheal tube tip till the glottic and subglottic area. The most common sites of stenosis are where the endotracheal cuff has been in contact with the tracheal wall and at the tracheal stoma site following a tracheostomy [8]. As a result, stenosis occurs most commonly following the two types of airway intubation: endotracheal intubation and tracheostomy [9].

Causative factor of stenosis is the pressure exerted by the cuff on the tracheal mucosa. At a cuff pressure of >30 mmHg, there is an increase in mucosal capillary perfusion pressure, which leads to mucosal ischemia and consequent inflammation of the tracheal cartilages. These pathological changes may eventually lead to fibrosis of circumferential lesions, resulting in progressive tracheal stenosis [10]. Ischemic injury can occur even within minutes after insufflation of the cuff and subsequent fibrotic changes within the following 3–6 weeks. Although the use of large-volume, low-pressure cuffs markedly reduces the occurrence of cuff injury, glottic stenosis continues to occur at a high frequency, with the incidence of postintubation tracheal stenosis in intensive care units being 6–21%, although only 1-2% of patients are symptomatic or have severe stenosis [3].

The diagnosis of laryngotracheal stenosis is often missed, and the related symptoms are generally evident only when stenosis of 30% of the original diameter of the trachea has occurred. Sometimes, the diagnosis may be delayed for as long as three months after the intubation [4]. Several risk factors of postintubation stenosis have been recognized thus far, including the size of the endotracheal

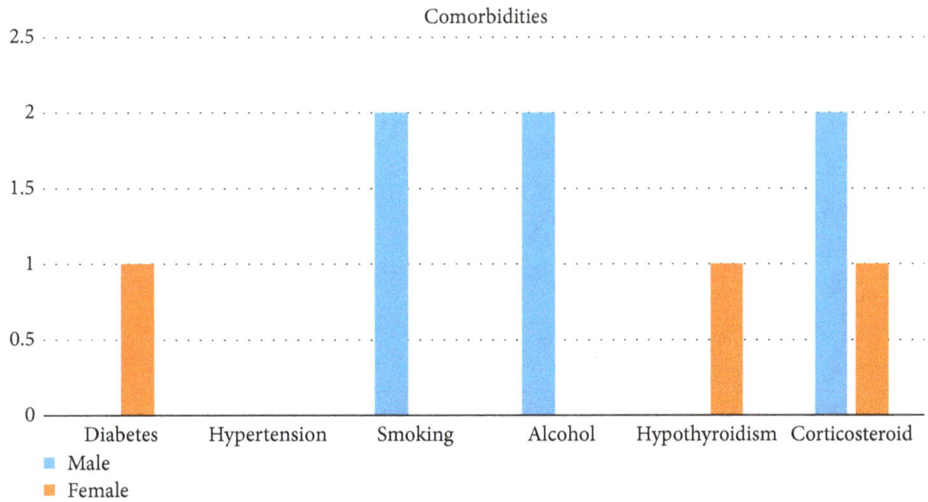

FIGURE 11: Comorbidities in males and females.

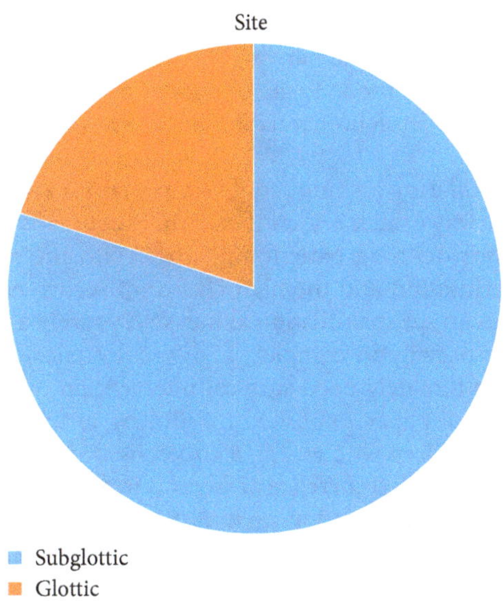

FIGURE 12: Site of stenosis.

TABLE 3: Characteristics of stenosis.

	Cases ($n = 5$)
Days with endotracheal tube	6.8 (7–10)
Days with tracheostomy	206.25 (14–900)
Distance from vocal cords (cm)	3.1 (2–7)
Distance from main carina (cm)	3.6 (3–5)
Length of stenosis (cm)	1.2 (0.5–2.5)
Percent of stenosis	78.5% (60–90%)

tube relative to the tracheal lumen, frequent replacement of the endotracheal tube, traumatic intubation, concurrent infection, blood pressure during the intubation period, female gender, estrogen effect, steroid administration, obesity, and smoking history [5, 6].

Intubation needed during treatment is the most likely cause of stenosis in the three cases. Development of stenosis following intubation has been reported to occur even with two days of intubation [9]. A period up to two weeks in adults and even longer in children is generally considered safe.

In the above 5 cases, patients were asymptomatic after discharge from their primary care and started showing symptoms of stenosis within 1 month.

The factors that are related to development of stenosis with shorter duration of intubations are large size of the tube, high pressure in cuff, not deflating cuff periodically, struggling or restless patient, traumatic intubation, multiple intubation, and infection around the cuff site [9, 11, 12]. All these factors may play a role in development of stenosis.

The assessment of the degree of stenosis is an important step for each patient. Although several grading systems have been proposed, the universally accepted grading of subglottic stenosis was devised by Myer et al.: grade 1, <50% obstruction; grade 2, 51–70% obstruction; grade 3, 71–99% obstruction; and grade 4, no detectable lumen [13].

Galluccio et al. proposed classifying subglottic stenosis as either simple or complex [14]. They defined simple stenosis as lesions <1 cm in length with no associated tracheomalacia or loss of cartilaginous support. Complex lesions were >1 cm and had the greatest benefit from surgical intervention. This is significant for our study as our patients had complex lesions.

Complications of open surgical end-to-end anastomosis include restenosis, dehiscence, granulation, dysphagia, and RLN damage.

Granulation tissue formation occurs in proportion to the traction at the anastomosis site; choosing an appropriate type of suture is important, and we preferred polypropylene. Suture tension should be appropriate, and the suture knot should be formed outside the trachea to prevent formation of granulation tissue. Behrend and Klempnauer used three types of suture material (polypropylene, polydioxanone, and polyglactin) in tracheal surgery in sheep [15]. The results were similar in all three groups, but it was noted that the suture material should be of high tensile strength and should not be absorbed in under six months. The authors concluded that the

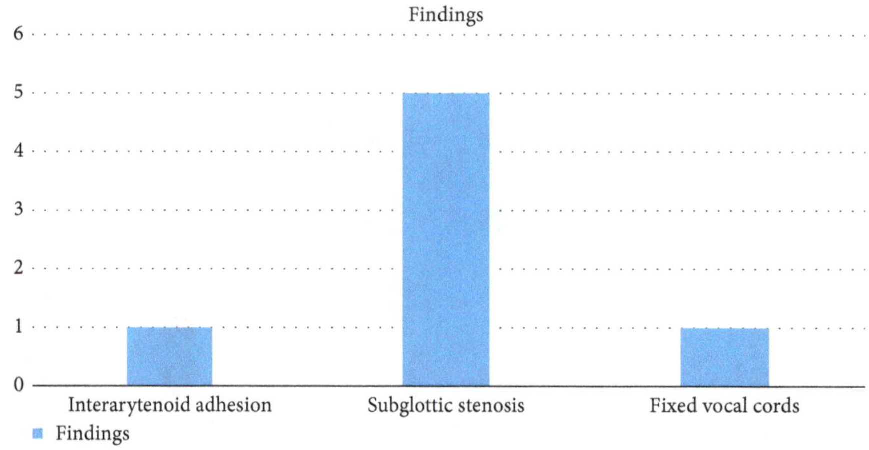

FIGURE 13: Findings/type of stenosis.

TABLE 4: Treatment modalities.

	Patients ($n = 5$)
Flexible bronchoscopy with dilation	1
Open surgical anastomosis	1
CO_2 laser-assisted cordotomy with removal of subglottic stenosis by laser	1
CO_2 laser-assisted resection with Montgomery tube stenting	1
Holmium laser-assisted resection of stenosis with balloon dilatation with application of mitomycin C	1

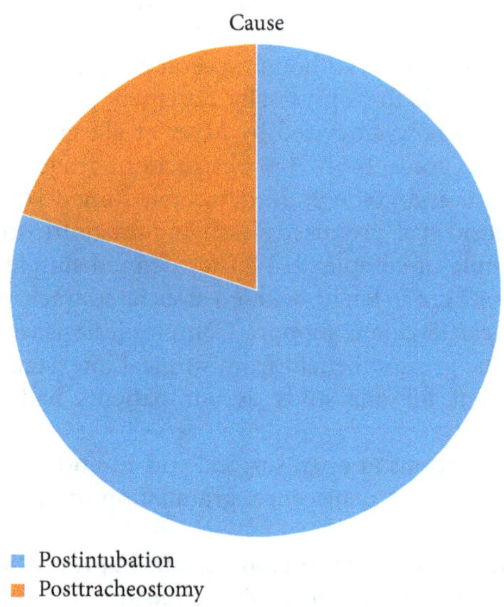

FIGURE 14: Main cause of trauma.

technical details (especially tension) are more important than the choice of suture material for postoperative results.

In case 1, the patient had previous history of 4 endoscopic dilations followed by stenting, and case 2 underwent dilation prior to laser excision; both patients were not relieved of their complaints. In case 4, the patient had undergone plain flexible bronchoscopy with dilation, and there was no evidence of recurrence postoperatively. Dilation is achieved with lubricated bougies of increasing diameter applying radial pressure circumferentially to the narrowed airway. Balloon dilation is an alternative method. Rigid bronchoscope can be used to perform blunt dissection and dilation of stenosed areas under direct vision.

For all dilating techniques, it is important that the path of the true airway lumen is identified [16]. Preoperative imaging is useful for defining patient anatomy. With the associated risk of perforation and the high chance of recurrence of stenosis, one can see that dilation alone is very rarely a definitive therapy (especially in complex, high-grade stenosis) and patients will ultimately need surgical intervention.

There is a paper published in 2014 by Ortiz et al., who treated 18 children with repeated endoscopic tracheal dilation [17]. There was no recurrence of stenosis in any of the patients (median follow-up duration: 36 months, range: 5–72 months). However, this finding may not be replicable in the adults. Children have more favourable results with tracheal dilation as their inflammatory response is less pronounced, and there is therefore less fibrous tissue formation, meaning they have a lower risk of restenosis. Ortiz et al. [17] applied mitomycin C as an antifibroblast agent to reduce the chance of recurrence. In case 5, mitomycin C was applied after laser excision and balloon dilatation. There was no evidence of recurrence after 6-month follow-up.

There is a lot of literature supporting the use of stents in treating benign and malignant laryngeal stenosis. Dass et al. [18] conducted a study between the year 2000 and 2010, where out of 111 patients with laryngotracheal trauma, 71 underwent tracheal T-stenting for laryngotracheal stenosis. It was concluded that the ideal treatment option should be individualized based on patient characteristics. Stenting remained a relatively conservative treatment, was successful in a proportion of cases, and does not preclude the possibility of future reconstructive surgery if it fails. In case 1, our patient who subsequently underwent open resection and anastomosis of the stenotic segment had history of stenting after multiple failed dilations which provided him with little improvement. In case 2, the patient who

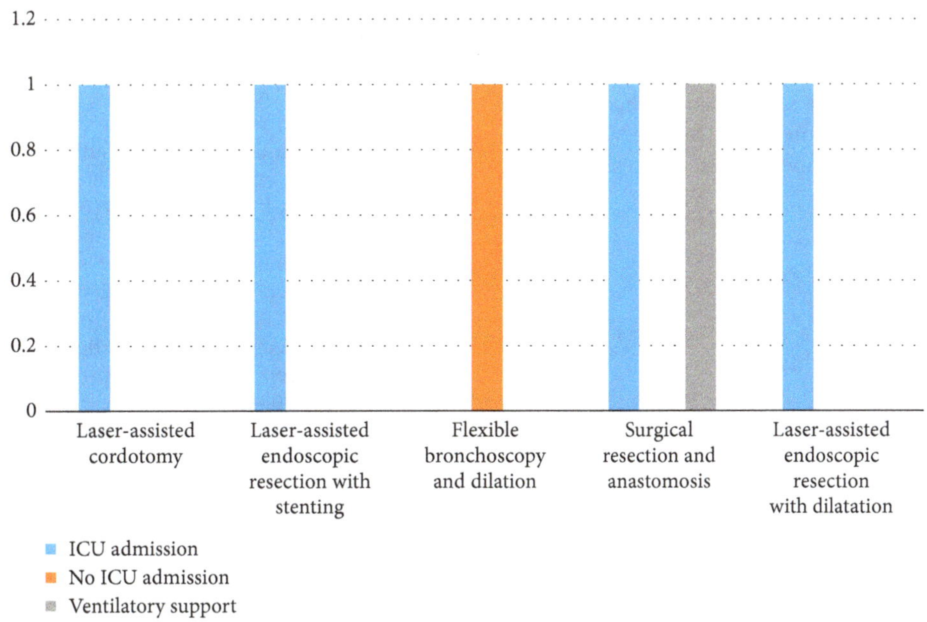

FIGURE 15: Patients requiring ICU/ventilatory support.

underwent laser-assisted resection was discharged with a stent, and there was no evidence of recurrence.

Another method of treatment for postintubation laryngotracheal stenosis is neodymium-doped yttrium aluminium garnet laser and cryotherapy. They have not been reported as being used in the treatment of postintubation laryngeal stenosis except in very small series or case reports with no long-term follow-up review.

In two of our cases (case 2 and 3), CO_2 diode laser was used for excision of the subglottic stenosis. In one of our cases (case 5), holmium laser was used for subglottic stenosis excision. In all the three cases of laser, there was improvement in airway and no evidence of stridor postoperatively.

It is seen that open surgical procedures involved certain potential risks not associated with endoscopic techniques including increased anaesthesia time and lengthy hospitalization. Because of these reasons, there has been a general tendency to treat laryngotracheal stenosis with endoscopic techniques. Addition of laser has offered new dimension in improving the conventional endoscopic technique in the management of laryngotracheal stenosis. Use of laser coupled to a rigid/flexible bronchoscope and ventilating bronchoscope allowed the surgeon to perform hands off endoscopic surgery such as scar excision or vaporization with increased precision. In our three cases treated by endoscopic laser, the patient could be decannulated after the procedure giving a fairly good success rate. Simpson et al. [19] successfully treated 1 of 5 (20%) patients having combined laryngeal and tracheal stenosis with endoscopic laser excision. Minimal pain, low levels of intraoperative and postoperative oedema, faster healing with less scar, and improved hemostasis are advantages of laser use.

There is a reduced risk of inadvertent injury to distal structures. A major advantage of the holmium laser is that it is capable of delivering energy to the target tissue through air, saline, or blood. Thus, it is particularly effective in wet environments such as the tracheobronchial tree. The ease of use with a fiber also enables this laser to be used endoscopically with flexible scopes. Hence, in case 5, holmium laser was preferred [20].

There is much evidence in the literature suggesting that for the treatment of subglottic stenosis, resection by endoscopy with laser and open surgical technique end-to-end anastomosis are the best available modality with regard to long-term results [21–24].

Our study supports this theory to perform resection for stenosis by end-to-end anastomosis or endoscopy with laser on patients who have had previous interventions.

5. Conclusion

Endotracheal intubation is life-saving when there is a need for artificial ventilation, but it is not without risk. Development of tracheal stenosis, that too of higher grade, is one of the most dreaded complications. However, such conditions can be managed with high degree of success.

Resection and primary anastomosis and laser-assisted excision of stenotic portion is a safe option for the treatment of subglottic stenosis following intubation in grade 3 or 4 stenosis without the need for repeated dilation. Collaboration is needed between thoracic and ENT surgeons to develop protocols for management of postintubation laryngotracheal stenosis as patients may present to both specialties.

Improved hemostasis, lesser pain, lesser postoperative oedema, and faster healing with less scar are advantages of laser, thus making it a safe option in management of tracheal stenosis.

Postoperative improvement in phonation was seen in surgical resection anastomosis, laser-assisted cordotomy, laser-assisted excision with dilation with mitomycin C application, and laser excision with stenting as compared to flexible bronchoscopy with dilation alone.

Given the high rates of recurrence, we cannot see a role for dilation alone in centres where specialised tracheal surgeons are available. Endoscopic dilation should be reserved for unfit patients or as a measure in nonequipped centres.

Conflicts of Interest

The authors declare that there are no conflicts of interest regarding the publication of this paper.

References

[1] H. C. Grillo, D. M. Donahue, D. J. Mathisen, J. C. Wain, and C. D. Wright, "Postintubation tracheal stenosis. Treatment and results," *Journal of Thoracic and Cardiovascular Surgery*, vol. 109, no. 3, pp. 486–492, 1995.

[2] V. K. Anand, G. Alemar, and E. T. Warren, "Surgical considerations in tracheal stenosis," *The Laryngoscope*, vol. 102, no. 3, pp. 237–243, 1992.

[3] H. Dutau, "Tracheal stenosis endoscopic treatment," in *Proceedings of the 12th World Congress for Bronchology*, pp. 83–88, Monduzzi Editore, Boston, MA, USA, June 2002.

[4] B. Papla, G. Dyduch, W. Frasik, and H. Olechnowica, "Post-intubation tracheal stenosis-morphological-clinical investigations," *Polish Journal of Pathology*, vol. 54, no. 4, pp. 261-266, 2003.

[5] E. Esteller-Moré, J. Ibañez, E. Matiñó, J. M. Ademà, M. Nolla, and I. M. Quer, "Prognostic factors in laryngotracheal injury following intubation and/or tracheotomy in ICU patients," *European Archives of Oto-Rhino-Laryngology*, vol. 262, no. 11, pp. 880–883, 2005.

[6] T. Vandemoortele, S. Laroumagne, O. Bylicki, P. Astoul, and H. Dutau, "Endobronchial treatment of complete tracheal stenosis: report of 3 cases and description of an innovative technique," *Annals of Thoracic Surgery*, vol. 95, no. 1, pp. 351–354, 2013.

[7] J. C. Wain, "Post intubation tracheal stenosis," *Chest Surgery Clinics of North America*, vol. 13, no. 2, pp. 231–246, 2003.

[8] S. A. Nouraei, E. Ma, A. Patel, D. J. Howard, and G. S. Sandhu, "Estimating the population incidence of adult post-intubation laryngotracheal stenosis," *Clinical Otolaryngology*, vol. 32, no. 5, pp. 411-412, 2007.

[9] N. Zias, A. Chroneou, M. K. Tabba et al., "Post tracheostomy and post intubation tracheal stenosis: report of 31 cases and review of the literature," *BMC Pulmonary Medicine*, vol. 8, no. 1, p. 18, 2008.

[10] N. Spittle and A. McCluskey, "Tracheal stenosis after intubation," *BMJ*, vol. 321, no. 7268, pp. 1000–1002, 2000.

[11] M. J. Cinnamond, "Stridor," in *Scott-Brown's Otolaryngology*, A. G. Kerr, J. Groves, and J. G. Evans, Eds., pp. 420–427, Butterworths & Co. Ltd., London, UK, 5th edition, 1987.

[12] K. Keshava, J. A. Weingarten, and H. B. Grosu, ""Benign" tracheal stenosis in an 18-year-old man," *Annals of the American Thoracic Society*, vol. 10, no. 6, pp. 701–703, 2013.

[13] C. M. Myer, D. M. O'Connor, and R. T. Cotton, "Proposed grading system for subglottic stenosis based on endotracheal tube sizes," *Annals of Otology, Rhinology & Laryngology*, vol. 103, no. 4, pp. 319–323, 1994.

[14] G. Galluccio, G. Lucantoni, P. Battistoni et al., "Interventional endoscopy in the management of benign tracheal stenoses: definitive treatment at long-term follow-up," *European Journal of Cardio-Thoracic Surgery*, vol. 35, no. 3, pp. 429–433, 2009.

[15] M. Behrend and J. Klempnauer, "Influence of suture material and technique on end-to-end reconstruction in tracheal surgery: an experimental study in sheep," *European Surgical Research*, vol. 33, no. 3, pp. 210–216, 2001.

[16] J. L. Bacon, C. M. Patterson, and B. P. Madden, "Indications and interventional options for non-resectable tracheal stenosis," *Journal of Thoracic Disease*, vol. 6, no. 3, pp. 258–270, 2014.

[17] R. Ortiz, E. Dominguez, C. Torre et al., "Early endoscopic dilation and mitomycin application in the treatment of acquired tracheal stenosis," *European Journal of Pediatric Surgery*, vol. 25, no. 1, pp. 39–45, 2014.

[18] A. Dass, N. M. Nagarkar, S. K. Singhal, and H. Verma, "Tracheal T-tube stent for laryngotracheal stenosis: ten year experience," *Iranian Journal of Otorhinolaryngology*, vol. 26, no. 74, pp. 37–42, 2014.

[19] G. T. Simpson, M. S. Strong, S. M. Shapsay, G. B. Healy, and C. W. Vaugham, "Predictive factors of success or failure in the endoscopic management of laryngeal and tracheal stenosis," *Annals of Otology, Rhinology & Laryngology*, vol. 91, no. 4, pp. 384–388, 1982.

[20] D. J. Verret, A. Jategaonkar, S. Helman et al., "Holmium laser for endoscopic treatment of benign tracheal stenosis," *International Archives of Otorhinolaryngology*, 2017.

[21] M. George, F. Lang, P. Pasche, and P. Monnier, "Surgical management of laryngotracheal stenosis in adults," *European Archives of Oto-Rhino-Laryngology*, vol. 262, no. 8, pp. 609–615, 2005.

[22] P. Marques, L. Leal, J. Spratley, E. Cardoso, and M. Santos, "Tracheal resection with primary anastomosis: 10 years experience," *American Journal of Otolaryngology*, vol. 30, no. 6, pp. 415–418, 2009.

[23] H. C. Grillo, D. M. Donahue, D. J. Mathisen, J. C. Wain, and C. D. Wright, "Postintubation tracheal stenosis," *Journal of Thoracic and Cardiovascular Surgery*, vol. 109, no. 3, pp. 486–492, 1995.

[24] F. H. Hassan, B. S. Goh, M. H. Kong, M. B. Marina, and A. Sani, "Tracheal resection and anastomosis: an 11 year management outcome," *Rawal Medical Journal*, vol. 38, no. 2, pp. 177–180, 2013.

15

Isolated Inferior Rectus Muscle Entrapment following Endoscopic Sinus Surgery

Scott Shapiro,[1] Jamie L. Schaefer,[2] Sumeet Gupta,[2] John Nguyen,[2] and Brian Kellermeyer[1]

[1]*Department of Otolaryngology, Head and Neck Surgery, West Virginia University, P.O. Box 9200, HSC Room 4520, Morgantown, WV 26506, USA*
[2]*Department of Ophthalmology, West Virginia University, P.O. Box 9193, One Medical Center Dr., Morgantown, WV 26506, USA*

Correspondence should be addressed to Brian Kellermeyer; bmkellermeyer@hsc.wvu.edu

Academic Editor: Rong-San Jiang

Orbital complications are known risks of endoscopic sinus surgery (ESS). The lamina papyracea and medial rectus muscle are the most commonly injured structures during ESS. Inferior rectus injury is more rare, with only one reported case of isolated inferior rectus injury in the literature. Guidelines for managing ESS-induced inferior rectus injury do not exist, and delayed intervention and management of adjacent sinuses may affect long-term outcomes such as persistent diplopia and disfigurement. In this report, we present a case of a 67-year-old man with diplopia due to isolated left inferior rectus muscle entrapment and injury from violation of the orbital floor during previous ESS. We postulate that an incomplete maxillary antrostomy contributed to scar band formation and entrapment of the inferior rectus muscle after the orbital floor was violated, and advocate early intervention with a wide, complete maxillary antrostomy if the orbital floor is injured during ESS.

1. Introduction

Endoscopic sinus surgery (ESS) is the standard of care for the treatment of medically resistant inflammatory sinus disease, as well as other pathology of, or anatomically related to, the paranasal sinuses. An inherent risk of ESS is injury to the thin bones of the medial orbital wall, and violation of the periorbita can pose significant danger to the extraocular muscle, fat, nerves, and globe. With over 19,000 ESS procedures performed in the US annually, fortunately ophthalmic complications remain rare, occurring in 0.3 to 3% of all procedures [1–4]. Risk factors for ophthalmic injuries include severity of sinonasal disease, surgeon experience, revision surgery, older age patient, and anatomical variations [4, 5]. Most involve injury to the medial rectus muscle via violation of the lamina papyracea, while the orbital floor and adjacent inferior rectus muscle is generally not considered a high-risk area [6]. Although injuries to the inferior rectus muscle have been reported, almost all have been associated with injuries to other orbital structures, usually the medial rectus, with only one reported case in the literature, where injury was isolated to the inferior rectus muscle [7]. There are few guidelines that exist on how to proceed if an orbital floor injury is noticed during ESS, and subsequent management may affect long-term outcomes such as persistent diplopia. In this report of a case, we (1) describe a patient who suffered orbital floor injury and isolated inferior rectus muscle damage from ESS, (2) endoscopically demonstrate the proximity of the orbital floor to the maxillary antrostomy site, and (3) discuss management of the floor and the adjacent sinuses if orbital floor injury is noticed intraoperatively.

2. Case Report

A 67-year-old Caucasian man presented to the ophthalmology clinic with persistent vertical diplopia on left and superior gaze for 8 months. He noticed diplopia upon waking from general anesthesia after an endoscopic sinus surgery which included

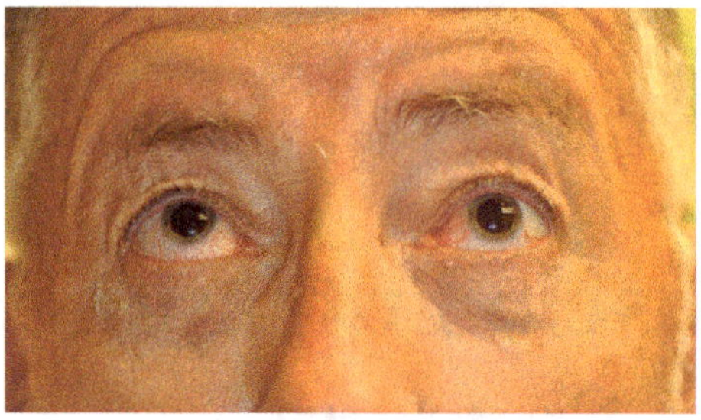

Figure 1: Frontal photograph during superior gaze. Limitation of left superior gaze.

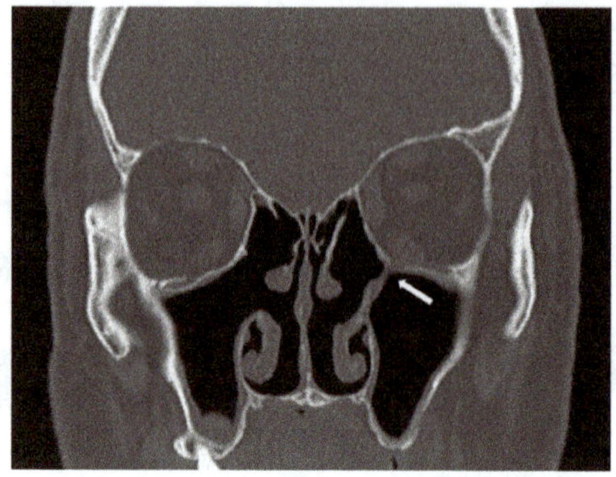

Figure 2: CT scan of the sinuses without contrast, frontal view. 5 mm defect in the posterior medial orbital floor with inferior displacement of the inferior rectus muscle into the defect. Soft tissue band was present from the defect to the remnant of the uncinate process (arrow).

bilateral ethmoidectomy and medial maxillary antrostomy for chronic sinusitis at an outside facility. Examination revealed restriction of superior gaze of the left eye (Figure 1). A CT scan revealed a 5 mm defect in the posterior medial orbital floor with inferior displacement of the inferior rectus muscle into the defect (Figure 2). A soft tissue band was present from the defect to the remnant of the uncinate process. He was referred to the otolaryngology clinic, and endoscopic examination revealed a small and posterior maxillary antrostomy, with a scar band connecting it to the orbital floor, but no obvious defects in the mucosa or exposed orbital contents.

He underwent revision endoscopic sinus surgery to revise the maxillary antrostomy, along with a transconjunctival orbitotomy to release the inferior rectus muscle and repair the orbital floor defect. Intraoperatively, there was a thick scar band tethering the inferior rectus muscle to the sinus mucosa through the defect on the orbital floor (Figure 3). After releasing of the scar band, a round bony defect was observed. From the nasal perspective, there was healthy sinonasal mucosa over the defect, but bulging of that mucosa could be seen when instrumented through the orbit (Figure 4). The forced duction test was free of restriction, and a smooth porous polyethylene implant was used to repair the orbital floor defect. Postoperatively, the left maxillary antrostomy did not develop scarring or restenosis based on surveillance via rigid nasal endoscopy in the office. His diplopia on superior gaze improved but did not resolve entirely 6 months after the revision surgery. He was offered but deferred additional treatment.

3. Discussion

Due to its proximity to the surgical field, the lamina papyracea is the most commonly violated boundary of the orbit, and damage to it represents the most common complication of sinus surgery [8–10]. The lamina is at risk during uncinectomy or ethmoidectomy, with the orbital floor at risk during maxillary antrostomy and sinusotomy [11], though the orbital floor is generally not considered a high-risk area during sinus surgery [6]. Although injuries to the inferior rectus muscle have been reported in association with injuries to other orbital structures, most commonly the medial rectus muscle [12], isolated inferior rectus injuries via orbital floor violation are rare with only one reported case in the literature [7]. In their reported case, the orbital defect was significantly larger than in our patient, the patient presented earlier (2 weeks versus our 8 months), and with diplopia on both superior and inferior gaze.

As demonstrated by these two cases, the proximity of the orbital floor to the site of maxillary antrostomy should be a concern during ESS. To prevent this complication, the antrostomy should be made just posterior to the hard lacrimal bone and at the level of the inferior aspect of the ethmoid bulla. Despite the rarity of this complication, it is not difficult to place to an antrostomy slightly posterior and superior which may result in injury to the orbital floor. In our case, it appeared the maxillary antrostomy was halted at this point and not fully opened, thus not connecting with the natural os of the maxillary sinus, as shown in Figure 2.

These two cases highlight some important aspects of management of iatrogenic orbital floor injury during ESS. Guidelines do not exist expressly for this entity, but to some degree, we may rely on guidelines from management of traumatic orbital fractures, which suggest emergent intervention if entrapment is present [13–16]. In ESS-induced injury to the orbital floor, management is complicated by the adjacent sinuses, which may be inflamed due to chronic sinusitis and/or surgery, and may be more likely to develop scarring, which occurred in our patient. We speculate that during the previous surgery, the orbital floor injury was noticed and the surgeon chose to not to complete the antrostomy for fear of causing further injury in this area. It is unknown whether persistent diplopia was the result of direct injury, subsequent scar formation, or both; however, this case does emphasize that if an orbital floor injury is made during antrostomy, and there are no acute complications such as orbital hemorrhage or hematoma, the maxillary antrostomy should be completed to prevent postoperative synechiae, which can contribute to postoperative orbital dysfunction. It may be beneficial to repair the orbital defect at the time of surgery if it is noticed. If it is not noticed intraoperatively, a patient who awakens with diplopia after ESS should elicit a high suspicion for orbital injury, and reexploration or imaging is considered. Delayed care likely

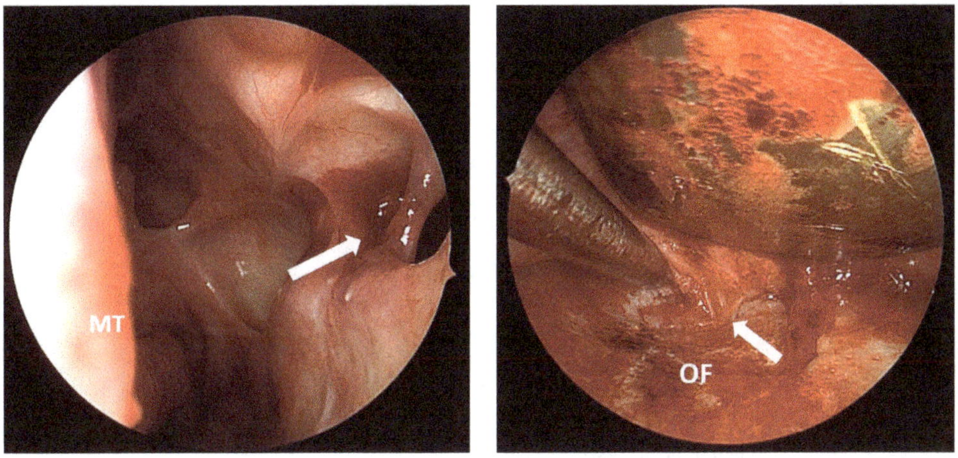

(a) (b)

FIGURE 3: Endoscopic view of left nasal cavity (a) and orbital floor (b). MT, middle turbinate. Arrow denotes scar band tethering the inferior rectus muscle to the sinus mucosa through the defect on the orbital floor (OF).

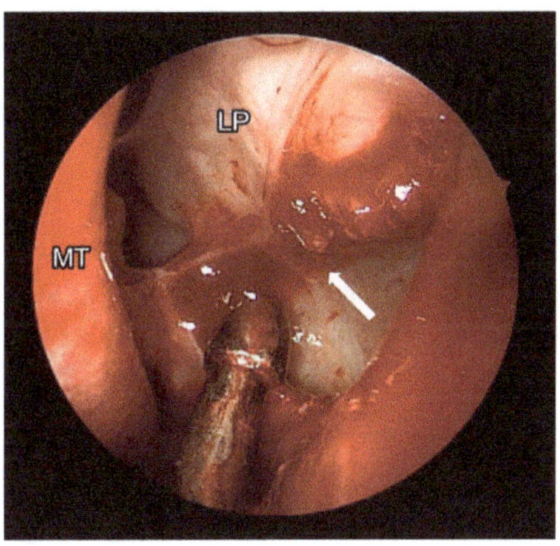

FIGURE 4: Endoscopic view of the left nasal cavity after revision ESS and uncinectomy. Bulging in nasal mucosa when instrumented through the orbital defect (arrow). LP, lamina papyracea.

contributed to persistent diplopia after surgical repair of the maxillary antrostomy and orbital floor. Perhaps, if our patient more urgently underwent ophthalmologic consultation, with subsequent orbital floor repair and revision sinus surgery, persistent diplopia could have been prevented.

In summary, the orbital floor is in close proximity to surgical field during maxillary antrostomy. Although very rare, orbital floor injury can result from a posteriorly or superiorly placed antrostomy. If orbital floor injury occurs, the floor should be repaired and the antrostomy should be completed to prevent postoperative synechiae which may contribute to postoperative orbital dysfunction.

Conflicts of Interest

The authors declare that there are no conflicts of interest regarding the publication of this article.

References

[1] A. Al-Mujaini, U Wali, and M. Alkhabori, "Functional endoscopic sinus surgery: indications and complications in the ophthalmic field," *Oman Medical Journal*, vol. 24, no. 2, pp. 70–80, 2009.

[2] M. Seredyka-Burduk, P. K. Burduk, M. Wierzchowska et al., "Ophthalmic complications of endoscopic sinus surgery," *Brazilian Journal of Otorhinolaryngology*, vol. 83, no. 3, pp. 318–323, 2017.

[3] V. L. Cumberworth, R. M. Sudderick, and I. S. Mackay, "Major complications of functional endoscopic sinus surgery," *Clinical Otolaryngology*, vol. 19, no. 3, pp. 248–253, 1994.

[4] J. G. Krings, D. Kallogjeri, A. Wineland et al., "Complications of primary and revision functional endoscopic sinus surgery for chronic rhinosinusitis," *Laryngoscope*, vol. 124, no. 4, pp. 838–845, 2014.

[5] M. T. Bhatti and J. A. Stankiewicz, "Ophthalmic complications of endoscopic sinus surgery," *Survey of Ophthalmology*, vol. 48, no. 4, pp. 389–402, 2003.

[6] T. Ohnishi, T. Tachibana, Y. Kaneko, and S. Esaki, "High-risk areas in endoscopic sinus surgery and prevention of complications," *Laryngoscope*, vol. 103, no. 10, pp. 1181–1185, 1993.

[7] A. Carton and S. Hislop, "Orbital floor injury with extraocular muscle entrapment following functional endoscopic sinus surgery," *British Journal of Oral and Maxillofacial Surgery*, vol. 38, no. 1, pp. 82-83, 2000.

[8] J. Rombout and N. de Vries, "Complications in sinus surgery and new classification proposal," *American Journal of Rhinology*, vol. 15, no. 6, pp. 363–370, 2001.

[9] M. May, H. L. Levine, S. J. Mester et al., "Complications of endoscopic sinus surgery: analysis of 2108 patients–incidence and prevention," *Laryngoscope*, vol. 104, no. 9, pp. 1080–1083, 1994.

[10] M. Vleming, R. J. Middelweerd, and N. de Vries, "Complications of endoscopic sinus surgery," *Archives of Otolaryngology-Head and Neck Surgery*, vol. 118, no. 6, pp. 617–623, 1992.

[11] M. T. Bhatti, I. M. Schmalfuss, and A. A. Mancuso, "Orbital complications of functional endoscopic sinus surgery: MR and

CT findings," *Clinical Radiology*, vol. 60, no. 8, pp. 894–904, 2005.

[12] H. Wu, T. Shen, J. Chen et al., "Long-term therapeutic outcome of ophthalmic complications following endoscopic sinus surgery," *Medicine*, vol. 95, no. 38, p. e4896, 2016.

[13] C. P. Back, N. R. McLean, P. J. Anderson et al., "The conservative management of facial fractures: indications and outcomes," *Journal of Plastic, Reconstructive and Aesthetic Surgery*, vol. 60, no. 2, pp. 146–151, 2007.

[14] F. S. Roth, J. C. Koshy, J. S. Goldberg et al., "Pearls of orbital trauma management," *Seminars in Plastic Surgery*, vol. 24, no. 4, pp. 398–410, 2010.

[15] N. Ela-Dalman, F. G. Velez, and A. L. Rosenbaum, "Importance of sagittal orbital imaging in evaluating extraocular muscle trauma following endoscopic sinus surgery," *British Journal of Ophthalmology*, vol. 90, no. 6, pp. 682–685, 2006.

[16] N. M. Thacker, F. G. Velez, J. L. Demer et al., "Strabismic complications following endoscopic sinus surgery: diagnosis and surgical management," *Journal of American Association for Pediatric Ophthalmology and Strabismus*, vol. 8, no. 5, pp. 488–494, 2004.

16

Combined Surgical Approach for Obstructive Sleep Apnea Patient

Mahmoud A. K. Ebrahim,[1] **Osamah AlSanea**,[2] **and Abdulmohsen E. Al-Terki**[3]

[1] *Al-Sabah Hospital, Ministry of Health, Kuwait City, Kuwait*
[2] *Department of Surgery Health, Medical Clinic Dammam, Saudi Arabia*
[3] *ENT Clinic, Dasman Diabetes Institute, Kuwait City, Kuwait*

Correspondence should be addressed to Abdulmohsen E. Al-Terki; q8ent@hotmail.com

Academic Editor: Dinesh K. Chhetri

Obstructive sleep apnea (OSA) is a disease that is associated with high morbidity and mortality and can significantly impact the quality of life in a patient. OSA is strongly associated with obesity, and literature showed that weight loss will lead to improvement in OSA. The gold standard treatment for OSA is continuous positive airway pressure (CPAP). However, other methods of treatment are available. One of these methods is multilevel sleep surgery (MLS). Literature showed that bariatric surgery can also improve OSA. A common question is which surgical procedure of these two should be performed first. We present a 5-year follow-up of a patient who underwent simultaneously bariatric surgery and MLS. His apnea-hypopnea index (AHI) decreased from 53 episodes per hour to 5.2 per hour within the first 18 months, which was measured via a level 3 polysomnography. Five years after the surgery, a repeat level 3 polysomnography showed an AHI of 6.8 episodes per hour, and the patient is asymptomatic. The patient maintained his weight and did not use CPAP after the combined surgery during the five-year period.

1. Introduction

Obstructive sleep apnea (OSA) is characterized by recurrent upper airway obstruction during sleep and presents as oxygen desaturation, hypercapnia, and sleep fragmentation, which occurs because of complete or partial upper airway obstruction [1]. The OSA prevalence is approximately 2%–4% in middle-aged adults [2]. OSA is related to major metabolic, cardiovascular, and neurocognitive morbidities because of hypoxemia, hypercapnia, and sleep disturbance [1]. Continuous positive airway pressure (CPAP) is the current treatment of choice for moderate-to-severe OSA [3]. In compliant patients, CPAP improves sleepiness and quality of life and reduces cardiovascular morbidity [4]. Surgery is a second-line treatment for patients who cannot tolerate CPAP or CPAP nonresponders [5]. Because OSA involves one or more upper airway levels, a multilevel single-stage procedure has been developed to treat OSA (success rate of 60%) [6]. We present the 5-year follow-up data of a patient who underwent combined multilevel surgery (MLS) and laparoscopic Roux-en-Y gastric bypass. To our knowledge, this is the first such case in the literature. The patient exhibited significantly reduced apnea-hypopnea index (AHI) values without CPAP use.

2. Case Presentation

A morbidly obese male patient (body mass index (BMI) of 39 kg/m^2) in his thirties, with a history of diabetes, hypertension, OSA, hypercholesterolemia, and hyperuricemia, consulted for excess body weight and sleep apnea; he had undergone many failed trials, including diets, exercise, and medication, to lose weight. He had experienced multiple episodes of apnea and gasping for air during sleep, snoring, and sleeping during the morning with headaches. He was put on CPAP but could not tolerate it and opted for an alternative treatment. Ear, nose, and throat examination revealed hypertrophied tonsils and inferior turbinates, with a redundant soft palate. His blood investigations were within normal range. Computed tomography of the paranasal sinuses revealed normal findings. His Epworth sleepiness scale (ESS) score was 18.

Preoperative level III polysomnography detected AHI of 53 episodes/h, indicating severe OSA. Sleep endoscopy showed that the tongue base did not fill the vallecula, but the lateral pharyngeal wall was collapsed where the palatine tonsils blocked the airway, plus at the level of the soft palate it showed a flaccid soft palate.

In June 2012, after easy intubation, the patient underwent MLS, which involved the insertion of five pillar palatal implants in the soft palate, followed by cold dissection tonsillectomy. Because the posterior end of the right inferior turbinate was blocking the posterior choanae, it was removed using zero-degree nasal endoscopy and a straight shaver. Bilateral blow-out fractures of the right and left inferior turbinates were performed to make the posterior nasal cavity patent. Once homeostasis was achieved, laparoscopic Roux-en-Y gastric bypass was immediately conducted. Postoperatively, the patient was admitted for 48 h intensive care unit monitoring and used CPAP for several days; he was discharged 4 days postoperatively.

At 18 months postoperatively, repeat level III polysomnography showed that AHI decreased from 53 to 5.2 episodes/h without CPAP use, and the patient was asymptomatic.

Five years later, follow-up level III polysomnography revealed AHI of 6.8 episodes/h, and the patient remains asymptomatic (current ESS score of 8 (versus 18 preoperatively); latest BMI, 27 kg/m^2).

3. Discussion

Most OSA patients have multilevel disease; hence, nasal, oropharyngeal and palatal, and hypopharyngeal treatment measures are required to improve the airway [7]. Waite et al. first presented a multilevel procedure in 1989 [8]. Staged surgery with multilevel treatment can be used to treat OSA [9]. The aim of successful surgery is to reduce AHI to <20 or by ≥50% of preoperative AHI, which occurred in our patient [10]. Additionally, improvement in daytime sleepiness and reduction in ESS score to <10 (reduced to 8 in our case) are expected [11]. Until 2010, 11 controlled studies and 32 case series investigated the effectiveness of MLS. Average AHI was reduced to 20.3 postoperatively from 43.9 preoperatively. However, it remains unclear which combination of MLS is superior and most effective [12]. A meta-analysis of 1978 patients showed that the overall success rate was 66.4% in patients with multilevel sleep apnea surgery involving at least two anatomical sites: nose, oropharynx, or hypopharynx [13]. Furthermore, patients receiving postoperative CPAP had lower AHI and ESS scores and higher SpO_2 [14]. Azbay et al. reported that approximately 48% of patients who cannot tolerate CPAP preoperatively can tolerate it postoperatively [14].

Two most important factors that determine postoperative AHI after multilevel surgery are preoperative AHI and tonsillectomy. Preoperative BMI is marginally significant, whereas age is not [15]. Tonsillectomy is proven to treat OSA [16]. MLS with tonsillectomy was effective in reducing AHI scores in 58% patients (versus 19% patients without tonsillectomy) similar to what has been previously reported [17]. Another important factor for maintaining the success rate of MLS postoperatively is sustained weight loss [18]. Neruntarat showed that, in most patients, MLS treatment failure was due to weight gain [19]. In our case, BMI was maintained even at 5 years postoperatively. Pillar implants are designed to reduce vibration or narrowing of the soft palate by increasing its stiffness and to decrease collapsibility of the airway [20–22] and have been reported to significantly decrease ESS and AHI [23, 24]; however, this finding is not definitive because only two of the studies reporting this result were placebo controlled [23, 24].

Obesity and OSA are known to be related [25]. Bariatric surgery can reduce many comorbidities, such as OSA, in obese people [26]. OSA prevalence in bariatric surgery patients is 64%–97%, with a strong male dominance [27]. Dixon et al. demonstrated that shorter sleep duration is associated with significant weight gain and high BMI, which can be attributed to reduced sleep efficiency and changes in sleep architecture [28]. Almost all studies in a meta-analysis reported reduction in AHI after bariatric surgery [29], but some studies stated that a longer follow-up period is associated with a larger relapse rate [30]. Conversely, a recent study showed that reduction in AHI can be maintained in the long term [31]. A meta-analysis by Buchwald et al. demonstrated that OSA resolved in 85.7%, patients assessed either subjectively or objectively (via postoperative polysomnography) [32]. Conversely, Greenburg et al. assessed OSA patients' AHI via polysomnography before and after bariatric surgery and detected significant residual OSA (AHI >15 events/h) in approximately 62% patients [33]. Holty et al. reported a huge reduction in ESS scores at 2 years after bariatric surgery in OSA patients [34]. Additionally, patients who underwent gastric bypass had greater improvement in AHI than patients who underwent laparoscopic adjustable gastric banding [35]. This can be explained by weight-dependent factors that decrease the mechanical force on the cervical region, upper airway, and diaphragm, as well as weight-independent metabolic effects such as bile flow alteration, restriction of gastric size, anatomical gut rearrangement and altered flow of nutrients, vagal manipulation, and enteric gut hormone modulation [35].

4. Conclusion

OSA affects multiple organ systems and can lead to significant morbidity and mortality. Although CPAP is the gold standard, several other methods, including surgery, have been developed to treat OSA. MLS is an alternative method for treating OSA, improving AHI, alleviating symptoms, and improving quality of life. This is a case report of a patient who underwent bariatric and sleep surgery simultaneously.

Five-year follow-up revealed significant improvement and sustainability of the reduction in AHI and symptoms.

Consent

The consent was taken from the patient before surgery and the same after surgery by the corresponding author.

Conflicts of Interest

The authors declare that there are no conflicts of interest regarding the publication of this article.

References

[1] A. S. Jordan, D. G. McSharry, and A. Malhotra, "Adult obstructive sleep apnoea," *The Lancet*, vol. 383, no. 9918, pp. 736–747, 2014.

[2] T. Young, M. Palta, J. Dempsey, J. Skatrud, S. Weber, and S. Badr, "The occurrence of sleep-disordered breathing among middle-aged adults," *New England Journal of Medicine*, vol. 328, no. 17, pp. 1230–1235, 1993.

[3] C. Holmdahl, I.-L. Schöllin, M. Alton, and K. Nilsson, "CPAP treatment in obstructive sleep apnoea: a randomised, controlled trial of follow-up with a focus on patient satisfaction," *Sleep Medicine*, vol. 10, no. 8, pp. 869–874, 2009.

[4] M. H. Sanders, J. M. Montserrat, R. Farre, and R. J. Givelber, "Positive pressure therapy: a perspective on evidence-based outcomes and methods of application," *Proceedings of the American Thoracic Society*, vol. 5, no. 2, pp. 161–172, 2008.

[5] K. Humphreys and W. P. Maddern, "Upper airway surgery for adult obstructive sleep apnoea: what is the evidence?," *ANZ Journal of Surgery*, vol. 79, no. 4, pp. 223-224, 2009.

[6] B. T. Kotecha and A. C. Hall, "Role of surgery in adult obstructive sleep apnoea," *Sleep Medicine Reviews*, vol. 18, no. 5, pp. 405–413, 2014.

[7] K. Ceylan, H. Emir, Z. Kizilkaya et al., "First-choice treatment in mild to moderate obstructive sleep apnea: single-stage, multilevel, temperature-controlled radiofrequency tissue volume reduction or nasal continuous positive airway pressure," *Archives of Otolaryngology–Head & Neck Surgery*, vol. 135, no. 9, pp. 915–919, 2009.

[8] P. D. Waite, V. Wooten, J. Lachner, and R. F. Guyette, "Maxillomandibular advancement surgery in 23 patients with obstructive sleep apnea syndrome," *Journal of Oral and Maxillofacial Surgery*, vol. 47, no. 12, pp. 1256–1261, 1989.

[9] N. R. Lee, C. D. Givens, J. Wilson, and R. B. Robins, "Staged surgical treatment of obstructive sleep apnea syndrome: a review of 35 patients," *Journal of Oral and Maxillofacial Surgery*, vol. 57, no. 4, pp. 382–385, 1999.

[10] A. E. Sher, K. B. Schechtman, and J. F. Piccirillo, "The efficacy of surgical modifications of the upper airway in adults with obstructive sleep apnea syndrome," *Sleep*, vol. 19, no. 2, pp. 156–177, 1996.

[11] E. Vicente, J. M. Marín, S. Carrizo, and M. J. Naya, "Tongue-base suspension in conjunction with uvulopalatopharyngoplasty for treatment of severe obstructive sleep apnea: long-term follow-up results," *Laryngoscope*, vol. 116, no. 7, pp. 1223–1227, 2006.

[12] T. Verse, R. Bodlaj, R. de la Chaux et al., "Guideline: treatment of obstructive sleep apnea in adults," *HNO*, vol. 57, no. 11, pp. 1136–1156, 2009.

[13] H. C. Lin, M. Friedman, H.-W. Chang, and B. Gurpinar, "The efficacy of multilevel surgery of the upper airway in adults with obstructive sleep apnea/hypopnea syndrome," *Laryngoscope*, vol. 118, no. 5, pp. 902–908, 2008.

[14] S. Azbay, A. Bostanci, Y. Aysun, and M. Turhan, "The influence of multilevel upper airway surgery on CPAP tolerance in non-responders to obstructive sleep apnea surgery," *European Archives of Oto-Rhino-Laryngology*, vol. 273, no. 9, pp. 2813–2818, 2016.

[15] J. T. Maurer, "Update on surgical treatments for sleep apnea," *Swiss Medical Weekly*, vol. 139, no. 43-44, pp. 624–629, 2009.

[16] T. Verse, B. A. Kroker, W. Pirsig, and S. Brosch, "Tonsillectomy as a treatment of obstructive sleep apnea in adults with tonsillar hypertrophy," *Laryngoscope*, vol. 110, no. 9, pp. 1556–1559, 2000.

[17] T. Verse, "Update on surgery for obstructive sleep apnea syndrome," *HNO*, vol. 56, no. 11, pp. 1098–1104, 2008.

[18] U. Andsberg and M. Jessen, "Eight years of follow-up–uvulopalatopharyngoplasty combined with midline glossectomy as a treatment for obstructive sleep apnoea syndrome," *Acta Oto-Laryngologica*, vol. 120, no. 543, pp. 175–178, 2000.

[19] C. Neruntarat, "Genioglossus advancement and hyoid myotomy: short-term and long-term results," *Journal of Laryngology & Otology*, vol. 117, no. 6, pp. 482–486, 2003.

[20] K. A. Franklin, H. Anttila, S. Axelsson et al., "Effects and side-effects of surgery for snoring and obstructive sleep apnea—a systematic review," *Sleep*, vol. 32, no. 1, pp. 27–36, 2009.

[21] S. M. Caples, J. A. Rowley, J. R. Prinsell et al., "Surgical modifications of the upper airway for obstructive sleep apnea in adults: a systematic review and meta-analysis," *Sleep*, vol. 33, no. 10, pp. 1396–1407, 2010.

[22] W. K. Ho, W. I. Wei, and K. F. Chung, "Managing disturbing snoring with palatal implants: a pilot study," *Archives of Otolaryngology–Head & Neck Surgery*, vol. 130, no. 6, pp. 753–758, 2004.

[23] D. L. Steward, T. C. Huntley, B. T. Woodson, and V. Surdulescu, "Palate implants for obstructive sleep apnea: multi-institution, randomized, placebo-controlled study," *Otolaryngology-Head and Neck Surgery*, vol. 139, no. 4, pp. 506–510, 2008.

[24] C. Neruntarat, "Long-term results of palatal implants for obstructive sleep apnea," *European Archives of Oto-Rhino-Laryngology*, vol. 268, no. 7, pp. 1077–1080, 2011.

[25] L. F. Drager, S. M. Togeiro, V. Y. Polotsky, and G. Lorenzi-Filho, "Obstructive sleep apnea: a cardiometabolic risk in obesity and the metabolic syndrome," *Journal of the American College of Cardiology*, vol. 62, no. 7, pp. 569–576, 2013.

[26] A. G. Tsai and T. A. Wadden, "In the clinic: obesity," *Annals of Internal Medicine*, vol. 159, no. 5, pp. ITC3-1–ITC3-15, 2013.

[27] P. Peromaa-Haavisto, H. Tuomilehto, J. Kössi et al., "Prevalence of obstructive sleep apnoea among patients admitted for bariatric surgery. A prospective multicentre trial," *Obesity Surgery*, vol. 26, no. 7, pp. 1384–1390, 2016.

[28] J. B. Dixon, L. M. Schachter, and P. E. O'Brien, "Predicting sleep apnea and excessive day sleepiness in the severely obese: indicators for polysomnography," *Chest*, vol. 123, no. 4, pp. 1134–1141, 2003.

[29] M. Quintas-Neves, J. Preto, and M. Drummond, "Assessment of bariatric surgery efficacy on obstructive sleep apnea (OSA)," *Revista Portuguesa de Pneumologia*, vol. 22, no. 6, pp. 331–336, 2006.

[30] D. C. Cowan and E. Livingston, "Obstructive sleep apnoea syndrome and weight loss: review," *Sleep Disorders*, vol. 2012, Article ID 163296, 11 pages, 2012.

[31] A. Obeid, J. Long, M. Kakade, R. H. Clements, R. Stahl, and J. Grams, "Laparoscopic Roux-en-Y gastric bypass: long term clinical outcomes," *Surgical Endoscopy*, vol. 26, no. 12, pp. 3515–3520, 2012.

[32] H. Buchwald, Y. Avidor, E. Braunwald et al., "Bariatric surgery: a systematic review and meta-analysis," *Journal of the American Medical Association*, vol. 292, no. 14, pp. 1724–1737, 2004.

[33] D. L. Greenburg, C. J. Lettieri, and A. H. Eliasson, "Effects of surgical weight loss on measures of obstructive sleep apnea: a meta-analysis," *American Journal of Medicine*, vol. 122, no. 6, pp. 535–542, 2009.

[34] J. E. Holty, N. Parimi, M. Ballesteros et al., "Does surgically induced weight loss improve daytime sleepiness?," *Obesity Surgery*, vol. 21, no. 10, pp. 1535–1545, 2011.

[35] K. Sarkhosh, N. J. Switzer, M. El-Hadi, D. W. Birch, X. Shi, and S. Karmali, "The impact of bariatric surgery on obstructive sleep apnea: a systematic review," *Obesity Surgery*, vol. 23, no. 3, pp. 414–423, 2013.

17

Maxillary Swing Approach for Removal of Palatal Carcinoma

Tsutomu Nomura,[1] **Megumi Kishimoto**,[2] **Hirohisa Iwaki**,[2] **Atsushi Ochi**,[2] **and Seiji Kishimoto**[3]

[1]*Department of Otorhinolaryngology, Saitama Medical Center, Saitama, Japan*
[2]*Department of Otorhinolaryngology, Kameda Medical Center, Kamogawa, Japan*
[3]*Department of Head and Neck Surgery, Kameda Medical Center, Kamogawa, Japan*

Correspondence should be addressed to Tsutomu Nomura; t-nomura@bc5.so-net.ne.jp

Academic Editor: Yuh Baba

Introduction. We report a modification of the maxillary swing approach to remove a palatal tumor while preserving the anterior alveolar area. *Methods.* Case report using clinical records. *Results.* The patient was a 54-year-old male. TNM grade was T4bN0M0, and invasion to the base of the pterygoid process was seen. Two courses of induction chemotherapy were administered prior to the operation. Because there was no evidence of anterior maxillary invasion, the maxillary swing approach was chosen. The left anterior maxilla was cut and swung laterally, preserving the blood supply. After removal of the palatal tumor, the maxilla was repositioned and the defect was restored with an anterior lateral thigh flap. Postoperative course was typical, and facial appearance, speech, and masticatory function were satisfactory. *Conclusions.* This technique is particularly useful for preserving appearance as well as speech and mastication.

1. Introduction

In surgical treatment for tumors invading to the pterygoid fossa, complete resection with adequate surgical margins is challenging because of the anatomic complexity of the maxillofacial region. To overcome this issue, Wei et al. [1] developed the maxillary swing (MS) approach to the nasopharyngeal area; this was later modified by Sumi et al. [2] into the partial maxillary swing approach. A further modified version of the technique was reported by Shimoda et al. [3]. Here, we used an anteriorly modified form of MS to preserve the anterior alveolar area while removing a palate tumor invading the pterygoid lesion.

2. Case Report

A 54-year-old man who had complained of ongoing pain in the palate was referred to our department with a diagnosis of a palatal squamous cell carcinoma. The stage T4bN0M0 tumor had formed an ulcer in the palate and invaded the posterior portion of the inferior nasal turbinate. The pharyngeal orifice of the auditory tube was intact (Figure 1). Coronal view CT showed that the tumor had invaded the base of the pterygoid process without cranial base invasion (Figure 2(b)). After two courses of induction chemotherapy, the tumor was found to have disappeared from this area.

Because there was no evidence of anterior maxillary invasion, the maxillary swing approach was chosen. The surgical technique was as follows: a skin incision was made along the Weber–Fergusson incision, as in the original maxillary swing technique, and widened minimally to enable osteotomy. In order to preserve the blood supply to the maxilla, the skin was kept attached to the maxilla. An upper right incisor was missing, and bridge work had been done. The bridge was removed, and cuts were made along this line. The infraorbital nerve was sacrificed, and osteotomy was performed with a thin oscillating saw. The red lines in Figure 2 show the osteotomy lines. The resulting bone flap was then elevated (Figure 3(a)).

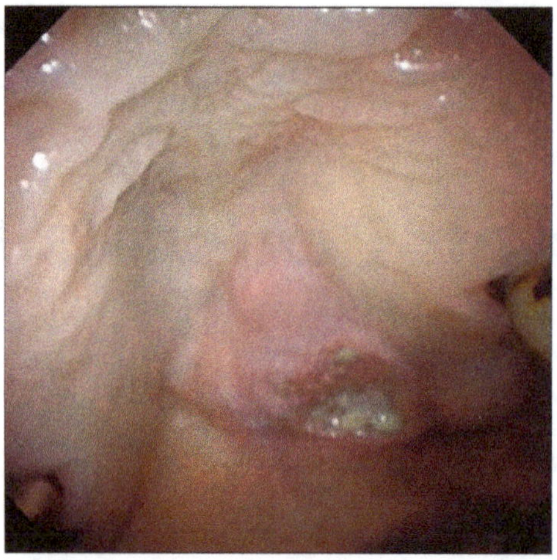

(a)

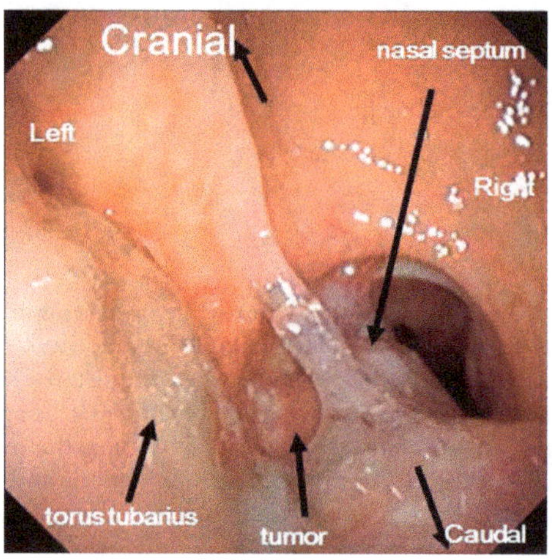

(b)

Figure 1: (a) Oral view of the palatal tumor. (b) Posterior nasal aperture view. Fiberscope was inserted from mouth and turned to posterior nasal aperture via uvula. Fiberscope tip was turned upside down, and posterior nasal aperture view was taken. Tumor can be seen in the left posterior nasal meatus area and is clearly invading the nasal septum. Right torus tubarius is intact.

After the flap was elevated, the tumor outline was visualized and the posterior sections of the maxilla and pterygoid process were resected (Figure 3(b)). The cut surfaces of bone were smoothed, and a frozen section was examined for pathology and found to be negative.

Reconstruction was then performed using an anterior lateral thigh (ALT) flap (Figure 3(c)). The maxilla flap was repositioned and fixed with a miniplate (Figure 3(d)). The total operation time was 10 hours 54 minutes, and blood loss was 1200 ml.

Mock surgery was performed on a 3D printer-generated model prior to the operation (Figure 4). The lines to be cut were identified on the 3D model. The white area represents the swung anterior maxilla, and the blue area (inferior part of the zygomatic arch) represents the area removed for visualization purposes. The red area represents the dissected area. The actual operation was performed while referencing

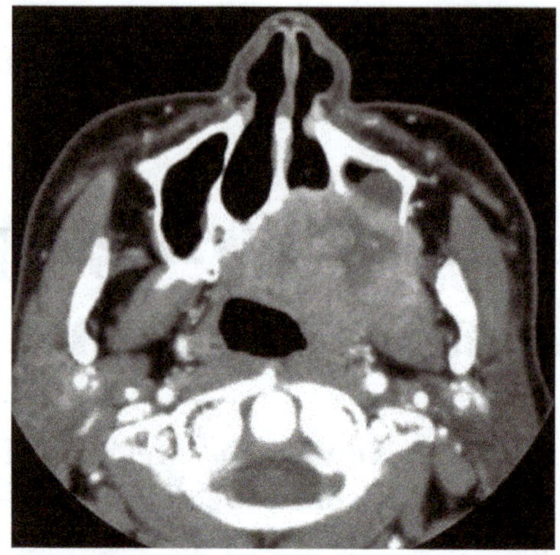

(a)

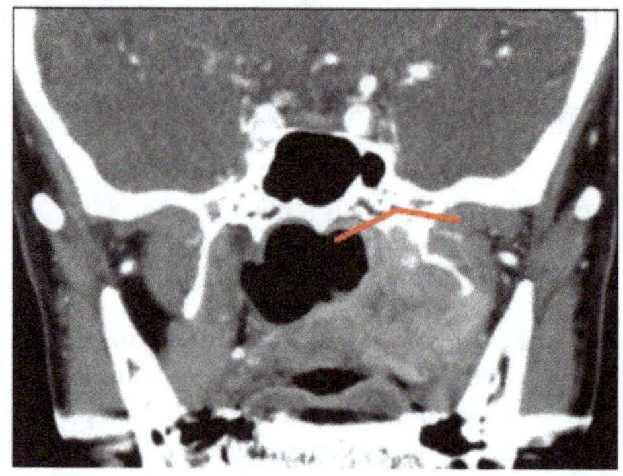

(b)

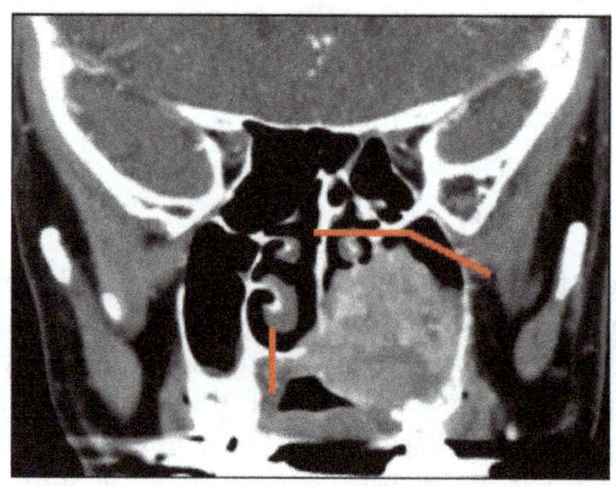

(c)

Figure 2: CT views. (a) Axial view: tumor invading the left posterior maxillary sinus but not the anterior area. (b) Coronal view: tumor invading the base of the pterygoid process. (c) Tumor not invading the orbital fossa or cranial bone. Red lines are dissection lines.

this model and using the same techniques employed during the mock surgery.

Figure 5 shows a frontal view of the patient two months after surgery. Buccal deformity was minimal and acceptable. Five months after surgery, bilateral neck and retropharyngeal metastasis occurred, and bilateral neck dissection and postoperative radiation were performed.

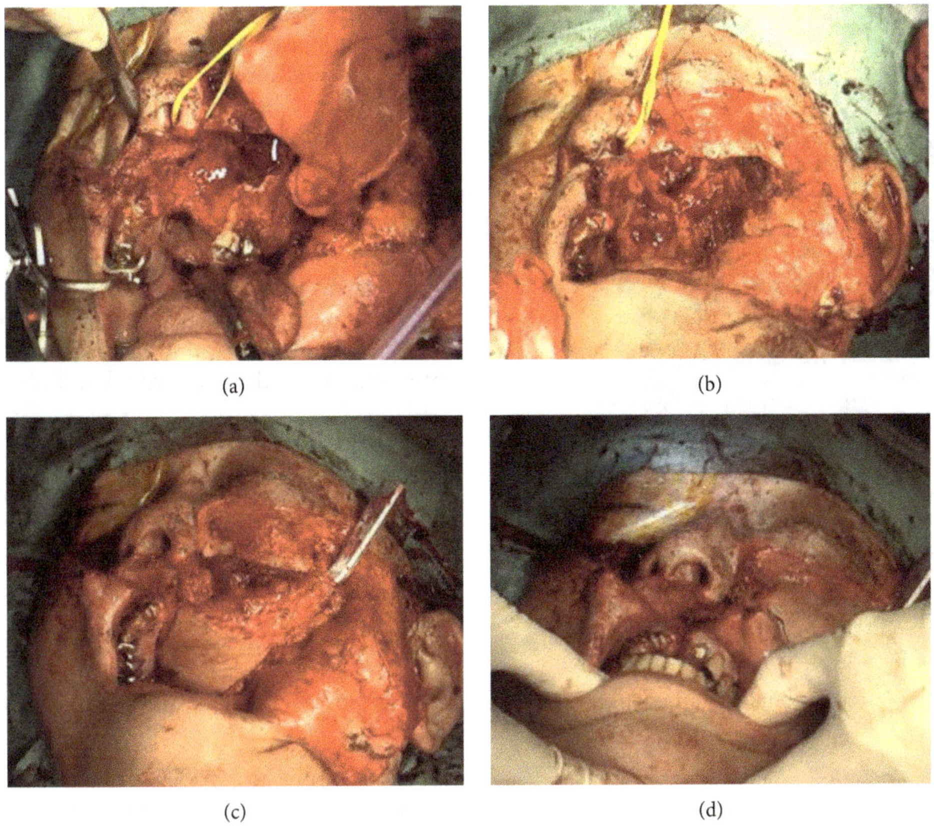

FIGURE 3: Surgical procedure of the modified partial swing approach. (a) Weber–Fergusson incision was made, and an anterior maxillary flap was elevated. (b) Tumor was excised. (c) Reconstruction was performed with an ALT flap. (d) The maxilla flap was repositioned and fixed with miniplate.

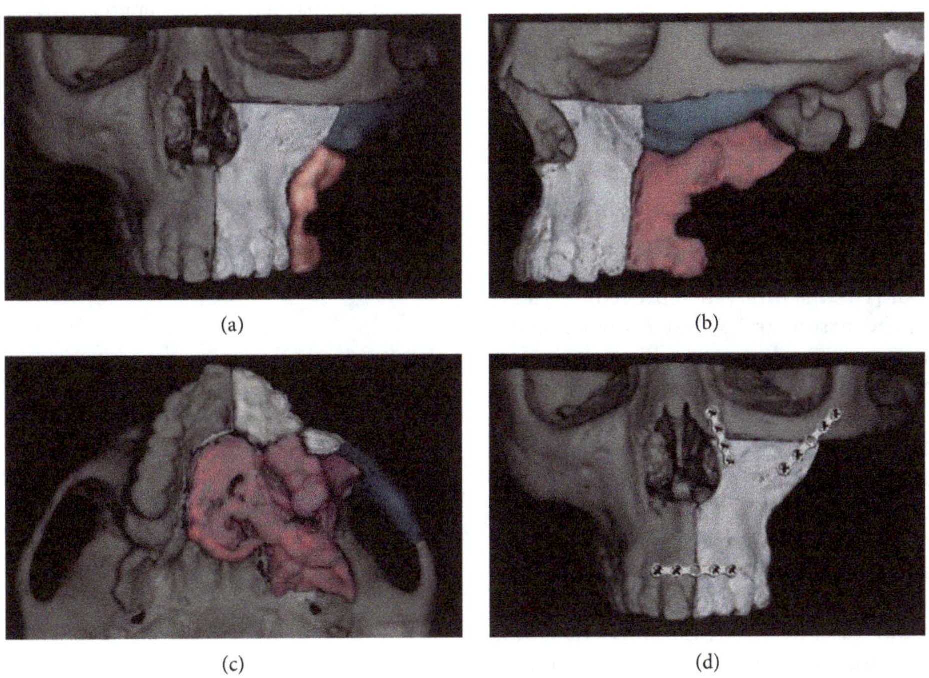

FIGURE 4: (a) Frontal view of model surgery. (b) Lateral view of model surgery. (c) Look-up view of model surgery. (d) View after tumor was resected, and the anterior maxilla flap was fixed with three miniplates.

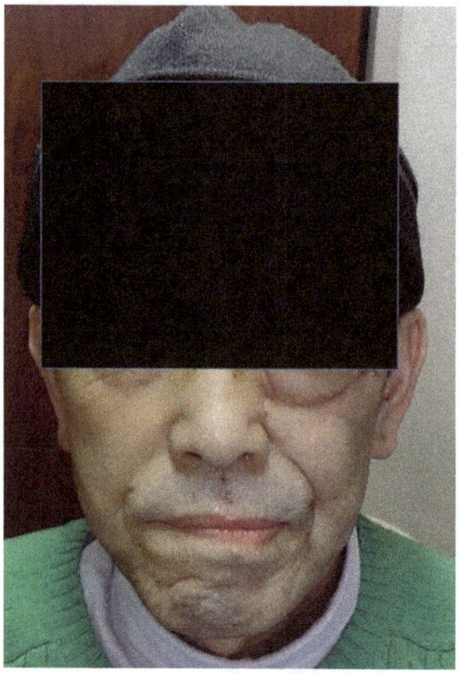

Figure 5: Frontal view two months after surgery.

3. Discussion

Since midface and cranial base bone areas are anatomically very complicated, adequate visualization for tumor resection is needed. Additionally, since severe complications occur if large incisions are made, the selection of the surgical approach and reconstruction are very important. For facial translocation of the cranial base, Janecka et al. [4] presented the basic concept of the approach to be used in this area.

Palatal tumors, especially those invading to the pterygoid fossa, are difficult to dissect and reconstruct after total resection. Total resection of the maxilla and pterygoid area is a good radical procedure, but it results in large defects and causes functional and esthetic problems. The LeFort I approach is not indicated for this area because the incision line overlaps the tumor.

To overcome these issues, the original MS was introduced by Wei et al. [1]. This innovative procedure yields an excellent view of the nasopharynx, but it does include a total maxillotomy. In cases such as ours, this technique is not indicated because of concerns surrounding tumor separation.

The partial MS reported by Sumi et al. [2] features a modified maxillectomy line that is more anterior to the hard palate. With this technique, retropharyngeal areas can be resected, but the palate is not preserved. Shimoda et al. [3] reported another modified MS procedure in which osteotomy is performed on the anterior wall of the maxilla and zygomatic bone. In our case, however, this was unsuitable because the palate tumor could not be resected without sacrificing the alveolar bone.

Thus, we developed our own version of the modified partial MS that was more anterior than the previous versions. We also created an anterior maxilla and alveolar ridge flap. As this area is crucial for both esthetic reasons and mastication purposes, the blood supply to the flap is a major concern. Careful setup and maintenance of the flap enabled us to preserve its blood supply.

For reconstruction, we used an ALT flap due to its many advantages (e.g., low donor site morbidity and tissue versatility). Parkes et al. [5] showed the utility of ALT in cranio-orbitofacial reconstruction, and ALT reconstruction was extremely useful in our MS approach.

In terms of functional results, postoperative mastication and swallowing functions were good. Speech function was also good, and esthetic appearance was acceptable due to our preservation of the infraorbital and alveolar frame.

4. Conclusion

The maxillary swing approach can be applied not only to the nasopharynx and retromaxillary area but also to palatal tumors. This technique is particularly useful for preserving appearance as well as speech and mastication.

Conflicts of Interest

The authors declare that they have no conflicts of interest.

References

[1] W. I. Wei, K. H. Lam, and J. S. Sham, "New approach to the nasopharynx: the maxillary swing approach," *Head and Neck*, vol. 13, no. 3, pp. 200–207, 1991.

[2] T. Sumi, A. Tsunoda, S. Shirakura et al., "Partial maxillary swing approach for removal of the tumors in the retromaxillary area," *Auris Nasus Larynx*, vol. 36, no. 5, pp. 567–570, 2009.

[3] H. Shimoda, K. Yonezawa, H. Shinomiya et al., "Modified partial maxillary swing approach for myxofibrosarcoma in pterygopalatine fossa," *Head and Neck*, vol. 38, no. 12, pp. E2519–E2522, 2016.

[4] I. P. Janecka, C. N. Sen, L. N. Sekhar, and D. W. Nuss, "Facial translocation for cranial base surgery," *Keio Journal of Medicine*, vol. 40, no. 4, pp. 215–220, 1991.

[5] W. J. Parkes, H. Krein, R. Heffelfinger, and J. Curry, "Use of the anterolateral thigh in cranio-orbitofacial reconstruction," *Plastic Surgery International*, vol. 2011, Article ID 941742, 6 pages, 2011.

18

Metastasis to Paranasal Sinuses from Carcinoma of Prostate

Elio Bittar Barbosa,[1] Evaldo César Macau Furtado Ferreira,[1] Fernanda Viviane Mariano,[2] Albina Messias de Almeida Milani Altemani,[2] Emerson Taro Inoue Sakuma,[3] and Eulalia Sakano[1]

[1]*Department of Ophthalmology and Otorhinolaryngology, Faculty of Medical Sciences, University of Campinas, Campinas, SP, Brazil*
[2]*Department of Pathology, Faculty of Medical Sciences, University of Campinas, Campinas, SP, Brazil*
[3]*Department of Radiology, Faculty of Medical Sciences, University of Campinas, Campinas, SP, Brazil*

Correspondence should be addressed to Elio Bittar Barbosa; eliobb2006@gmail.com

Academic Editor: Richard T. Miyamoto

Metastasis from distant primary tumors is extremely rare in the paranasal sinuses with few hundred cases in the literature. Metastatic carcinoma of the prostate is even rarer, despite being one of the most common tumors, with only 24 cases published. In this article, we report a case of a 58-year-old male presenting with epistaxis and nasal obstruction as initial symptoms of a metastatic prostate carcinoma in the ethmoid cells and maxillary sinus.

1. Introduction

Paranasal sinus cancer represents a small portion of the head and neck cancer, approximately 5% of all head and neck tumors [1]. These tumors may arise from multiple tissues present in the nose and paranasal sinuses [2] or more rarely be a metastasis from a distant primary cancer.

Prostate adenocarcinoma is the most prevalent malignant cancer in the male population. In Europe, the incidence rate is 214 cases per 1000 men [3]. Metastases from prostate tumors are a major determinant of survival rates, and prostate-specific antigen tests decrease the incidence of metastatic disease at diagnosis [4].

In this article, we presented the rare case of a patient with a distant metastasis in the right ethmoid cells from a prostate adenocarcinoma.

2. Case Report

A 58-year-old male patient was referred to the Otolaryngology Emergency Service because of important unilateral epistaxis, the third episode in the previous month. He also presented with ipsilateral nasal obstruction and diplopia with a three-month evolution. In his medical report, there was a record of penile squamous cell carcinoma treated with surgery and radiotherapy in 2014 and stage IV prostate adenocarcinoma (iliac, lumbar, and encephalic metastasis) refractory to hormone therapy and chemotherapy, submitted to palliative radiotherapy one month earlier.

During endoscopy, a polypoid, papilloma-like mass originated from the middle meatus was visible, occupying the entire right nasal fossa. No other abnormality was seen in the left nasal fossa. The epistaxis was controlled; the patient was stabilized and referred to biopsy.

The computed tomography (CT) and magnetic resonance imaging (MRI) showed soft tissue density lesion in the right nasal fossa, ethmoid cells, and maxillary sinus with extension into the inferior portion of the orbit through the lamina papyracea and posteriorly to the pterygomaxillary fissure (Figures 1 and 2).

The biopsy resulted in adenocarcinoma (Figures 3(a) and 3(b)). Since the patient had a medical report of prostate

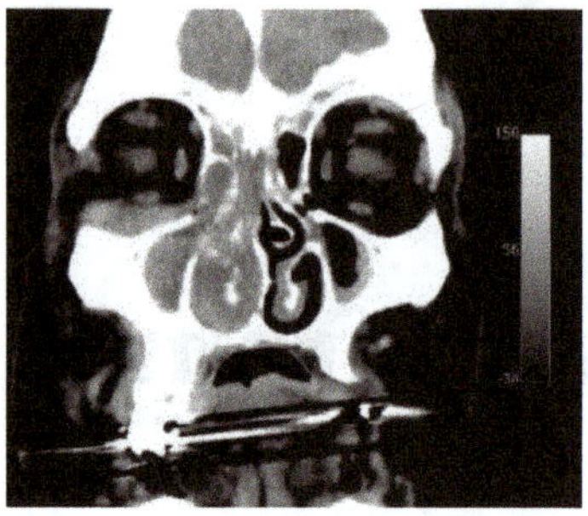

Figure 1: CT demonstrates lesion occupying ethmoid cells, nasal cavity, and maxillary sinus and extending through the lamina papyracea.

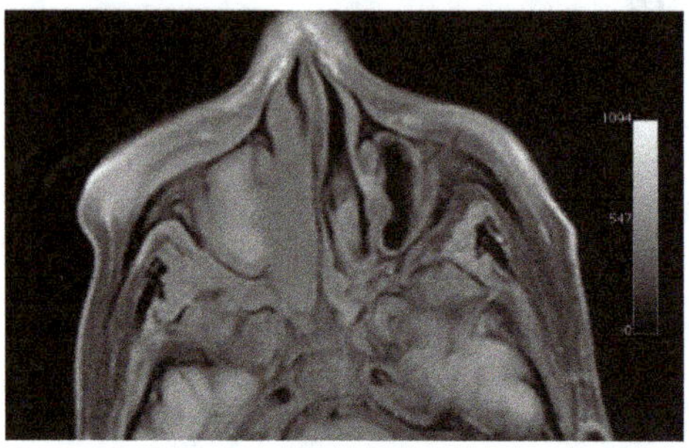

Figure 2: T1-weighted MRI with fat suppression demonstrates the lesion extending to the pterigomaxillary fissure.

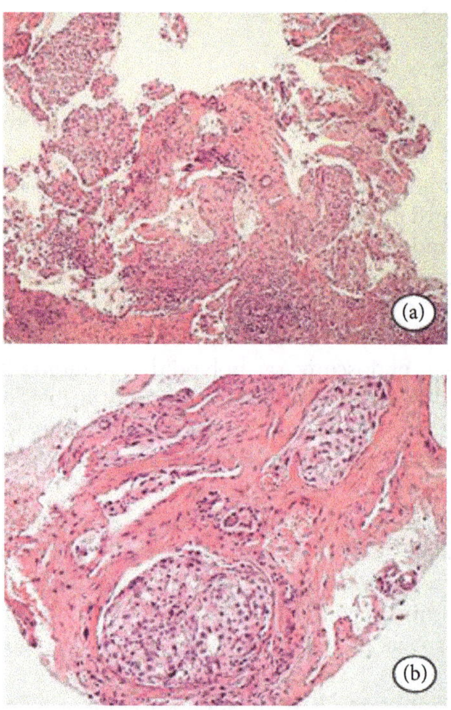

Figure 3: (a) Neoplasia infiltrating surrounding tissue with irregular margins (H&E stain). (b) Atypical epithelial islands with ductal characteristics resembling adenocarcinoma (H&E stain).

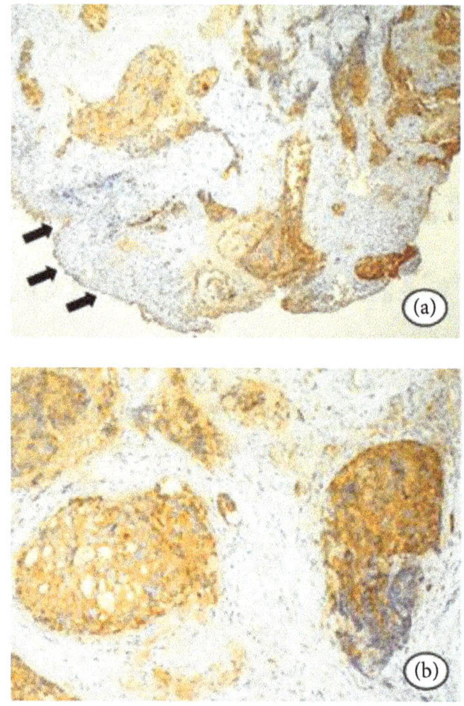

Figure 4: (a) Positive reaction to the PSA antigen in the epithelial islands, and there is no reaction in the superficial epithelium. (b) Strong expression of the PSA antigen in the ductal cells.

adenocarcinoma, the sample was submitted to an immunohistochemical panel. The prostate-specific antigen (PSA) was highly positive, and the diagnosis was confirmed as metastatic prostate adenocarcinoma (Figures 4(a) and 4(b)).

Because of the clinical status of the patient, a few symptoms presented, and the fact that he was already submitted to radiotherapy at the same field, it was opted for a clinical follow-up. After two months of the diagnosis, the patient deceased.

3. Discussion

Paranasal sinuses are a complex anatomic area, surrounding important structures such as the orbit and skull base. The most incident tumors are the squamous cell carcinoma, followed by adenocarcinoma and adenoid cystic carcinoma [5].

In a review, Prescher and Brors reported 169 cases of metastatic tumor to the paranasal sinuses [6]. Most cases originated from the kidney, followed by the lung, breast, thyroid, and prostate. Prescher and Brors also reported that the maxillary sinus was the most affected, followed by the sphenoid, ethmoid, and frontal sinuses [6]. These data are similar to those published by Bernstein [7]. In 77% of the cases, just one paranasal sinus was affected [6].

The nonspecific symptoms are similar to those of primary tumors. The nasal symptoms are usually nasal mass, nasal obstruction, facial deformity, and epistaxis. Orbital

Table 1: Prostate metastasis to the paranasal sinuses.

Author	Age	Sinus	Symptoms	Treatment	Survival
Barrs et al. [15]	61	Sphenoid	Diplopia	Unknown	Died 2 years after presentation
Barrs et al. [15]	57	Sphenoid	Diplopia, decreased visual acuity, ptosis, and numbness of the left face	Unknown	Died 2 years after presentation
McClatchey et al. [16]	54	Sphenoid	Frontal headache and blurring of the right eye	Radiotherapy	Alive 1 year after presentation
Leduc et al. [17]	75	Sphenoid	Diplopia and ptosis of the right eye	Pulpectomy	Alive 19 months after presentation
Matsumoto et al. [18]	79	Sphenoid	Headache and diplopia	Orchiectomy	Unknown
Har-el et al. [19]	77	Maxillary	Exophthalmos of the right eye	Orchiectomy and hormonal block	Unknown
Mickel and Zimmerman [20]	67	Sphenoid	Diplopia and numbness on the right side of the nose	Radiotherapy	Died 2 and a half months after presentation
Saleh et al. [21]	71	Sphenoid	Bilateral exophthalmos and hemoptysis	None	Died 1 month after biopsy
Fortson et al. [22]	50	Ethmoid	Nasal obstruction, diplopia, proptosis, and blurred vision	Chemotherapy and radiotherapy	Died 7 months after presentation
Telera et al. [23]	61	Sphenoid	Ptosis and diplopia of the right eye	Radiotherapy	Died 13 months after presentation
Oliver et al. [8]	72	Maxillary, frontal, and ethmoid	Frontal headache and retro-orbital pain	Hormonal block	Alive three months after presentation
Hunt et al. [11]	76	Sphenoid	Unknown	Radiotherapy and hormonal block	Alive 14 months after presentation
Lavasani et al. [24]	67	Sphenoid	Decreased visual acuity	Radiotherapy	Alive 6 months after presentation
Başeskioglu et al. [25]	69	Maxillary	Sinus fullness	Radiotherapy	Died 32 months after diagnosis
Ibarguren et al. [26]	64	Maxillary and frontal	Ptosis, proptosis, and facial numbness	Hormonal block and chemotherapy	Alive 8 months after presentation
El Khatib et al. [27]	57	Maxillary	Facial swelling	Pulpectomy and hormonal block	Died 9 months after presentation
Viswanatha [28]	68	Ethmoid and frontal	Facial swelling and epistaxis	Radiotherapy	Lost to follow-up after 3 months of presentation
Tunio et al. [29]	65	Ethmoid	Nasal obstruction, diplopia, and proptosis	Radiotherapy and hormonal block	Alive until article publication
Azarpira et al. [30]	74	Maxillary	Nasal obstruction	Chemotherapy and radiotherapy	Died 11 months after presentation
Petersson et al. [31]	55	Sphenoid	Headache, diplopia, and blurred vision	Hormonal block	Unknown
Puche-Sanz et al. [32]	56	Sphenoid	Decreased visual acuity and facial numbness	Radiotherapy and hormonal block	Alive 5 years after presentation
Akdemir et al. [33]	73	Frontal and ethmoid	Headache and exophthalmos	Hormonal block	Unknown
Evarts et al. [34]	59	Maxillary and ethmoid	Cheek numbness, headache, decreased visual acuity, nasal obstruction, and drainage	Chemotherapy	Died 2 months after biopsy
Lechien et al. [35]	67	Frontal	Diplopia, facial pain, and headache	Hormonal block	Died a few months after presentation
Present case	58	Ethmoid and maxillary	Epistaxis, nasal obstruction, and diplopia	None	Died 2 months after diagnosis

symptoms may also occur, such as proptosis, ptosis, decreased vision, and diplopia. Occasionally, these symptoms may be the first presentation of an occult primary tumor [8, 9].

The most frequent sites involved in prostate metastasis are the bone (90%), lung (46%), and liver (25%) [10]. The head and neck are rare locations for metastasis, and it occurs more frequently in the brain, dura, and lymph nodes [11]. The treatment may be hormone therapy, chemotherapy, radioisotopes, and radiotherapy [12].

Metastasis may reach the paranasal sinuses by hematogenous, lymphogenous, or vertebral venous plexus pathways. First postulated by Batson [13], this low-pressure valveless system is a connection between deep pelvic veins, intercostal veins, vena cava, and the azygos system. A rise in the abdominal pressure might redirect the blood flux from the vena cava system to the vertebral venous plexus. This flux alteration can allow the tumor to reach the paranasal sinuses [14].

This is the twenty-fifth reported case of metastatic prostate adenocarcinoma in the paranasal sinuses. The majority of cases involved patients with known prostate cancer, with a mean age of 63.15 years, and the most affected sinus was the sphenoid (44.5%). Radiotherapy was the preferred treatment option (40.7%). In Table 1, we describe the cases reported in full text, available online so far.

Imaging is not able to differentiate a local tumor from a metastasis; however, it is essential to determine location and extension and for surgical planning. CT may show enhancement, bone erosion, remodeling, and invasion. Magnetic resonance imaging (MRI) has an important role to help, defining leptomeningeal and orbital invasion [13]. Positron emission tomography (PET-CT) might be useful in the primary occult tumor.

Histopathology has an essential role in the diagnosis. When metastasizing to the paranasal sinuses, normally prostate carcinoma is not well differentiated. Immunohistochemical panel is also important, with positivity of prostate-specific antigen, prostate acid phosphatase, EpCam, NKX3.1, and prostein [36].

Usually, the diagnosis of a metastasis to the paranasal sinuses means a poor prognosis. An important factor that can be crucial is whether the metastasis is isolated or part of a widespread disease.

Normally, the treatment involving the metastasis to the paranasal sinuses is palliative, with the exception of an isolated metastasis, for which the radical surgery may be a viable option. The patient's quality of life should be a priority. The main goal is pain relief and bleeding prevention. Management has not changed greatly over the years, and therapy options include radiotherapy, chemotherapy, immunotherapy, and, more recently, endoscopic surgery [37].

Endoscopic surgery may provide symptom relief faster, with lower systemic and local side effects [37]. Tabaee et al. suggested three criteria to help in the decision of the surgery: reasonable expectation of improvement, possible prolongation of life, and survivability after anesthesia [38].

4. Conclusion

Despite being a rare entity, metastatic prostatic tumor in the paranasal sinuses should always be part of the differential diagnosis in patients with known prostatic tumor and recently developed nasal or orbital symptoms.

References

[1] P. Bossi, D. Farina, G. Gatta, D. Lombardi, P. Nicolai, and E. Orlandi, "Paranasal sinus cancer," *Critical Reviews in Oncology/Hematology*, vol. 98, pp. 45–61, 2016.

[2] L. Barnes, J. W. Eveson, P. Reichart, and D. Sidransky, *World Health Organization Classification of Tumours, Pathology and Genetics, Head and Neck Tumours*, IARC Press, Lyon, France, 2005.

[3] A. Jemal, R. Siegel, and E. Ward, "Cancer statistics, 2008," *CA: A Cancer Journal for Clinicians*, vol. 58, no. 2, pp. 71–96, 2008.

[4] B. Carlotta, A. Auvinen, M. J. Roobol et al., "Metastatic prostate cancer incidence and prostate-specific antigen testing: new insights from the European randomized study of screening for prostate cancer," *European Urology*, vol. 68, no. 5, pp. 885–890, 2015.

[5] V. J. Lund, H. Stammberger, P. Nicolai et al., "European position paper on endoscopic management of tumours of the nose, paranasal sinuses and skull base," *Rhinology Supplement*, vol. 22, no. 1, pp. 1–143, 2010.

[6] A. Prescher and D. Brors, "Metastases to the paranasal sinuses: case report and review of the literature," *Laryngo-rhinootologie*, vol. 80, no. 10, pp. 583–594, 2001, in German.

[7] J. M. Bernstein, W. W. Montgomery, and K. Balogh Jr., "Metastatic tumors to the maxilla, nose, and paranasal sinuses," *Laryngoscope*, vol. 76, no. 4, pp. 621–650, 1966.

[8] V. J. Oliver, A. L. Valdés, A. D. Morillo et al., "Frontal ethmoid metastases of prostatic carcinoma. Report of one case and review of the literature," *Acta Otorrinolaringológica Española*, vol. 52, no. 2, pp. 151–154, 2001.

[9] S. M. Lee, Y. M. Kim, and B. M. Kim, "Epistaxis as the first manifestation of silent renal cell carcinoma: a case report with relevant literature review," *Iran Journal of Radiology*, vol. 13, no. 1, p. e31208, 2016.

[10] L. Bubendorf, A. Schopfer, U. Wagner et al., "Metastatic patterns of prostate cancer: an autopsy study of 1,589 patients," *Human Pathology*, vol. 31, no. 5, pp. 568–583, 2000.

[11] J. L. Hunt, J. E. Tomaszewski, and K. T. Montone, "Prostatic adenocarcinoma metastatic to the head and neck and the workup of an unknown epithelioid neoplasm," *Head and Neck*, vol. 26, no. 2, pp. 171–178, 2004.

[12] C. Gilson, T. Manickavasagar, and S. Chowdhury, "Treatment of metastatic prostate cancer," *Trends Urology & Men Health*, vol. 6, no. 4, pp. 7–12, 2015.

[13] O. V. Batson, "The function of the vertebral veins and their role in the spread of metastases," *Annals of Surgery*, vol. 112, no. 1, pp. 138–149, 1940.

[14] F. Lopéz, K. O. Devaney, E. Y. Hanna, A. Rinaldo, and A. Ferlito, "Metastases to nasal cavity and paranasal sinuses," *Head and Neck*, vol. 38, no. 12, pp. 1847–1854, 2016.

[15] D. M. Barrs, T. J. McDonald, and J. P. Whisnant, "Metastatic tumors to the sphenoid sinus," *Laryngoscope*, vol. 89, no. 8, pp. 1229–1243, 1979.

[16] K. D. McClatchey, R. V. Lloyd, and J. D. Schaldenbrand, "Metastatic carcinoma to the sphenoid sinus. Case report and review of the literature," *Archives Otorhinolaryngology*, vol. 241, no. 3, pp. 219–224, 1985.

[17] D. Leduc, C. Massot, G. Crouzet et al., "Metastase spheno-caverneuse d'un cancer prostatique," *La Revue de Medécine Interne*, vol. 7, no. 1, pp. 70–73, 1986, in French.

[18] I. Matsumoto, M. Furusato, L. Inomaia, T. Wada, and S. Aizawa, "Prostatic cancer presenting as metastatic adenocarcinoma of sphenoid sinus," *Acta Pathologica Japonica*, vol. 36, no. 11, pp. 1753–1756, 1986.

[19] G. Har-el, I. Avidor, A. Weisbord, and J. Sidi, "Carcinoma of the prostate metastatic to the maxillary antrum," *Head and Neck*, vol. 10, no. 1, pp. 55–58, 1987.

[20] R. A. Mickel and M. C. Zimmerman, "The sphenoid sinus—a site for metastasis," *Otolaryngology-Head and Neck Surgery*, vol. 102, no. 6, pp. 709–716, 1990.

[21] H. A. Saleh, P. O'Flynn, and N. S. Jones, "Prostatic metastases in the nose and paranasal sinuses," *Journal of Laryngology Otology*, vol. 107, no. 7, pp. 629–632, 1993.

[22] J. K. Fortson, Z. L. Bezmalinovic, and D. L. Moseley, "Bilateral ethmoid sinusitis with unilateral proptosis as an initial manifestation of metastatic prostate carcinoma," *Journal of*

the National Medical Association, vol. 86, no. 12, pp. 945–948, 1994.

[23] S. Telera, S. Carloia, D. Cavallotti, S. Bosco, M. Manni, and L. Cecconi, "Sphenoidal metastasis from prostate carcinoma. Case report and review of literature," *Neurochirurgie*, vol. 47, no. 1, pp. 61–65, 2001.

[24] L. Lavasani, P. E. Zapanta, N. Tanna, and N. Sadeghi, "Metastasis of prostatic adenocarcinoma to the sphenoid sinus," *Annals of Otology, Rhinology & Laryngology*, vol. 115, no. 9, pp. 690–693, 2006.

[25] B. Başeskioglu, S. Esklçorapçi, S. Ekici, D. E. Baydar, S. Kendi, and H. Özen, "Maxillary sinus metastasis of prostate cancer: a case report," *Turkish Journal of Cancer*, vol. 36, no. 2, pp. 79–81, 2006.

[26] R. L. Ibarguren, J. G. Rodríguez, A. V. Mateos, I. A. Arin, I. O. Grasa, and C. P. Peña, "Metástasis en senos paranasales secundaria a adenocarcinoma prostático," *Archivos Españoles de Urología*, vol. 60, no. 9, pp. 1137–1140, 2007, in Spanish.

[27] K. El Khatib, K. Moufid, A. Abouchadi, M. Nassih, and A. Rzin, "Maxillary metastasis revealing a prostate cancer," *Revue Stomatologie Chirurgie Maxillo-Faciale*, vol. 108, no. 5, pp. 468-469, 2007, in French.

[28] B. Viswanatha, "Prostatic carcinoma metastatic to the paranasal sinuses: a case report," *Ear Nose Throat Journal*, vol. 87, no. 9, pp. 519-520, 2008.

[29] M. A. Tunio, M. Rafi, R. Mohsin, A. Hashmi, S. Raza, and M. Mubarak, "Ipsilateral ethmoid sinuses metastasis and proptosis: rare presentation of metastatic prostate cancer," *Pakistan Journal of Medical Sciences*, vol. 27, no. 1, pp. 212-213, 2011.

[30] N. Azarpira, M. J. Ashraf, B. Khademi, and N. Asadi, "Distant metastases to nasal cavities and paranasal sinuses case series," *Indian Journal of Otolaryngology Head Neck Surgery*, vol. 64, no. 4, pp. 349–352, 2011.

[31] F. Petersson, T. S. Hui, D. Loke, and T. C. Putti, "Metastasis of occult prostatic carcinoma to the sphenoid sinus: report of a rare case and a review of the literature," *Head and Neck Pathology*, vol. 6, no. 2, pp. 258–263, 2012.

[32] I. Puche-Sanz, F. Vázquez-Alonso, J. F. Flores-Martín, H. Almonte-Fernández, and J. M. Cózar-Olmo, "Sphenoid sinus metastasis as the presenting manifestation of a prostatic adenocarcinoma: case report and overview of the literature," *Case Reports in Oncological Medicine*, vol. 2012, Article ID 819809, 4 pages, 2012.

[33] F. Akdemir, M. Aldemir, H. Çakar, and G. Güler, "Metastasis of prostate adenocarcinoma to the frontal and ethmoid sinus," *Turkish Journal of Urology*, vol. 42, no. 4, pp. 299–302, 2016.

[34] M. Evarts, R. A. Schuster, M. Steehler, and K. Steehler, "Metastasis of prostate carcinoma to the paranasal sinuses: a case study," *Journal of Case Reports in Medicine*, vol. 5, pp. 1-3, 2016.

[35] J. R. Lechien, J. Doyen, M. Khalife, and S. Saussez, "Prostatic carcinoma metastatic to frontal and cavernous sinuses: a case report," *Brazilian Journal of Otorhinolaryngology*, 2016. In press.

[36] M. B. Amin, J. I. Epstein, T. M. Ulbright et al., "Best practices recommendations in the application of immunohistochemistry in the prostate: report from the International Society of Urologic Pathology consensus conference," *American Journal of Surgical Pathology*, vol. 38, no. 8, pp. 1017–1022, 2014.

[37] J. M. Roberts, C. Brook, and S. Parnes, "Palliative endoscopic surgery for sinonasal metastases: a case report and literature review," *Ear Nose Throat Journal*, vol. 94, no. 2, pp. 24–26, 2015.

[38] A. Tabaee, G. Nyquist, V. K. Anand, A. Singh, A. Kacker, and T. H. Schwartz, "Palliative endoscopic surgery in advanced sinonasal and anterior skull base neoplasms," *Otolaryngology-Head and Neck Surgery*, vol. 142, no. 1, pp. 126–128, 2010.

19

A Very Rare Case of Hypereosinophilic Syndrome Secondary to Natural Killer/T-Cell Lymphoma

Takanori Yamamoto,[1] Atsushi Kamijo,[1,2] Tadao Nakazawa,[3] Kei Nakajima,[4] Keita Kirito,[4] Norio Komatsu,[5] and Keisuke Masuyama[1]

[1]*Department of Otorhinolaryngology and Head & Neck Surgery, University of Yamanashi, Yamanashi, Japan*
[2]*Department of Otorhinolaryngology and Allergy Center, Saitama Medical University, Saitama, Japan*
[3]*Department of Pathology, University of Yamanashi, Yamanashi, Japan*
[4]*Department of Hematology and Oncology, University of Yamanashi, Yamanashi, Japan*
[5]*Department of Hematology, Juntendo University School of Medicine, Tokyo, Japan*

Correspondence should be addressed to Takanori Yamamoto; beatstick@yahoo.co.jp

Academic Editor: Rong-San Jiang

Hypereosinophilic syndrome (HES) is a systemic disease characterized by an increased peripheral blood eosinophil count accompanied by systemic organ dysfunction. HES is classified into idiopathic HES, primary (neoplastic) HES (HES_N), and secondary (reactive) HES (HES_R). In this case report, a patient who developed peripheral blood eosinophilia and granulation tissue in the pharynx and paranasal sinus, which was initially diagnosed as chronic eosinophilic leukemia (CEL), categorized as HES_N, but was eventually identified after the patient had died as natural killer/T-cell (NK/T) lymphoma, nasal type (ENKL), categorized as HES_R, is presented. ENKL-induced HES is very rare but must be considered.

1. Introduction

Hypereosinophilic syndrome (HES), organ dysfunction due to eosinophilia, has various etiologies. In this case report, a patient diagnosed as having chronic eosinophilic leukemia (CEL) because FIP1-like-1-platelet-derived growth factor receptor α (*FIP1L1-PDGFRA*: FP) chimeric gene was initially detected by reverse transcription polymerase chain reaction (RT-PCR) expression analysis is described. However, the patient was refractory to treatment and subsequently died, after which the diagnosis was revised to nasal-type NK/T-cell lymphoma. NK/T-cell lymphoma is rarely the cause of HES and can be difficult to diagnose. It is therefore essential to consider the possibility of this disease to make a correct diagnosis.

2. Case Report

The patient was a 23-year-old woman who was referred to our hospital in mid-June of XXXX (day 1) with a chief complaint of nasal congestion. Before visiting our hospital, the patient had been diagnosed by her local otolaryngologist with rhinosinusitis and was taking oral antimicrobial drugs, but her condition did not improve, and she developed a fever (38°C) at the beginning of June. The patient had a previous history of systemic lupus erythematosus (SLE) for which she had undergone treatment from the age of 15 years. However, the SLE was well controlled with 5 mg/day of oral prednisolone.

Nasal fiberscopy findings showed that the nasal cavity and nasopharynx were filled with a viscous exudate and granulation tissue (Figure 1(a)). Computed tomography (CT) scans demonstrated space-occupying lesions in the bilateral ethmoid and sphenoid sinuses and a soft tissue lesion from the nasopharynx to the oropharynx (Figures 1(b) and 1(c)). Hematology findings showed a C-reactive protein (CRP) count of 7.32 mg/dl and a peripheral blood white blood cell (WBC) count of 14,000/μl, consisting of a neutrophil count of 9,660/μl (69%) and eosinophil count of 2,940/μl (21%), indicating eosinophilia without blasts. Lactate dehydrogenase (LDH) was slightly elevated at 313/IU,

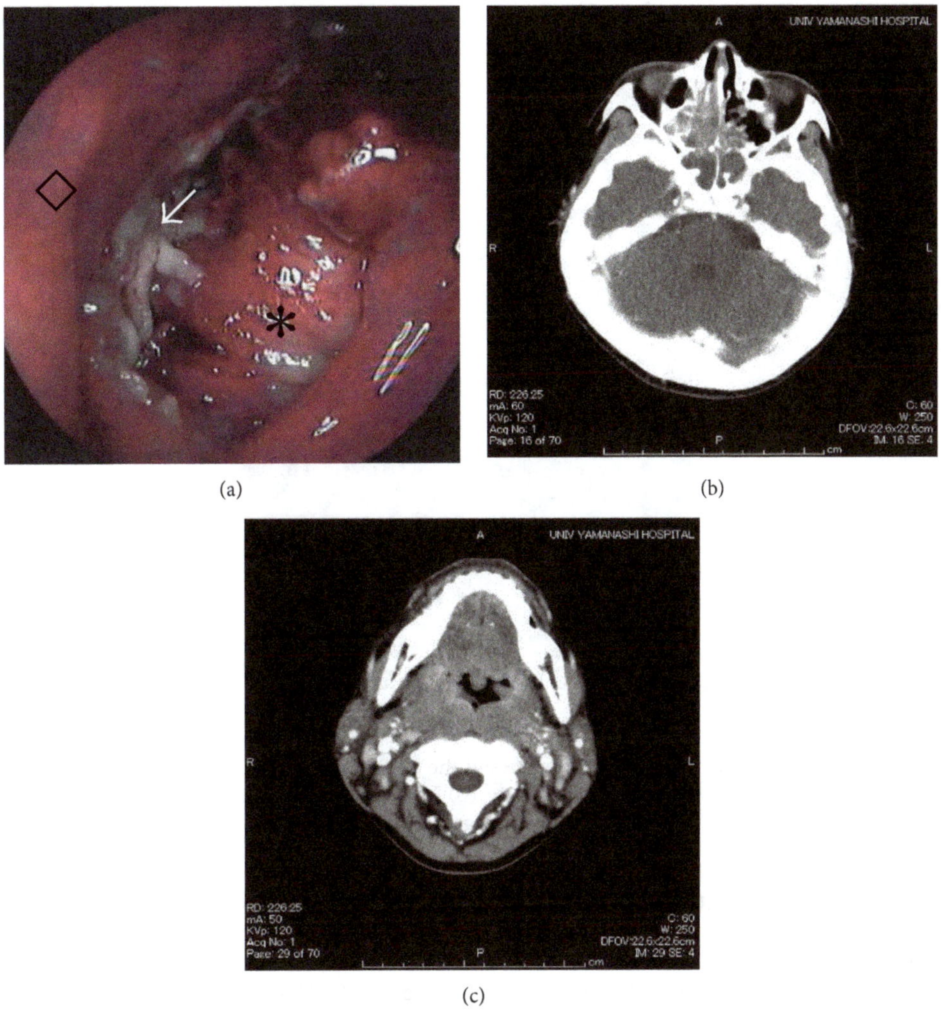

(a) (b) (c)

Figure 1: Scope image and computed tomography (CT) findings. (a) Scope image of the left nasal cavity. White granulation tissue is observed (arrow). *: inferior turbinate and ◇: nasal septum. (b) Axial CT with contrast demonstrating soft tissue lesions or effusions in the ethmoid and sphenoid sinuses. (c) Axial CT with contrast demonstrating mucosal and tissue swelling in the pharynx.

and soluble interleukin-2 receptor (sIL-2R) was also high at 2200 U/ml.

Infection was initially suspected, but antimicrobial treatment was ineffective. The results of subsequent biopsies of tissue from the nasal cavity and pharynx led to a diagnosis of granulation tissue with significant eosinophil infiltration, for which steroid pulse therapy was given. The patient's eosinophil count decreased transiently, but it then increased again, so bone marrow aspiration was performed. The results did not indicate any blasts in the bone marrow; they only showed that mature eosinophils comprised half of the infiltrating cells. The results of Giemsa- (G-) banded chromosome analysis performed at that time did not show any abnormalities. Abdominal ultrasound showed hepatosplenomegaly. However, RT-PCR expression analysis was positive for the *FIP1L1-PDGFRA* chimeric gene. The patient was therefore diagnosed with chronic eosinophilic leukemia (CEL). From day 60, the patient was started on oral therapy with the tyrosine kinase inhibitor imatinib (100 mg/day), after which her eosinophil count decreased from 21,366/μl to 12,079/μl the next day. However, the swelling in the patient's larynx and neck worsened, so the imatinib dose was increased to 400 mg/day. The eosinophil count decreased transiently again, but it increased on day 65 to 27,424/μl. On day 75, the imatinib was switched to oral hydroxyurea (1500 mg/day), but it was ineffective, and she died on day 85.

The fact that the patient did not improve on imatinib therapy despite testing positive for the *FIP1L1-PDGFRA* fusion gene led to testing for the imatinib-resistant PDGFRA-T674I mutant, but the results were negative. Retesting for the FP chimeric gene was then requested at another facility after the patient died, but all test results were negative. Reanalysis of pathology specimens yielded positive results for Epstein–Barr virus-encoded early small RNA (EBER), cluster of differentiation 3 (CD3), CD4, and granzyme A, and negative results for CD56 (Figures 2(a)–2(c)), leading to an eventual diagnosis of nasal-type extranodal NK/T-cell lymphoma (ENKL).

3. Discussion

A case of nasal-type ENKL with concomitant HES was described. Since the initial PCR detected the *FIP1L1-PDGFRA*

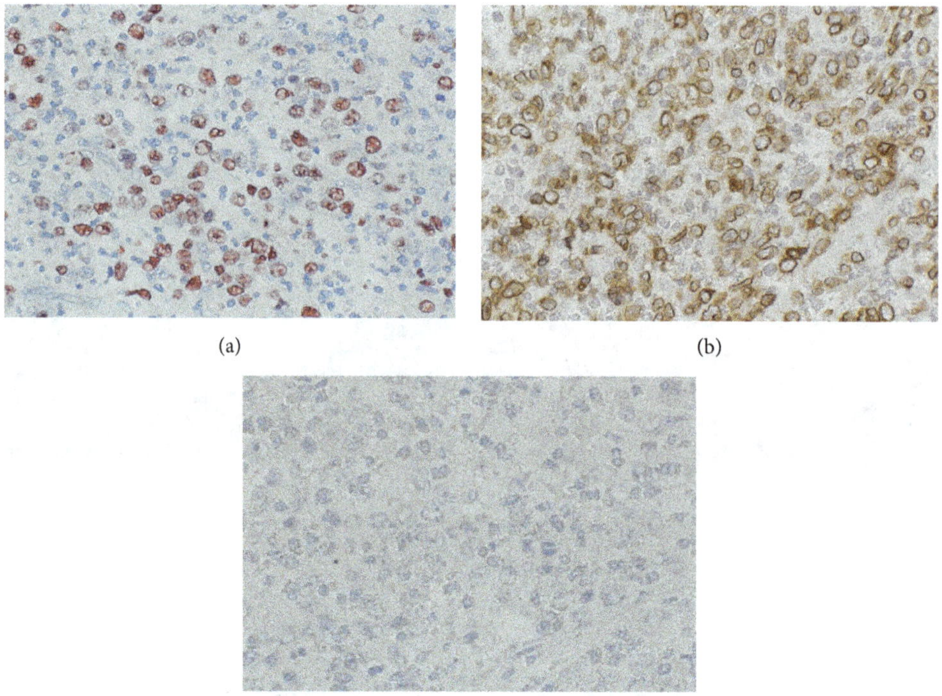

Figure 2: Morphological and immunohistochemical characteristics of the lymphoma (×200). (a) In situ hybridization with EBER showing strong Epstein–Barr virus expression by a large atypical lymphocyte. (b) Immunohistochemical staining with CD3 showing strong positive staining. (c) Immunohistochemical staining with CD56 showing negative staining.

chimeric gene and a pathological diagnosis of NK/T-cell lymphoma was not made, there was a delay in providing appropriate treatment, which led to an unfortunate outcome.

The Working Conference on Eosinophilic Disorders and Syndromes proposed a classification of HES in 2011 [1]. This classification defines hypereosinophilia (HE) as a peripheral blood eosinophil count $\geq 1500/\mu l$ recorded on at least two occasions with a minimum interval of four weeks, or as extensive tissue infiltration by eosinophils. Depending on the cause, HE is classified as (1) familial variant HE, HE_{FA}; (2) HE of undetermined significance (no clear underlying cause and no clinical symptoms), HE_{US}; (3) primary (clonal/neoplastic), HE_N; and (4) secondary (associated with lymphoma, etc.), HE_R. HE accompanied by organ dysfunction due to eosinophilia is defined as HES, which is classified as either idiopathic HES, primary (neoplastic) HES (HES_N), or secondary (reactive) HES (HES_R). Although this patient was seen in 2007 before this classification was proposed, if this classification was to be applied retrospectively, then the patient would have initially been diagnosed with HES_N and finally with HES_R. According to the 2016 World Health Organization (WHO) classification [2], eosinophilic leukemia with no existing gene mutation, with blasts in the bone marrow or blood, and with clonal eosinophilia is classified as "chronic eosinophilic leukemia, not otherwise specified" (CEL, NOS). Separate from this classification, pathological conditions based on four molecular abnormalities, namely, PDGFRA, PDGFRbeta (PDGFRB), fibroblast growth factor receptor 1 (FGFR1), and *PCM1-JAK2* (fusion gene resulting from a t(8;9)(p22;p24) chromosomal translocation), are classified as myeloid/lymphoid tumors, all of which belong to the HES_N variant.

In 2003, Cools et al. identified the FP chimeric gene in nine of 16 HES patients [3]. Patients who carry this fusion gene are eligible for treatment with the tyrosine kinase inhibitor imatinib, which has been reported to be very effective [3, 4]. However, treatment with imatinib proved to be ineffective in this patient. Imatinib tolerance in individuals with the FP fusion gene is often caused by the T674I mutation occurring in the adenosine triphosphate- (ATP-) binding region, but it is also known to occur in those with S601P/L629P and D842V kinase domain mutations. Examination for the T674I mutation was performed in the present patient, but it was not detected. FP fusion gene searches typically use RT-PCR analysis, and this method was also used in reaching the initial diagnosis of eosinophilia due to myeloproliferative neoplasms involving the *FIP1L1-PDGFRA* chimeric gene. However, Sada et al. [5] reported that when performing RT-PCR with commonly used primer sets, an artificial splicing mechanism in the PCR process causes the FP chimeric gene to form even in the gene samples of healthy individuals. Diagnosis combining the use of fluorescence in situ hybridization (FISH) technique encompassing the three regions of the 4q12 cleavage site is therefore currently recommended.

After the patient's death, the cause of the eosinophilia was attributed to nasal-type extranodal NK/T-cell lymphoma (ENKL). All types of lymphomas are reportedly capable of triggering eosinophilia [6], but nasal-type NK/T-cell lymphoma is very rare in HES patients. The only case, a 21-year

Bolivian woman with hemophagocytic syndrome-associated NK/T-cell lymphoma, was reported in English literature [7]. In addition to ENKL, the lymphocyte variant HE is also reported to accompany chronic active Epstein–Barr virus (CAEBV) infection, with EBV-infected TV beta 5.1 T-cell clones identified as causing the overproduction of Th2 cytokines [8]. The involvement of EBV has also been demonstrated in the onset of NK/T-cell lymphoma, so eosinophilia is believed to occur secondary to the abnormal secretion of cytokines induced by EBV-infected NK/T tumor cells.

Most cases of ENKL are NK cell-derived lymphomas expressing the CD3− CD56+ phenotype without T-cell receptor gene rearrangement. The present patient expressed the CD3+ CD56− phenotype, which appears to be relatively rare in ENKL. Wang et al. [9] reported that approximately 20% of 288 early-stage ENKL patients were categorized as CD56−. They also found that the complete remission rate was significantly lower in CD56− ENKL than in CD56+ ENKL (60.8% versus 80.6%) and that the overall survival was significantly lower in CD56− ENKL, stating that CD56 expression is an independent predictor of survival.

In addition, Li et al. compared nasal ENKL and ENKL of the extranasal upper aerodigestive tract and found that CD56-negative lymphomas are more common in the latter (16.7% and 53.6%, resp.) [10].

ENKL lesions consist mainly of necrotic tissue, which often complicates pathological diagnosis and can necessitate several biopsies. Although rare, ENKL must also be considered as a potential etiology of HES.

4. Conclusion

A patient who developed peripheral blood eosinophilia and granulation tissue in the pharynx and paranasal sinus, which was initially diagnosed as CEL, but which was eventually identified as ENKL after the patient had died, was presented. Since various diseases present with peripheral blood eosinophilia, correct differential diagnosis, though challenging, followed by appropriate treatment is essential.

Acknowledgments

The authors would like to thank Dr. Luba Wolchuk with Forte Science Communications, Tokyo, Japan, for editorial assistance and Junichi Tamaru for assisting in pathological diagnosis.

References

[1] P. Valent, A. D. Klion, H. P. Horny et al., "Contemporary consensus proposal on criteria and classification of eosinophilic disorders and related syndrome," *Journal of Allergy and Clinical Immunology*, vol. 130, no. 3, pp. 607–612, 2012.

[2] D. A. Arber, A. Orazi, R. Hasseriian et al., "The 2016 revision to the World Health Organization classification of myeloid neoplasms and acute leukemia," *Blood*, vol. 127, no. 20, pp. 2391–2405, 2016.

[3] J. Cools, D. J. Deangelo, J. Gotlib et al., "A tyrosine kinase created by fusion of the PDGFRA and FIP1L1 genes as a therapeutic target of imatinib in idiopathic hypereosinophilic syndrome," *New England Journal of Medicine*, vol. 348, no. 13, pp. 1201–1214, 2003.

[4] A. MS. Muller, U. M. Martens, S. C. Hofmann, L. Bruckner-Tuderman, R. Mertelsmann, and M. Lübbert, "Imatinib mesylate as a novel treatment option for hypereosinophilic syndrome: two case reports and a comprehensive review of the literature," *Annals of Hematology*, vol. 85, no. 1, pp. 1–16, 2006.

[5] A. Sada, Y. Katayama, K. Yamamoto et al., "A multicenter analysis of the FIP1L1-αPDGFR fusion gene in Japanese idiopathic hypereosinophilic syndrome: an aberrant splicing skipping the αPDGFR exon 12," *Annals of Hematology*, vol. 86, no. 12, pp. 855–863, 2007.

[6] A. D'Souza, A. Pardanani, and A. Tefferi, "Lymphoma-associated versus lymphocytic-variant hypereosinophilia," *Leukemia and Lymphoma*, vol. 53, no. 11, pp. 2103-2104, 2012.

[7] E. R. Fernández, J. R. P. Pardo, A. Doyle, M. C. Albendea, and A. R. de la Rúa, "Hemophagocytic syndrome associated NK/T nasal type lymphoma presenting as hypereosinophilic syndrome: a case report and literature review," *Leukemia Research*, vol. 35, no. 7, pp. e97–e99, 2011.

[8] A. D. Klion, R. Mejia, E. W. Cowen et al., "Chronic active Epstein-Barr virus infection: a novel cause of lymphocytic variant hypereosinophilic syndrome," *Blood*, vol. 121, no. 12, pp. 2364–2366, 2013.

[9] L. Wang, Z. Wang, Z. Xia, Y. Lu, H. Huang, and Y. Zhang, "CD56-negative extranodal NK/T cell lymphoma should be regarded as a distinct subtype with poor prognosis," *Tumor Biology*, vol. 36, no. 10, pp. 7717–7723, 2015.

[10] Y. X. Li, H. Wang, X. L. Feng et al., "Immunophenotypic characteristics and clinical relevance of CD56+ and CD56− extranodal nasal-type natural killer/T-cell lymphoma," *Leukemia and Lymphoma*, vol. 52, no. 3, pp. 417–424, 2011.

20

Gradenigo's Syndrome and Labyrinthitis: Conservative versus Surgical Treatment

Ahmad Al-juboori [1,2] **and Amira Nasser Al Hail** [1,2]

[1] *Otorhinolaryngology, Head & Neck Surgery (ORL-HNS) Department, Al Wakra Hospital, Hamad Medical Corporation, Doha, Qatar*
[2] *Weill Cornell Medical College, Ar-Rayyan, Qatar*

Correspondence should be addressed to Ahmad Al-juboori; ahmednas2005@yahoo.com

Academic Editor: Kamal Morshed

Background. Extracranial intratemporal complications of chronic suppurative otitis media (CSOM) are extremely rare. Gradenigo's syndrome is defined as a clinical triad of otitis media, severe pain originating from the trigeminal nerve, and ipsilateral sixth cranial nerve palsy. *Case Report.* A 61-year-old man presented with chronic left ear discharge, left-sided headache, diplopia associated with vertigo, tinnitus, and hearing impairment. MRI with contrast showed asymmetrical signal changes in the bilateral petrous bone with reduced enhancement on the left with high suspicion of petrositis; in the context of chronic tympanomastoiditis, there was a 10 × 4 mm enhancing lesion in the left internal auditory meatus involving the 7th-8th nerve complex. The patient was treated conservatively with local and systemic antimicrobial agents, he had satisfactory response and improvement regarding symptoms of ear discharge, vertigo, and diplopia, but there is no remarkable response regarding hearing loss and tinnitus. *Conclusion.* Although there is little evidence to support the use of conservative treatment in the treatment of Gradenigo's syndrome resulting from chronic ear disease, we here demonstrate successful conservative treatment of Gradenigo's syndrome.

1. Introduction

Chronic suppurative otitis media (CSOM) is characterized by recurrent or persistent ear discharge (otorrhoea) over 12 weeks through a perforation of the tympanic membrane [1]. The complications of CSOM have been greatly reduced because of the development of antibiotics. Complications of CSOM are classified into intracranial and extracranial complications. Extracranial complications can be further divided into intratemporal and extratemporal complications. Different prevalence rates for extracranial complications of CSOM have been reported to date [2–4]. There are still a number of patients, who develop acute mastoiditis, subperiosteal abscess, facial palsy, and intracranial complication due to recent increase of antibiotic-resistant bacteria [5], and other very rare complications like labyrinthitis and petrositis are also encountered. In 1907, Guisseppe Gradenigo described a symptom complex of suppurative otitis media, pain in the distribution of the trigeminal nerve, and abducens (6th) nerve palsy [6]. Gradenigo's syndrome (GS) is defined as a clinical triad of otitis media, severe pain originating from the trigeminal nerve, and ipsilateral sixth cranial nerve palsy. The syndrome is an exceedingly rare complication of CSOM in the era of the widespread use of antibiotics and easily accessible health-care services. Petrositis diagnosis requires imaging studies, namely, computed tomography (CT), magnetic resonance imaging (MRI), or nuclear imaging techniques, to identify the petrous apex as the site of the inflammatory process [3]. The treatment of Gradenigo's syndrome is not consensual and should be managed on an individual basis [7].

Here, we reported a case of acute labyrinthitis and Gradenigo's syndrome following CSOM, treated successfully with conservative therapy with antibiotics, and there was also accidental finding of an internal auditory canal lesion most likely acoustic neuroma.

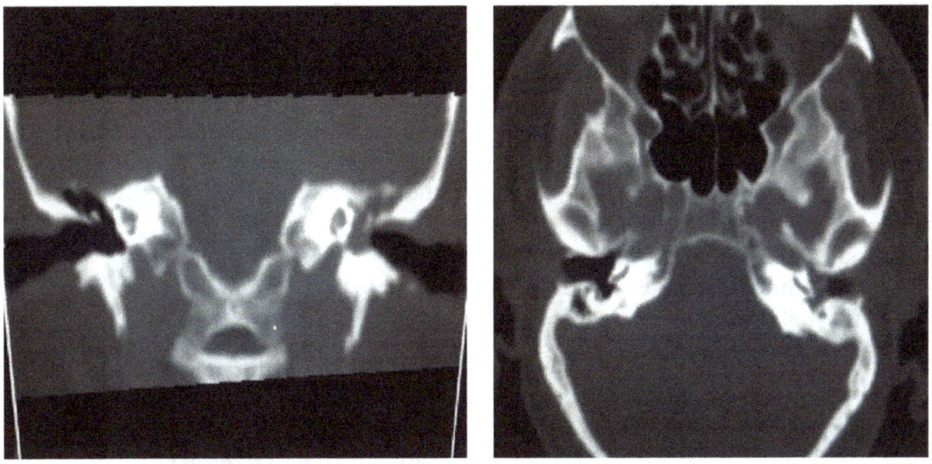

(a) (b)

FIGURE 1: CT scan of temporal bone showing features of tympanomastoiditis and soft tissue shadow involving the middle ear and attic areas. (a) Coronal. (b) Axial.

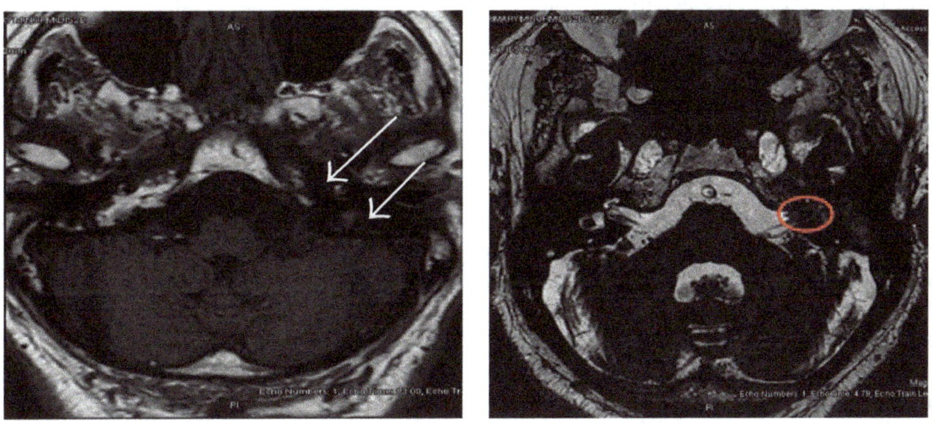

(a) (b)

FIGURE 2: (a) MRI with contrast showing asymmetrical signal changes in the bilateral petrous bone with reduced enhancement on the left with high suspicion of petrositis. (b) Contrast showing an enhancing lesion in the internal auditory meatus involving the 7th-8th nerve complex most likely acoustic neuroma (red circle).

2. Case Report

A 61-year-old man referred from the emergency department to the ear, nose, and throat (ENT) clinic in Al Wakra Hospital because of vertigo and left ear discharge. The vertigo is rotatory in nature and is associated with hearing impairment and tinnitus as well as nausea and vomiting. Ear discharge was purulent, odorless, and intermittent for the last few years, but it became profuse and continuous for the last few days. The described symptoms were associated with severe left-sided headache and diplopia, and there were associated medical comorbidities (diabetic and hypertensive patient). On examination, the patient was conscious, oriented, and not feverish. Left ear examination showed pulsating purulent discharge with granulation tissue filling the middle ear cavity, the tympanic membrane was perforated, and the fistula test was negative. There was left beating nystagmus with left sixth cranial nerve palsy. Other ENT and neurological examinations were not remarkable. Pure tone audiometry showed left-sided severe mixed deafness, and left ear swab for microbiological study for culture and sensitivity was negative. Urgent CT scan was done to rule out intracranial complications, and it showed features of tympanomastoiditis and soft tissue shadow involving the middle ear and attic areas (Figures 1(a) and 1(b)).

MRI with contrast showed asymmetrical signal changes in the bilateral petrous bone with reduced enhancement on the left with high suspicion of petrositis, in the context of chronic tympanomastoiditis (Figure 2(a)).

In addition to the mentioned pathology, there was a 10×4 mm enhancing lesion in the internal auditory meatus involving the 7th-8th nerve complex most likely acoustic neuroma, and there was no extension to the cerebellopontine angle (Figure 2(b)). Conservative treatment started with local and parenteral antimicrobial agents with labyrinthine sedative drugs. After ten-day treatment with good monitoring of blood sugar, the patient had satisfactory response and improvement regarding symptoms of ear discharge, vertigo, and diplopia, but there is no remarkable response regarding hearing loss and tinnitus. The patient continued on conservative treatment for the coming two months, he developed symptomatic response regarding vertigo, diplopia, and ear discharge, and further appointment given for exploration of mastoid and middle ear. Exploration of the mastoid and middle ear showed tympanomastoiditis with a lot of granulation tissue in the middle ear, mastoid, and attic; canal wall down procedure was done with successful result after postoperative follow-up.

3. Discussion

The prevalence of CSOM is estimated at 2.5–29.5% [8]. Complications of CSOM can cause grave morbidity and even mortality even though there are intratemporal and/or intracranial complications. Infectious ear diseases have become rarer with the advent of broad-spectrum antibiotics. Gradenigo's syndrome (GS) is an uncommon but life-threatening complication of otitis media. The typical presentation of GS comprises a sixth cranial nerve palsy, otorrhoea, headache, and pain along the distribution of the trigeminal nerve. In our patient, there were more than one complication of CSOM, and they were extracranial intratemporal, that is, petrositis and labyrinthitis. MRI and CT are required to identify the deep seated petrous apex as the site of the inflammatory process [9]. While CT scans may demonstrate opacification of the air cells of the petrous apex with cortical bone erosion, MRI is very useful for assessing inflammatory soft tissue lesions around the petrous apex [10]. Both CT and MRI are essential to establish opacification of air cells in the petrous apex under suspicion, as opposed to asymmetric pneumatization. In our patient, both the CT scan and MRI were done, but MRI was more helpful in the diagnosis of petrositis; otherwise, the labyrinthitis in both facilities would not show any remarkable findings. This is probably because there was circumscribe labyrinthitis, and there was no involvement of bony and membranous labyrinth. Cases of GS as a complication of acute otitis media have usually been successfully treated with broad-spectrum antibiotics, even in cases of petrous abscess formation [11]. In the treatment of chronic ear disease, most authors support surgical intervention as primary management to ensure adequate petrous and mastoid drainage [12, 13]. However, a case of successful conservative treatment of GS associated with chronic otitis media was reported with the use of antibiotic therapy [14, 15]. Our case involved GS and labyrinthitis as complications of chronic ear disease, in which symptoms and sign responded primarily, completely, and successfully to antibiotics therapy. However, the patient explored later on for tympanomastoiditis disease. Regarding the hearing loss and tinnitus, there was no remarkable response, and the explanation could be related to pressure due to pathology that cause an enhancing lesion in the internal auditory meatus involving the 7th-8th nerve complex most likely acoustic neuroma.

4. Conclusion

Although there is little evidence to support the use of medical therapy in the treatment of Gradenigo's syndrome resulting from chronic ear disease, we here demonstrate successful conservative treatment of Gradenigo's syndrome and labyrinthitis.

Consent

The patient's consent was obtained for the publication of the case report and the figures.

Conflicts of Interest

All authors declare no financial or personal relationships with other people or organizations.

References

[1] J. A. Smith and C. J. Danner, "Complications of chronic otitis media and cholesteatoma," *Otolaryngologic Clinics of North America*, vol. 39, no. 6, pp. 1237–1255, 2006.

[2] A. Ceylan, Y. Bayazit, M. Yilmaz et al., "Extracranial complications of chronic otitis media," *Journal of International Advanced Otology*, vol. 5, no. 1, pp. 51–55, 2009.

[3] J. Kangsanarak, S. Fooanant, K. Ruckphaopunt, N. Navacharoen, and S. Teotrakul, "Extracranial and intracranial complications of suppurative otitis media. report of 102 cases," *Journal of Laryngology and Otology*, vol. 107, pp. 999–1004, 1993.

[4] U. Osma, S. Cureoglu, and S. Hosoglu, "The complications of chronic otitis media: report of 93 cases," *Journal of Laryngology and Otology*, vol. 114, no. 2, pp. 97–100, 2000.

[5] M. B. Benito and B. P. Gorricho, "Acute mastoiditis: increase in the incidence and complications," *International Journal of Pediatric Otorhinolaryngology*, vol. 71, no. 7, pp. 1007–1011, 2007.

[6] G. Gradenigo, "Ueber die paralyse des Nervus abducens bei Otitis," *Archiv für Ohrenheilkunde*, vol. 774, no. 1, pp. 149–187, 1907.

[7] L. Gibier, V. Darrouzet, and V. Franco-Vidal, "Gradenigo syndrome without acute otitis media," *Pediatric Neurology*, vol. 41, no. 3, pp. 215–219, 2009.

[8] Philippine Society of Otolaryngology Head and Neck Surgery, Inc., *Clinical Practice Guidelines on Chronic Suppurative Otitis Media in Adults*, Philippine Society of Otolaryngology Head and Neck Surgery, Pasig City, Philippines, 2006.

[9] A. H. Yeung, "Skull base, petrous apex infections," 2006, http://www.emedicine.com/ent/byname/skull-base-petrous-apex-infection.htm.

[10] R. A. Chole and P. J. Donald, "Petrous apicitis, clinical considerations," *Annals of Otology, Rhinology, and Laryngology*, vol. 92, no. 6, pp. 544–551, 1983.

[11] M. brahim, G. Shah, and H. Parmar, "Diffusion-weighted MRI identifies petrous apex abscess in Gradenigo syndrome," *Journal of Neuro-Ophthalmology*, vol. 30, no. 1, pp. 34–36, 2010.

[12] R. Marianowski, S. Rocton, J. L. Ait-Amer, M. P. Morisseau-Durand, and Y. Manach, "Conservative management of

Gradenigo syndrome in a child," *International Journal of Pediatric Otorhinolaryngology*, vol. 57, no. 1, pp. 79–83, 2001.

[13] A. M. Minotti and S. E. Kountakis, "Management of abducens palsy in patients with petrositis," *Annals of Otology, Rhinology, and Laryngology*, vol. 108, no. 9, pp. 897–902, 1999.

[14] B. J. Burston, P. M. Pretorius, and J. D. Ramsden, "Gradenigo's syndrome: successful conservative treatment in adult and paediatric patients," *Journal of Laryngology and Otology*, vol. 119, no. 4, pp. 325–329, 2005.

[15] Y. Plodpai, S. Hirunpat, and W. Kiddee, "Gradenigo's syndrome secondary to chronic otitis media on a background of previous radical mastoidectomy: a case report," *Journal of Medical Case Reports*, vol. 8, no. 1, p. 217, 2014.

21

Two Cases of Cartilaginous Choristoma—Not Chondroma of the Bony External Auditory Canal

Kohei Yamahara[1] **Yuki Katsura,**[1] **Yuki Egawa,**[2] **Kana Lee,**[3] **and Satoshi Ikegami**[1]

[1]*Department of Otolaryngology, Head and Neck Surgery, Shizuoka City Shizuoka Hospital, Shizuoka City, Shizuoka 420-8630, Japan*
[2]*Department of Pathology, Shizuoka City Shizuoka Hospital, Shizuoka City, Shizuoka 420-8630, Japan*
[3]*Department of Otolaryngology, Shin-Suma General Hospital, Kobe, Hyogo 654-0048, Japan*

Correspondence should be addressed to Kohei Yamahara; k_yamahara@ent.kuhp.kyoto-u.ac.jp

Academic Editor: M. Tayyar Kalcioglu

The presence of a cartilaginous mass on the bony external auditory canal is an unusual finding. Currently, two different diagnoses have been used to describe this type of mass: chondroma and cartilaginous choristoma. There is currently no consensus on which diagnosis is appropriate for this type of lesion. Choristoma is defined as a tumor-like growth of normal tissue occurring in an abnormal location. Histological examination alone cannot be used to distinguish between cartilaginous choristoma and chondroma, as both lesions comprise normal mature hyaline cartilage. To diagnose a mass as cartilaginous choristoma on the bony external auditory canal, it is necessary to confirm that it does not originate from the underlying periosteum. Here, we present the cases of two patients with typical cartilaginous masses on the bony external auditory canal, in which the surgical findings showed that the masses were not in contact with the underlying periosteum, indicating that cartilaginous choristoma—not chondroma—is an appropriate diagnosis for these mass lesions. The clinical findings (characteristic appearance and location) reported here may aid clinicians in the diagnostic and surgical management of these cartilaginous masses.

1. Introduction

The presence of a cartilaginous mass on the bony external auditory canal (EAC) is an unusual finding, with as few as 53 cases reported in the literature [1–7]. Previously, authors referred to these masses as *chondromas* in their reports [1, 2, 4, 7]. However, in 2005, Lee proposed that these masses should be diagnosed as *cartilaginous choristomas* (CC) rather than chondromas [3]. Nevertheless, nearly all reports continue to refer to these lesions as chondromas [5, 6]; thus, there is currently no consensus regarding how to appropriately identify these masses. Choristoma is defined as a benign tumor-like growth of normal tissue occurring in an abnormal location [8, 9]. There have been numerous reports of various types of choristomas occurring within the head and neck. They include gastric mucosa in the tongue [10], salivary gland tissue in the middle ear [11], and osseous or cartilaginous masses in the intraoral soft tissues [9]. Histopathological examination alone cannot distinguish between CC and chondroma because both mass lesions are composed of normal mature hyaline cartilage. To diagnose a tissue mass as CC on the bony EAC, it is necessary to confirm that it does not originate from the bony EAC. In this report, we present the cases of two patients with typical cartilaginous masses on the bony EAC, in which the surgical findings showed that the masses were not in contact with the underlying periosteum of the bony EAC, indicating that CC is an appropriate diagnosis for these types of lesions.

2. Case Presentations

Here, we report the cases of one 73-year-old woman (Case 1) and one 55-year-old man (Case 2). Both patients did not have a history of swimming in cold water or taking saunas.

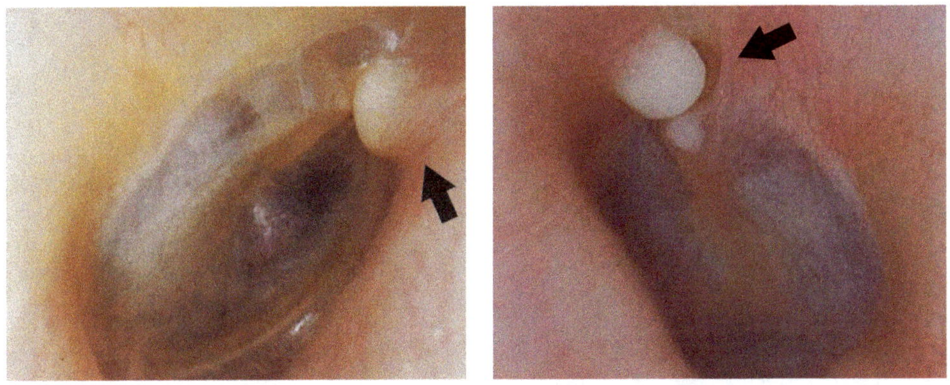

(a) (b)

Figure 1: Otoscopic view of the right ear in Case 1 (a), and the left ear in Case 2 (b). Masses were discovered at the medial portion of the anterior wall of the bony EAC just in front of the short process of the malleus. Arrows indicate the masses.

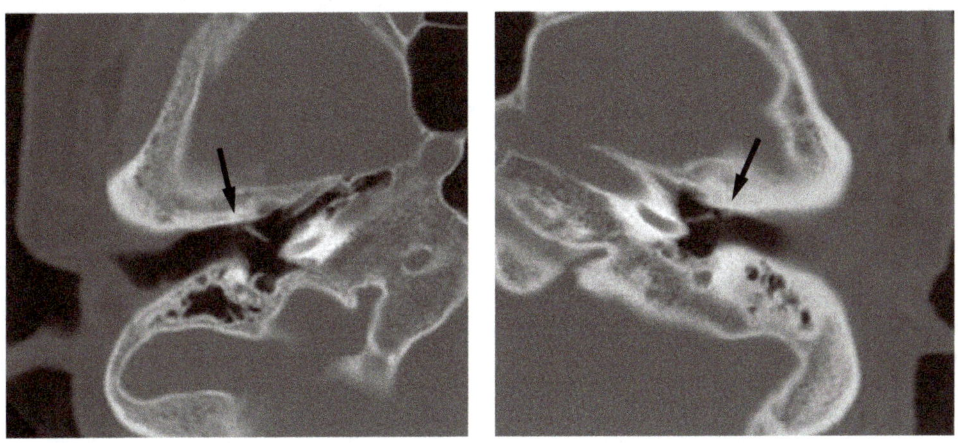

(a) (b)

Figure 2: CT images of the temporal bone in Case 1 (a) and Case 2 (b). CT imaging shows a lesion emanating from the anterior bony EAC in both cases. In each case, the EAC appears flat with well-defined boundaries. Arrows indicate the masses.

They each presented with a mass, discovered incidentally on routine examination, at the medial portion of the anterior wall of the bony EAC just in front of the short process of the malleus (Figures 1(a) and 1(b)). The mass was located in the right ear in Case 1 and in the left ear in Case 2; they did not touch the tympanic membranes, which were found to be normal in both patients. These masses were about 2 mm in diameter and were noted to be firm and white, somewhat mobile, and covered with normal appearing epithelium. Palpation using a Rosen needle revealed that these lesions were firm and nontender, suggesting that they were osseous or cartilaginous masses instead of soft tumors (i.e., cholesteatoma, keratoma, etc.). A CT scan of the temporal bone revealed a lesion emanating from the anterior bony EAC in both cases (Figures 2(a) and 2(b)). Additionally, CT imaging showed that the bony EAC was flat and had well-defined boundaries, suggesting that it had not been invaded. Although both patients were asymptomatic and the masses did not show any enlargement in size during the follow-up period (ranging from 3 to 4 years), both patients wanted the masses removed, and they were excised via the transcanal approach using a Rosen needle. The masses were located between the squamous epithelium and periosteum of the bony EAC, and they separated very easily—again indicating that masses were not in contact with the periosteum. On gross examination, the excised masses appeared round with a smooth surface (Figure 3(a)). After the masses were removed, the periosteum of the bony EAC just beneath the surgical site was found to be normal in both cases. The operation was completed without curettement of the underlying periosteum or bone cortex. Pathologic examination demonstrated that the excised masses consisted of mature hyaline cartilage formed by normal chondrocytes (Figure 3(b)). Based on information from the intraoperative report, the pathologist was informed that the masses did not arise from the periosteum, though they were on the surface of the bony EAC. Thus, based on these histological and intraoperative findings, we obtained the diagnosis of CC on the bony EAC—not chondroma. The postoperative courses of both patients were uneventful, and no recurrences were

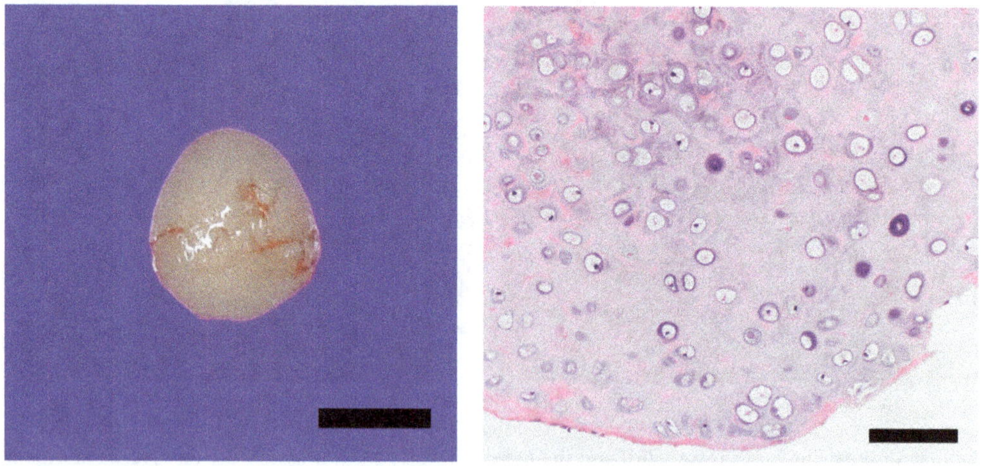

(a) (b)

Figure 3: Gross and pathologic examination of the excised mass of Case 2. (a) The masses appear round with a smooth surface (bar represents 1 mm). (b) Pathologic examination shows the excised masses comprising mature hyaline cartilage formed by normal chondrocytes (bar represents 100 μm).

found during follow-up at 1 to 2 years postoperatively. Both patients described here provided written informed consent for the publication of this case report.

3. Discussion

Only 53 cases of a cartilaginous mass on the bony EAC have been documented in the literature [1–7]. However, with heightened awareness, an increasing number of such lesions were detected in our hospital, suggesting that this lesion is not as rare as previously thought. All but two of these reports have described patients of Asian ethnicity. Additionally, there appears to be an equal distribution between male and female patients, with an average age of 31.5 years at the time of diagnosis [5]. These lesions typically present as a single, white, hard, and round mass with a smooth surface and a diameter of 2 mm; moreover, they frequently occur in the medial portion of the anterior wall of the bony EAC, just in front of the short process and handle of the malleus. Although these masses may meet the criteria for CC, they are still frequently described as chondromas in the literature [5, 6]. In this report, we assessed the clinical and histological features of two consecutive cases of such lesions and confirmed the diagnoses these masses as CC—as suggested by Lee.

Chondromas can be classified into several types, depending on the sites in which they originate. When a cartilaginous mass is found at the surface of the bony EAC, just as in our cases, "periosteal" chondroma is considered in the differential diagnosis of CC [3]. Periosteal chondroma is a benign hyaline cartilage neoplasm of the bone surface that arises from the periosteum [12] and has the potential to grow [13]. Initially, this lesion is small and is located on the surface of the bone. As it enlarges, it erodes the underlying cortex, and in some cases, the periosteal chondroma can reach a diameter of 6 cm [13]. Because both the periosteal chondroma and CC consist of mature hyaline cartilage formed by normal chondrocytes, they cannot be distinguished based on pathological examination alone. Thus, intraoperative findings are essential for distinguishing between the two diagnoses; the underlying periosteum and cortex should be eroded in cases of periosteal chondroma [14], whereas the periosteum and cortex should be normal in cases of CC [3]. In the cases reported here, the masses did not appear to be in contact with the underlying periosteum, and there was no evidence of erosion in the periosteum of the bony EAC just beneath the masses, indicating that they did not originate from the periosteum. These findings led us to conclude that these masses were CC and not periosteal chondroma, a diagnosis which has been frequently reported in studies of cartilaginous masses of the bony EAC [1, 2, 4–7]. However, these reports also described that these masses were removed very easily with a pick, needle, or curette, just as in our cases, further suggesting that they may have been CCs rather than periosteum chondromas. On the other hand, there is only one report describing the case of a chondroma that involved the bone cortex of the bony EAC, and it was accompanied by facial nerve paralysis [7]. Considering the bony involvement of the mass, we can assume that the diagnosis of chondroma for that case was appropriate. Thus, chondromas arising from EAC may be far rarer than previously thought. The ability to distinguish between CC and periosteum chondroma, preoperatively or intraoperatively, is important. It is not only a matter of terminology, but the diagnosis also determines the extent of mass excision; in cases of CC, successful treatment is obtained by simple excision of the lesion, whereas in cases of periosteum chondroma, complete excision of lesion with curettement of the underlying bone is required to avoid recurrence. Because CC is not a well-known lesion and there are no histological differences between CC and chondroma, pathologists frequently diagnose the cartilaginous masses on the bony EAC as simple chondromas if they are not provided with any additional clinical or intraoperative information. Therefore, to obtain a more accurate pathological diagnosis, surgeons should provide information to the pathologist concerning whether the masses were in contact with the periosteum or whether the underlying periosteum was eroded.

The pathogenesis of CC is thought to be due to the migration of embryological cartilage cells [3]. It is speculated that the mass develops from heterotopic cartilaginous embryonic rests of Meckel's or Reichert's cartilage of the first or second branchial arch. The cartilage precursor cells mistakenly migrate into the primitive external ear canal during invagination of the first pharyngeal cleft and grow deep in the ear canal. However, their true origin remains unclear.

When the lesion occurs at the typical site (i.e., the medial portion of the anterior wall of the bony EAC), the differential diagnosis can be narrowed by first categorizing the lesion into two groups: soft mass (cholesteatoma, keratoma, etc.) or firm mass (CC, chondroma, chondrosarcoma, etc.). This step could be easily achieved by palpation of the mass using a tool, such as a Rosen needle. If the lesion is found to be a firm mass, a CT scan could be useful in distinguishing between CC, periosteum chondroma, and a malignant tumor; the characteristic radiographic feature of periosteum chondroma is erosion of the underlying cortex [14]. In both cases described in this report, a CT scan showed no apparent erosion of the cortex, suggesting the possibility of CC. However, sometimes CT imaging cannot clearly detect these masses, as they are usually very small. Additionally, if the mass is in the early stages of periosteum chondroma formation, the cortex may not yet be eroded, making it nearly impossible for a CT scan to distinguish between CC and periosteal chondroma based on this characteristic.

In the literature, the majority of reported CCs on the bony EAC were removed surgically; however, several authors have described that CCs have low growth potential and have not been reported to undergo malignant transformation. In consideration of this, observation is an appropriate strategy. Nonetheless, one study reported that a single CC enlarged in size and touched the tympanic membrane, resulting in conductive hearing loss [4]. Furthermore, it is very difficult to distinguish between CC and periosteal chondroma, preoperatively. Thus, watchful observation is needed, even in asymptomatic patients.

4. Conclusion

In this case study, the cartilaginous masses on the bony EAC were appropriately diagnosed as CC and not chondromas. Preoperative examination, which included palpation and CT imaging, and intraoperative findings were useful in obtaining a proper pathological diagnosis for these lesions.

Acknowledgments

We would like to thank Shinya Hori for his excellent scientific advice and Editage (http://www.editage.jp) for English language editing.

References

[1] H. Kobayashi, A. Suzuki, and Y. Nomura, "Chondroma of the external ear canal," *Otology Japan*, vol. 5, no. 2, pp. 127–131, 1995.

[2] I. J. Johnson, M. H. Tadpatrikar, and J. F. Sharp, "Chondroma of the external auditory canal," *Journal of Laryngology and Otology*, vol. 112, no. 3, pp. 278-279, 1998.

[3] F.-P. Lee, "Cartilaginous choristoma of the bony external auditory canal: a study of 36 cases," *Otolaryngology-Head and Neck Surgery*, vol. 133, no. 5, pp. 786–790, 2016.

[4] K. Gyo, S. Kawakita, J. Kobayashi, N. Hakuba, and S. Matsumoto, "Chondroma of the bony external auditory canal attached to the short process of the malleus," *International Journal of Pediatric Otorhinolaryngology*, vol. 68, no. 11, pp. 1441–1444, 2004.

[5] T. Tanigawa, S. Inafuku, and M. Nakayama, "Five cases of chondroma involving the external auditory canal," *Auris Nasus Larynx*, vol. 35, no. 4, pp. 559–561, 2008.

[6] C. R. Graves and M. C. Thorne, "A case of external auditory canal chondroma," *International Journal of Pediatric Otorhinolaryngology Extra*, vol. 8, no. 4, pp. 147-148, 2013.

[7] M. Nagaba, Y. Koike, and F. Hishinuma, "Facial nerve involvement in chondroma of the externalauditory meatus," *Otolaryngology*, vol. 46, no. 3, pp. 199–204, 1974.

[8] S. M. Sheridan, "Osseous choristoma: a report of two gases," *British Journal of Oral and Maxillofacial Surgery*, vol. 22, no. 2, pp. 99–102, 1984.

[9] R. K. Wesley and R. J. Zielinski, "Osteocartilaginous choristoma of the tongue: clinical and histopathologic considerations," *Journal of Oral Surgery*, vol. 36, no. 1, pp. 59–61, 1978.

[10] M. J. Ortiz, J. T. Fay, and G. T. Weir, "Heterotopic gastric mucosa of the tongue," *Journal of Oral and Maxillofacial Surgery*, vol. 40, no. 10, pp. 667–670, 1982.

[11] P. J. Moore, B. N. P. Benjamin, and A. E. Kan, "Salivary gland choristoma of the middle ear," *International Journal of Pediatric Otorhinolaryngology*, vol. 8, no. 1, pp. 91–95, 1984.

[12] D. R. Lucas and J. A. Bridge, "Chondromas: enchondroma, periosteal chondroma, and enchondromatosis," in *World Health Organization Classification of Tumours: Pathology and Genetics of Tumours of Soft Tissue and Bone*, C. D. M. Fletcher, K. K. Unni, and F. Mertens, Eds., pp. 237–240, IARC Press, Lyon, France, 2002.

[13] A. Greenspan and W. Remagen, "Tumors of cartilaginous origin," in *Differential Diagnosis of Tumors and Tumor-like Lesions of Bones and Joints*, A. Greenspan and W. Remagen, pp. 123–133, Lippincott-Raven Publishers, Philadelphia, NY, USA, 1st edition, 1997.

[14] S. Kirchner, H. Pavlov, R. Heller, and J. Kaye, "Periosteal chondromas of the anterior tibial tubercle: two cases," *American Journal of Roentgenology*, vol. 131, no. 6, pp. 1088-1089, 1978.

22

An Unusual Case of Pinna Squamous Cell Carcinoma Arising Shortly after Resection of Atypical Fibroxanthoma

Eugene Omakobia,[1] **Ahmad Orabi**,[1] **and Richard Knights**[2]

[1]*Department of ENT, Calderdale Royal Hospital, Halifax, UK*
[2]*Department of Histopathology, Calderdale Royal Hospital, Halifax, UK*

Correspondence should be addressed to Eugene Omakobia; eugeneomakobia@doctors.org.uk

Academic Editor: Abrão Rapoport

Objective. To report a unique case of pinna squamous cell carcinoma (SCC) arising shortly after resection of atypical fibroxanthoma (AFX) at the same site. *Case report.* An 81-year-old gentleman presented with a nodular right pinna lesion. This was excised, and histology confirmed AFX. Ten weeks later, an ulcerative lesion appeared at the resection site. This was confirmed to be SCC. Comparative analysis revealed no morphological resemblance between the initial AFX and new SCC lesion, and there was no evidence of initial misdiagnosis. *Conclusion.* SCC is the most common cancer involving the pinna. Whilst prolonged sun exposure is an important risk factor for SCC, chronic inflammation and wounds are other potential sources. We postulate whether SCC could have arisen from the previous scar tissue in a manner similar to Marjolin's ulcer. This would be a highly unusual finding in the pinna and to our knowledge unprecedented in the English literature.

1. Introduction

Atypical fibroxanthoma (AFX) is a rare, superficial fibrohistiocytic skin tumour composed predominantly of fusiform, epithelioid, spindle, and pleomorphic cells [1]. It is usually regarded as a benign tumour associated with a good prognosis, but rarely, recurrence and metastasis can occur [2]. It has been suggested that tumours with adverse histological features or extension into subcutaneous fat have a low-to-intermediate malignant potential and should be reclassified as pleomorphic dermal sarcomas rather than AFX [3]. AFX classically presents as a solitary ulcerated nodule on the sun-damaged areas of the head and neck of elderly adults. The pathological differential diagnosis includes pleomorphic dermal sarcoma, spindle cell squamous cell carcinoma, malignant melanoma, and leiomyosarcoma [4].

Poorly differentiated spindle cell neoplasms pose a diagnostic challenge to histopathologists because of a lack of specific morphologic features on standard histopathology. Further characterisation with immunohistochemical studies is always required [5]. AFX can be a particularly difficult diagnosis to make as there are no common guidelines for diagnosis and management [3]. We present a unique case of moderately differentiated squamous cell carcinoma (SCC) arising at the resection site of an AFX of the right pinna. To our knowledge, this is the first reported case of this type in the English literature.

2. Case Report

An 81-year-old gentleman presented to our ENT department with a two-year-history of a nodular right pinna lesion. There had been no recent increase in size. The patient reported that the lesion had actually decreased in size over the past two months with the use of topical steroids and fusidic acid.

His past medical history included hypertension, transient ischaemic attack, and prostate malignancy treated with transurethral resection. He also wore bilateral hearing aids for presbyacusis. His regular medications included clopidogrel, simvastatin, and antihypertensives. There was no family history of head and neck malignancy. He was a retired police officer with no history of excessive sun exposure. He was an ex-smoker having stopped smoking 40 years ago and a teetotaller.

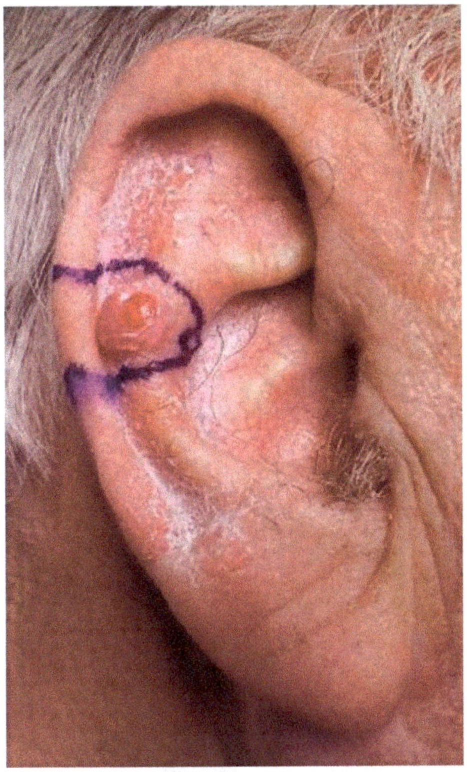

FIGURE 1: Clinical photograph showing a one-centimetre nodular lesion on the right upper pinna.

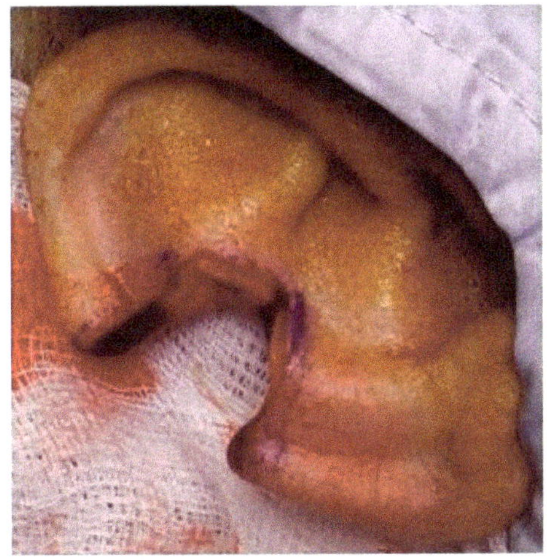

FIGURE 2: Clinical photograph showing appearance of the right upper pinna following wedge excision of the initial one-centimetre nodular lesion with 4-millimetre resection margins.

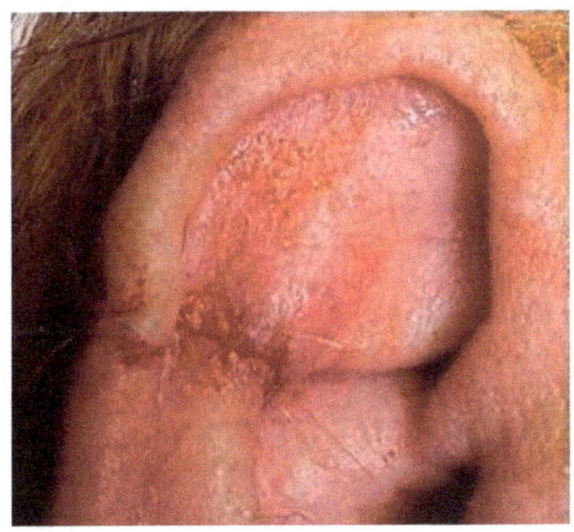

FIGURE 3: Clinical photograph showing right pinna after wedge excision of the initial nodular lesion and primary wound closure.

On examination, he was skin type II on the Fitzpatrick scale. There was a one-centimetre nodular lesion on the right upper pinna (Figure 1). There was no evidence of ulceration or associated cervical lymphadenopathy, and no other skin lesions were noted. The lesion was not tender to palpation, but there was a history of contact bleeding after irritation from his hearing aid.

Two weeks after initial presentation, a wedge excision of the lesion was performed under local anaesthesia with 4-millimetre resection margins (Figures 2 and 3). Histological analysis revealed a dermal spindle cell lesion exhibiting marked pleomorphism and brisk mitoses (Figure 4). Immunohistochemically, the lesion showed focal staining with CD68. Other markers (AE1AE3, S100, HMB45, SMA, and CD31/34) were negative. Morphologically and immunohistochemically, the features were consistent with atypical fibroxanthoma. The closest resection margin was found to be 3 millimetres located superiorly. Resected sleeves of cartilage at the inferior and superior margins were found to be free of disease.

One month later, a small fluctuant lesion was noted at the surgical wound site laterally. This was felt to be a small stitch abscess, but needle aspiration yielded no fluid. A decision was made to simply observe this, and the patient was brought back for review six weeks later. At this time, a one-centimetre raised, ulcerative, crusted lesion was seen at the upper margin of the incision site (Figure 5). Three-millimetre punch biopsies were taken which were subsequently discussed at the skin multidisciplinary team (MDT) meeting. The histological analysis showed full-thickness infiltration by a well-differentiated keratinising squamous cell carcinoma (Figure 6). There were no lymphovascular space permeation and no associated squamous hyperplasia. Remarkably, when this tumour was compared to the previous lesion (atypical fibroxanthoma), no morphological resemblance was seen. Immunohistochemistry of the biopsy confirmed squamous cell carcinoma (positive with AE1AE3 and p63 and negative with CD10).

The recommendation from the skin MDT (multidisciplinary team) was for wide excision and full-thickness skin grafting. This was performed three weeks later with 5-millimetre resection margins. The underlying cartilage was also excised, and a local full-thickness skin graft was raised from the right neck level II region to cover the skin defect (Figure 7). Subsequent histological and immunohistochemical analyses confirmed moderately differentiated squamous cell carcinoma with no invasion of the underlying cartilage or subcutaneous fat. There was no perineural or lymphovascular invasion, and the lesion was 4.5 millimetres thick (Figures 8 and 9(a)–9(c)). The margins were deemed

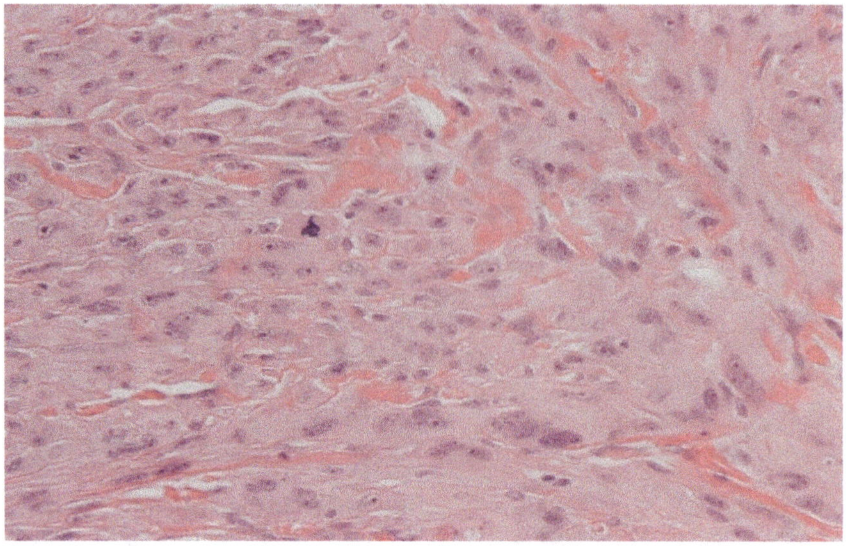

(a)

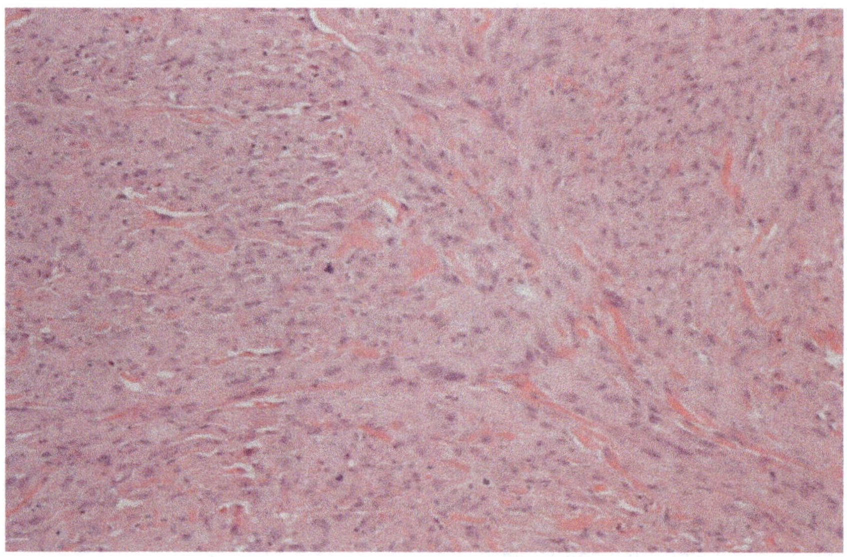

(b)

FIGURE 4: Photomicrograph of excised nodular lesion (H&E stain) showing a dermal spindle cell lesion exhibiting marked pleomorphism and brisk mitoses. Immunohistochemically, focal staining with CD68 was seen. Morphologically and immunohistochemically, the features are consistent with AFX. (a) ×40 magnification. (b) ×20 magnification.

acceptable following further discussion at the skin MDT meeting, and an ultrasound scan of the neck was organised, which showed normal cervical lymph nodes. To date, no local or regional recurrence has been noted at his most recent 4-month follow-up, and the wound has healed well with successful grafting (Figure 10).

3. Discussion

We have reported an unusual case of moderately differentiated pinna SCC arising at the resection site of AFX. This is unprecedented in the world literature. We conducted a literature search to gain further insight into how this may have arisen.

It is widely reported that diagnostic difficulties can exist particularly in the distinction between poorly differentiated cutaneous spindle cell squamous cell carcinoma (scSCC) and AFX [3, 5, 6]. This is due to the fact that AFX is generally accepted as a diagnosis of exclusion based on negativity for a broad panel of immunohistochemical markers, including multiple cytokeratins and melanocytic, muscle, and vascular markers [6]. A recent review article has suggested that the most important immunomarkers for differential diagnoses are cytokeratins (to exclude sarcomatoid or spindle cell SCC), S-100 and melanogenesis markers (to exclude melanoma), and desmin, actin, and H-caldesmon (to exclude leiomyosarcoma) [3]. As cytokeratins can also be occasionally lost in scSCC, this can pose diagnostic challenges. However, in our reported case, the second tumour was a moderately differentiated squamous cell carcinoma, which was not of the spindle cell variant, thereby reducing

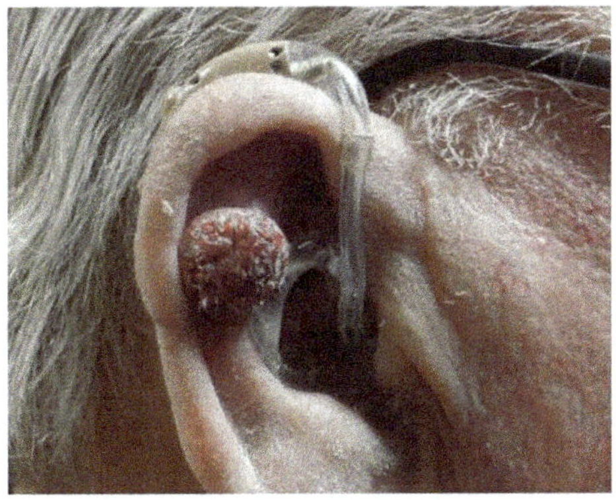

FIGURE 5: Clinical photograph showing the right pinna with a one-centimetre raised, ulcerative, crusted lesion at the upper margin of the previous incision site.

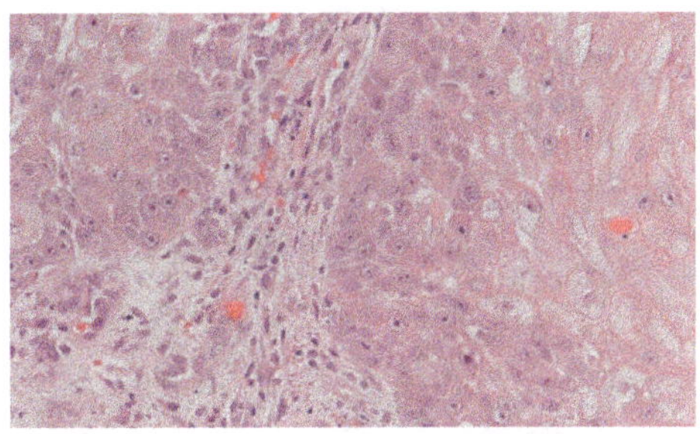

(a)

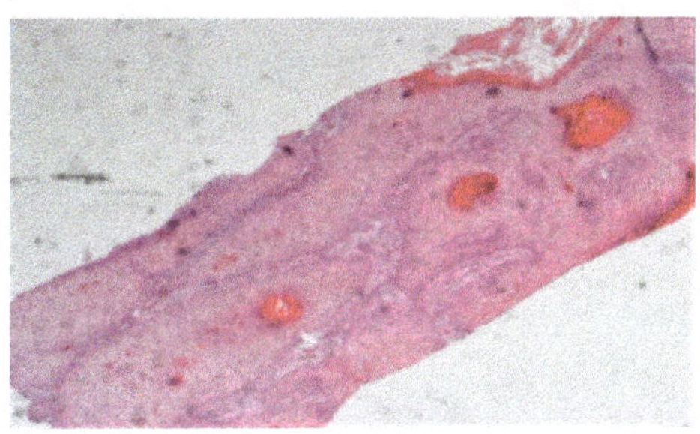

(b)

FIGURE 6: Photomicrograph of punch biopsy from the second ulcerative lesion (H&E stain). This demonstrates full-thickness infiltration by a well-differentiated keratinising SCC. (a) ×20 magnification. (b) ×2.5 magnification.

diagnostic uncertainty. Moreover, when the subsequently occurring SCC was compared to the previous AFX lesion, no morphological resemblance was seen.

In cases of poorly differentiated or spindle cell variants of invasive SCC, immunohistochemical studies for p63 are widely regarded as useful in confirming squamous differentiation, with particular utility in the diagnostic differentiation from AFX and melanoma [7, 8]. Hence, p63 is a useful addition to the standard immunohistochemical panel for cutaneous spindle cell neoplasms. Strong expression of p63 suggests scSCC and argues against the diagnosis of AFX.

AFX is usually a low-risk tumour, but as stated, care must be taken in diagnosis with exclusion of the more aggressive scSCC using immunohistochemical studies. We considered that a misdiagnosis of AFX which has been previously reported [5] may have been related to the subsequent development of SCC. However, in our reported case, the SCC was moderately differentiated and not of a spindle cell pattern. Comparative analysis revealed no similarities between the initial AFX and the new SCC lesion. Initial misdiagnosis is therefore highly unlikely. The case reiterates the importance of always considering a recurrent or new primary tumour at surgical resection sites.

Another factor to be considered is the possibility of metachronous (consecutive) development of AFX and SCC at the same site. This is plausible since UV radiation is known to be the major causative factor for cutaneous SCC, and both clinical and molecular data suggest that UV radiation is also a triggering factor for AFX [4].

We further speculated on whether the SCC arose from the previous scar tissue in a similar fashion to Marjolin's ulcer. Marjolin's ulcer classically occurs following previous trauma to tissue such as chronic inflammation, burns, or within any form of scar tissue, including postsurgical scars. It

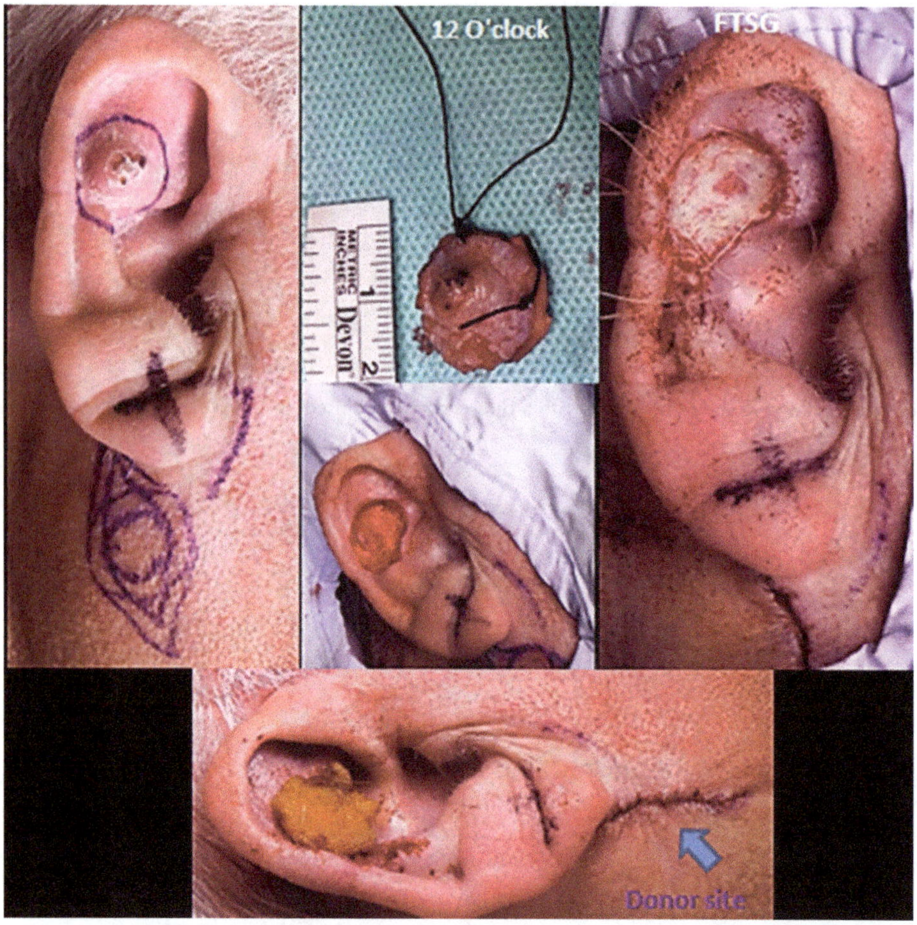

Figure 7: Clinical photographs showing wide excision (with 5-millimetre resection margins) of the right pinna ulcerative, crusted lesion and full-thickness skin grafting (FTSG). The underlying cartilage has also been excised, and a local full-thickness skin graft was raised from the right level II region to cover the skin defect. Primary closure of the donor site is also illustrated in the lower image.

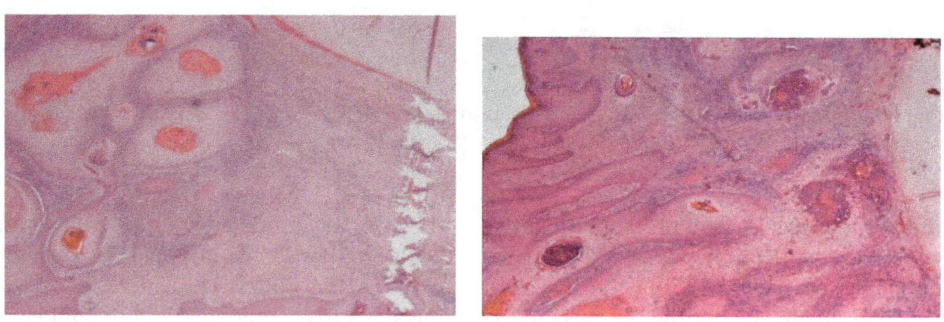

(a) (b)

Figure 8: Photomicrograph of excised ulcerative, crusted lesion (H&E stain). This demonstrates moderately differentiated SCC. (a) ×10 magnification. (b) ×2.5 magnification.

tends to be a more aggressive form of SCC which is usually well differentiated when biopsied [9]. There is commonly a delay between the initial tissue insult and the development of malignancy. This time period has been defined as latency and ranges between 11 and 75 years [10]. However, there have been reports of "acute" Marjolin's ulcer occurring after months or even weeks [11]. Marjolin's ulcer is not an uncommon finding in the lower limbs but is vanishingly rare in the head and neck site. Indeed, there is only one similar report in the literature of Marjolin's ulcer occurring in the postauricular region nine months after cortical mastoidectomy [11]. However, there are no reports of this pathology occurring in the pinna; hence, this would be a novel case. In the reported case, there was a short 10-week latency period after the initial surgery, making Marjolin's ulcer unlikely but not impossible. Due to the more aggressive nature of these

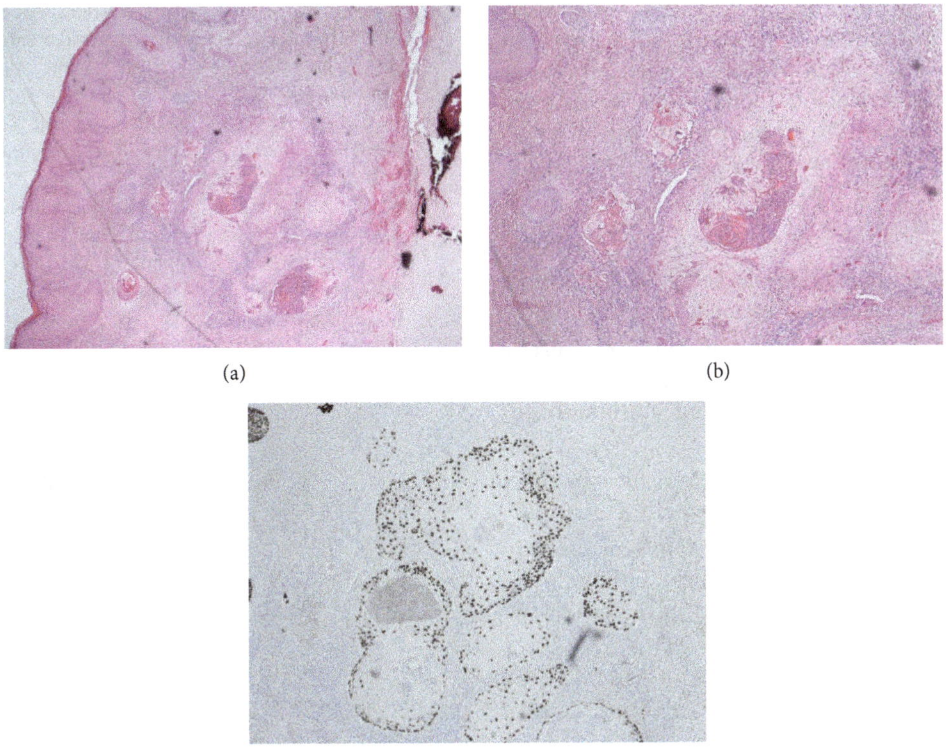

(a) (b) (c)

Figure 9: (a) Photomicrograph of wide locally excised ulcerative, crusted lesion (H&E stain) at ×2 magnification. Nests of squamous cell carcinoma are seen infiltrating the dermal tissue without involvement of the underlying cartilage (cartilage is seen in the right-hand field). (b) ×4 magnification of the same area; this demonstrates infiltrating nests of keratinising squamous cell carcinoma associated with a host inflammatory response. (c) p63 immunohistochemistry confirms the squamous phenotype of the tumour (nuclear positivity).

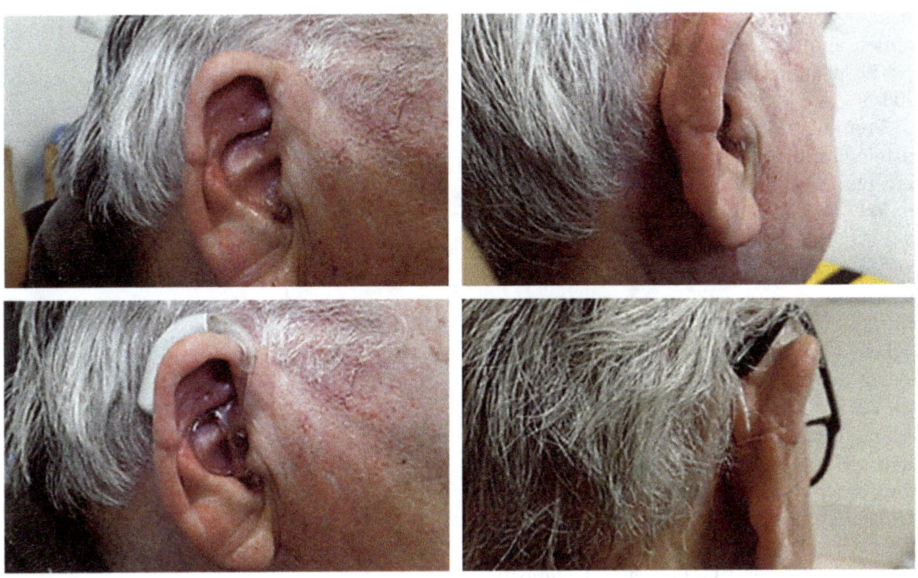

Figure 10: Clinical photographs showing the right pinna appearance at the most recent 4-month follow-up. The wound has healed well with successful grafting. The patient is comfortably able to wear his hearing aids and spectacles.

tumours, it is imperative to monitor Marjolin's ulcers for metastasis and recurrence. This is an important management consideration, and as in our case report, we would advocate the inclusion of baseline neck ultrasonography to assess cervical lymph nodes for involvement.

4. Conclusion

The finding of pinna SCC arising shortly after resection of AFX is extremely rare and, to our knowledge, unprecedented in the world literature. This finding does not appear to be related to an initial misdiagnosis of AFX. It is conceivable that the SCC could represent a metachronous tumour or a form of Marjolin's ulcer. Whilst this has been previously reported in the postauricular region, it has never been documented at the site of the pinna, making this a highly intriguing clinical presentation.

Additional Points

(i) Poorly differentiated spindle cell neoplasms pose a diagnostic challenge to histopathologists.

(ii) AFX is usually a low-risk tumour, but care must be taken in diagnosis with exclusion of the more aggressive spindle cell SCC using immunohistochemical studies.

(iii) It is crucial to consider a recurrent or new primary tumour at surgical resection sites.

(iv) SCC could have arisen from previous scar tissue in a similar fashion to Marjolin's ulcer, although this has not been previously reported in the pinna.

(v) Due to the more aggressive nature of these tumours, we would advocate the inclusion of baseline neck ultrasonography to assess cervical lymph nodal involvement.

References

[1] C. M. Nguyen, K. Chong, and D. Cassarino, "Clear cell atypical fibroxanthoma: a case report and review of the literature," *Journal of Cutaneous Pathology*, vol. 43, no. 6, pp. 538–542, 2016.

[2] M. Koch, A. Dimmler, and C. Alexiou, "Recurrent and metastasizing atypical fibroxanthoma," *HNO*, vol. 56, no. 10, pp. 1046–1051, 2008.

[3] M. Koch, A. J. Freundl, A. Agaimy et al., "Atypical fibroxanthoma–histological diagnosis, immunohistochemical markers and concepts of therapy," *Anticancer Research*, vol. 35, no. 11, pp. 5717–5735, 2015.

[4] M. R. A. Hussein, "Atypical fibroxanthoma: new insights," *Expert Review of Anticancer Therapy*, vol. 14, no. 9, pp. 1075–1088, 2014.

[5] A. Benoit, J. Wisell, and M. Brown, "Cutaneous spindle cell carcinoma misdiagnosed as atypical fibroxanthoma based on immunohistochemical stains," *JAAD Case Reports*, vol. 1, no. 6, pp. 392–394, 2015.

[6] S. A. Henderson, C. A. Torres-Cabala, J. L. Curry et al., "p40 is more specific than p63 for the distinction of atypical fibroxanthoma from other cutaneous spindle cell malignancies," *American Journal of Surgical Pathology*, vol. 38, no. 8, pp. 1102–1110, 2014.

[7] L. A. Compton, G. F. Murphy, and C. G. Lian, "Diagnostic immunohistochemistry in cutaneous neoplasia: an update," *Dermatopathology*, vol. 2, no. 1, pp. 15–42, 2015.

[8] B. C. Gleason, K. B. Calder, T. L. Cibull et al., "Utility of p63 in the differential diagnosis of atypical fibroxanthoma and spindle cell squamous cell carcinoma," *Journal of Cutaneous Pathology*, vol. 36, no. 5, pp. 543–547, 2009.

[9] B. Pekarek, S. Buck, and L. Osher, "A comprehensive review on Marjolin's ulcers: diagnosis and treatment," *Journal of the American College of Certified Wound Specialists*, vol. 3, no. 3, pp. 60–64, 2011.

[10] E. Copcu, A. Aktas, N. Sisman, and Y. Oztan, "Thirty-one cases of Marjolin's ulcer," *Clinical and Experimental Dermatology*, vol. 28, no. 2, pp. 138–141, 2003.

[11] K. A. Alhysoni, S. M. Bukhari, and M. F. Hajjaj, "Acute Marjolin's ulcer in a postauricular scar after mastoidectomy," *Case Reports in Otolaryngology*, vol. 2016, Article ID 2046954, 5 pages, 2016.

23

Primary Hyperparathyroidism due to Parathyroid Adenoma Originated from Supernumerary Gland

Fernando Mendoza-Moreno,[1] Ángel Rodriguez-Pascual,[1] María Rocío Díez-Gago,[2] Marina Pérez-González,[1] Laura Jiménez-Alvárez,[1] Isabel Furtado-Lobo,[1] Manuel Díez-Alonso,[1] and Fernando Noguerales-Fraguas[1]

[1]*Department of General and Digestive Surgery, Príncipe de Asturias Teaching Hospital, Alcalá de Henares, Madrid, Spain*
[2]*Department of Emergency Medicine, Príncipe de Asturias Teaching Hospital, Alcalá de Henares, Madrid, Spain*

Correspondence should be addressed to Fernando Mendoza-Moreno; khoril@hotmail.com

Academic Editor: Kyung Tae

Introduction. The variability of the location of the parathyroid glands is directly related to the events that occur during embryonic development. The impact that an individual submits more than four parathyroid glands is close to 13%. However the presentation of a parathyroid adenoma in a supernumerary gland is an uncommon event. *Case report.* A 30-year-old man diagnosed with primary hyperparathyroidism with matching findings on ultrasonography and scintigraphy for parathyroid adenoma localization lower left regarding the thyroid gland. A cervicotomy explorer showed four orthotopic parathyroid glands. The biopsy of the inferior left gland was normal. No signs of adenoma were seen in the biopsy. Following mobilization of the ipsilateral thyroid lobe, fifth parathyroid gland was found increased significantly in size than proceeded to remove, confirming the diagnosis of adenoma. After the excision, the levels of serum calcium and parathyroid hormone were normalized. *Conclusions.* The presentation of a parathyroid adenoma in a supernumerary gland is a challenge for the surgeon. The high sensitivity having different imaging techniques has been a key to locate preoperatively the pathological parathyroid gland. Analytical or clinical persistence of primary hyperparathyroidism after parathyroid surgery can occur if the location of the adenoma is a supernumerary or ectopic gland location.

1. Introduction

Primary hyperparathyroidism (pHPT) is the most frequent cause of increased serum calcium levels. The main cells of the parathyroid glands are responsible for secreting the parathormone (pHPT) which is involved in the reabsorption of calcium at the level of the distal tubule of the nephron, stimulating osteoclasts to promote bone resorption and catalyze the conversion of vitamin D3 in its active form [1].

The incidence of pHPT is 4 inhabitants per 1,000. It is twice as frequent as in postmenopausal women and in the fifth decade of life [2]. It is the most frequent cause of hypercalcemia. Among the etiology of pHPT, the parathyroid adenoma is the most frequent cause (80%) followed by other pathologies such as endocrine disorders of multiple neoplasia (MEN 1 and MEN 2A), hyperplasia of the parathyroid glands, or even carcinoma (1%) [3].

We present the case of a 30-year-old male with a history of primary hyperparathyroidism originated in a supernumerary parathyroid gland of ectopic location.

2. Case Report

A total of 376 patients diagnosed with pHPT were operated on in our service from January 2000 to December 2013.

We present the case of a 30-year-old male patient who referred to our clinic with the diagnosis of primary hyperparathyroidism. The patient had a history of stage IV-B non-Hodgkin lymphoma diagnosed in 2005 and treated with radiochemotherapy, currently in remission. Our patient presented with polydipsia and polyuria without associated bone pain. The laboratory tests showed a serum calcium of 12.7 mg/dl (laboratory range 8.7–10.4 mg/dl), phosphorus 2.4 mg/dl (2.4–5.1 mg/dl), hormone intact parathyroid (PTH) 216 pg/ml (11–80 pg/ml), 25-hydroxyvitamin D 23 ng/ml (30–100 ng/ml), alkaline phosphatase 102 U/l (45–129 U/l), 980 mg calciuria in 24 hours, and preserved renal function. Cervical ultrasound performed preoperatively showed a hyperechogenic nodule of 9 mm adjacent to the left lower thyroid pole. A scintigraphy with Tc99m sestamibi (MIBI) was performed in which a pathological hypercaptation was observed at the level of the left inferior thyroid.

In view of these findings, the patient underwent an exploratory cervicotomy using a classic Kocher incision. During surgery, a normal-appearing thyroid parenchyma without nodules was observed. A slightly enlarged left lower parathyroid gland that was excised under the suspicion that adenoma was evidenced. The left superior gland was of normal appearance and macroscopic characteristics although a biopsy was performed. The intraoperative PTH levels did not decrease (PTH at the beginning of the surgery of 333 pg/ml, PTH after 20 minutes of its extraction of 366 pg/ml). The intraoperative result of both biopsies was of parathyroid tissue without histological alterations. It was decided to explore the right side finding, an upper and lower gland of normal macroscopic appearance and orthotopic localization. The left inferior thyroid lobe was mobilized, finding an extracapsular supernumerary gland adjacent to the common carotid artery with a maximum diameter of 15 mm that was excised (Figure 1). The decrease in PTH to 22.1 pg/ml and biopsy confirmed the diagnosis of a paratiorial adenoma.

The patient presented an immediate postoperative period normal, with evidence of a decrease in PTH and normalization of calcium levels. During twenty months of follow-up, the patient has not shown data of recurrence or persistence of hyperparathyroidism with calcemia and PTH within laboratory ranks.

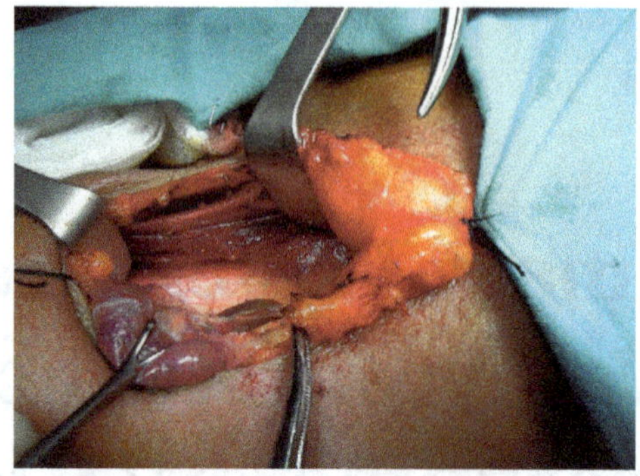

Figure 1: Parathyroid adenoma on the ectopic gland and its relationship with the left common carotid artery.

3. Discussion

The first identification of the parathyroid glands was made by Sir Richar Owen in 1850 in the Indian rhinoceros [4]. Later, the medical student, Ivar Sandström, identified it on a corpse in 1877 [5]. However, it was not until the beginning of the 20th century, in 1925, when Félix Mandl performed the first parathyroidectomy, almost 30 years before the laboratory isolation of parathyroid hormone [6].

Approximately 80–97% of individuals have 4 parathyroid glands. About 2% of the subjects have 5 parathyroid glands.

Supernumerary parathyroid glands are called those glands coinciding in the same subject with four others. Its meaning is of clinical importance since it can be a cause of persistent hyperparathyroidism. Their number can vary between 5 and 11 as described by Akersröm in his series of 503 autopsies [7]. Its incidence is variable, presenting between 2.5 and 22%. Chiu et al. in their work consisting of the dissection of 160 corpses reported an incidence of 1.8% for individuals with 5 glands and 0.6% for those who had up to 6 parathyroids [8].

The supernumerary glands can be rudimentary, small, and close to a nonpathological gland (2%), divided, two very close glands divided by a thin septum of adipose tissue (6%), or separated from the rest without any of the above characteristics (13%) The rudimentary and divided glands may be a consequence of the stimulation of certain chronic situations such as uremia, reaching pathological significance.

Cervical exploration of the four glands has been considered as the gold standard in those patients who are going to undergo pHPT and whose location of the pathological gland does not show coincidences in the preoperative imaging tests. However, the increase in the sensitivity of some of them for their location has allowed us to perform a surgical approach aimed at performing a minimally invasive surgery consisting of selective cervicotomy with a small incision [9].

The previous history of exposure to radiotherapy in our patient may be related to the development of a posterior parathyroid adenoma. As with thyroid cancer, exposure to previous radiation is related to the development of hyperparathyroidism years later [10]. Rosen, in 1975, was the first to relate exposure to radiation with the development of tumors of the parathyroid gland [11]. It has been described that exposure to radiation in the head and neck or upper mediastinum is related to the development of a parathyroid adenoma up to 3 times more frequent than in the unexposed population [12]. This ratio is noticeably higher in patients exposed to high doses of radiation, such as that observed in workers who performed sealing tasks in the nuclear accident at Chernobyl in 1986 [10]. Woll et al. correlate both breast radiation with the development of a parathyroid adenoma and with the side on which it is located [13].

Among the imaging tests used for the preoperative localization of the adenoma, cervical ultrasound and MIBI are the most frequent. Cervical ultrasound, in addition to being an explorer-dependent test, represents the one with the lowest sensitivity (45–57%). MIBI, on the other hand, is usually useful for adenoma localization in most cases, reaching a sensitivity of up to 77–85% [14]. In our experience, we have 376 patients operated on for PPH from the year 2000 to 2013; these techniques had sensitivity similar to that reported in the published literature (cervical ultrasound sensitivity was approximately 37.5% and 71.5% for the MIBI). Some authors, like us, opt for a selective cervicotomy if both tests coincide in the location of the parathyroid adenoma while an exploratory cervicotomy is performed if they are discordant.

In our series, this case represents the first described case of parathyroid adenoma in a supernumerary gland with a cervical location. Only between 0.5–1% of the pHPT are by a fifth gland, and it is usually located in the mediastinum [3].

Currently, the MIBI is the test that is usually performed preoperatively. The performance of SPECT preoperatively in patients who are going to be operated on for the first time of PPH is controversial despite that the SPECT has a sensitivity close to 88%, and even combined with magnetic resonance imaging (MRI) or axial tomography (CT) (SPECT-NMR or SPECT-TC, respectively), it can reach values close to 92–94% [15–17]. In our series, it is not performed preoperatively, reserving the case for patients who, after surgery, experience persistence or recurrence of pHPT.

The use of intraoperative determination of PTH has been shown to be of great help in confirming the removal of pathological parathyroid tissue. For them, in all our patients, we have used the determination of PTH in three moments during the surgery (at the beginning, when visualizing the gland suggestive of parathyroid adenoma and after about 15 minutes of extirpating it) by applying the Miami criteria to refer to healing [16].

Finally, some authors like Norman and colleagues have described radioguided surgery for minimally invasive accesses. In our experience, it has been shown to be useful in those cases in which MIBI and cervical ultrasound were not coincided, and a selective approach was insisted by cervicotomy [17, 18].

4. Conclusions

The most frequent causes of persistent pHPT are the unidentified adenoma in the first surgical intervention, the parathyroid adenoma with ectopic location, an incomplete parathyroidectomy in cases of polyglandular disease (double adenoma or hyperplasia). Less common causes are local recurrence of an adenoma or parathyroid carcinoma, hyperplasia of a remnant after subtotal parathyroidectomy, or a fifth hyperplastic gland after an apparently complete subtotal parathyroidectomy.

The only curative treatment of pHPT is surgery consisting in the removal of the pathological gland. The clinical or analytical persistence of primary hyperparathyroidism after parathyroid surgery can occur if the location of the adenoma is a supernumerary or ectopic gland that during surgery had gone unnoticed. The presentation of a parathyroid adenoma in a supernumerary gland is rare and a challenge for the surgeon expert in thyroid and parathyroid surgery.

The high sensitivity presented by different imaging techniques such as MIBI or SPECT have been a fundamental tool to preoperatively locate the pathological parathyroid gland. In addition, techniques such as the intraoperative determination of PTH allow the biochemical confirmation of the complete removal of all hyperfunctioning parathyroid tissue, with less invasive surgeries, more effective, and with lower morbidity.

Conflicts of Interest

The authors declare that they no conflicts of interest.

References

[1] E. M. Brown, "Extracellular Ca2+ sensing, regulation of parathyroid cell function, and role of Ca2+ and other ions as extracellular (first) messengers," *Physiological Reviews*, vol. 71, no. 2, pp. 371–411, 1991.

[2] S. Pallan and A. Khan, "Primary hyperparathyroidism Update on presentation, diagnosis, and management in primary care," *Canadian Family Physician*, vol. 57, no. 2, pp. 184–189, 2011.

[3] P. Emy, H. Combe, J.P. Marchand, A. Villeneuve, G. Sicre, and D. Chadenas, "Les adénomes parathyroïdiens médiastinaux sur 5ème glande ectopique. Deux observations, Mediastinal parathyroid adenomas on a 5th ectopic gland. Two cases," *Revue de Médecine Interne*, vol. 13, no. 6, pp. 423–426, 1992.

[4] R. Owen, "On the anatomy of the Indian Rhinoceros (Rh. Unicornis, L)," *Transactions of the Zoological Society of London*, vol. 4, p. 3, 1862.

[5] H. Johansson, "Parathyroid history and the Uppsala anatomist Ivar Sandström," *Medicina nei Secoli*, vol. 21, no. 1, pp. 387–401, 2009.

[6] F. Mandl, "Therapeutischer versuch bein einem falle von ostitis fibrosa generalisata mittels exstirpation eines epithelk orperchen tumors," *Zentralbl Chir*, vol. 5, p. 260, 1926.

[7] G. Akersröm, "Surgical anatomy of human parathyroid glands," *Surgery*, vol. 95, no. 1, pp. 14–21, 1984.

[8] C. Wang, "The anatomic basis of parathyroid surgery," *Annals of Surgery*, vol. 183, no. 3, pp. 271–275, 1976.

[9] S Nasiri, A. Soroush, A. Pejman et al., "Parathyroid adenoma Localization," *Medical Journal of the Islamic Republic of Iran*, vol. 26, no. 3, pp. 103–109, 2012.

[10] B. O. Boehm, S. Rosinger, D. Belyi, and J. W. Dietrich, "The parathyroid as a target for radiation damage," *New England Journal of Medicine*, vol. 365, no. 7, pp. 676–678, 2011.

[11] I. B. Rosen, H. G. Strawbridge, and J. Bain, "A case of hyperparathyroidism associated with radiation to the head and neck area," *Cancer*, vol. 36, no. 3, pp. 1111–1114, 1975.

[12] G. Ippolito, F. F. Palazzo, F. Sebag, and J. F. Henry, "Long-term follow-up after parathyroidectomy for radiation-induced hyperparathyroidism," *Surgery*, vol. 142, no. 6, pp. 819–822, 2007.

[13] M. L. Woll, H. Mazeh, B. M. Anderson, H. Chen, and R. S. Sippel, "Breast radiation correlates with side of parathyroid adenoma," *World Journal of Surgery*, vol. 36, no. 3, pp. 607–611, 2012.

[14] M. Uludag, "Supernumerary ectopic parathyroid glands. Persistent hyperparathyroidism due to mediastinal parathyroid adenoma localized by preoperative single photon emission computed tomography and intraoperative gamma probe application," *Hormones*, vol. 8, no. 2, pp. 144–149, 2009.

[15] D. Rubello, "An ectopic mediastinal parathyroid adenoma accurately located by a single-day imaging protocol of Tc-99m pertechnetate-MIBI substraction scintigraphy and

MIBI-SPECT- computed tomographic image fusion," *Clinical Nuclear Medicine*, vol. 27, no. 3, pp. 186–190, 2002.

[16] M. Díez, T. Ratia, M. J. Medrano et al., "Relationship between parathormone concentration during surgery and the post-operative outcome of primary hyperparathyroidism," *Cirugía Española*, vol. 89, no. 6, pp. 386–391, 2011.

[17] J. Norman, "Controversies in parathyroid surgery: the quest for a "mini" unilateral parathyroid operation seems to have gone too far," *Journal of Surgical Oncology*, vol. 105, no. 1, pp. 1–3, 2011.

[18] G. Scerrino, S. Castorina, G. I. Melfa et al., "The intraoperative use of the mini-gamma camera (MGC) in the surgical treatment of primary hyperparathyroidism technical reports and immediate results from the initial experience," *Annali Italiani di Chirurgia*, vol. 86, pp. 212–218, 2015.

24

Recurrent Desmoid Tumor of the Neck: A Case Report of a Benign Disease with Aggressive Behavior

Dionisios A. Klonaris,[1] **Alexander D. Karatzanis**,[1] **Stylianos G. Velegrakis**,[1] **Eleni D. Lagoudakis**,[2] **Emmanuel P. Prokopakis**,[1] **and George A. Velegrakis**[1]

[1]*Department of Otorhinolaryngology, University of Crete Medical School, Heraklion, Crete, Greece*
[2]*Department of Pathology, University of Crete Medical School, Heraklion, Crete, Greece*

Correspondence should be addressed to Dionisios A. Klonaris; daklonaris@yahoo.com

Academic Editor: Rong-San Jiang

We present a case of a desmoid tumor recurrence in a patient with a history of a resected desmoid tumor of the right neck area with free surgical margins six months earlier. The neoplasm was found to invade the parapharyngeal space, and wide excision was performed including most of the sternocleidomastoid muscle (SCM), the thrombosed internal jugular vein (IJV), and the infiltrated spinal accessory nerve (SAN). The histopathologic findings displayed free microscopic margins, with close margins at the site of the parapharyngeal space extension. After 3 months, there was no sign of tumor recurrence. After 6 months, local tumor recurrence was identified on clinical examination and imaging. The decision of the Oncology Board was further treatment with radiotherapy (RT). Response to treatment was satisfactory, and the patient was on close follow-up for twelve months. Desmoid tumors are very rare benign neoplasms of mesenchymal origin with negligible mortality but high morbidity, due to their high recurrence rates, local tissue infiltration, and unpredictable disease course and response to treatment. No universally acceptable treatment protocols have been introduced to date. Appropriate patient counseling and close follow-up are warranted in all cases.

1. Introduction

Desmoid tumors, also known as "well-differentiated non-metastasizing fibrosarcoma," "Grade I fibrosarcoma," and "aggressive fibromatosis," are very rare benign neoplasms of mesenchymal origin [1]. They arise from musculoaponeurotic structures throughout the body. Estimated overall incidence is 2–4 cases per million, and appearance in the head and neck region concerns only a small minority of cases. Despite their benign nature and typically slow growth rate, these tumors exhibit a locally aggressive infiltrative behavior. Thus, they frequently invade nearby structures and show a tendency for local recurrence [1]. In this report, we present a case of a desmoid tumor of the neck with locally aggressive behavior requiring combined modality treatment for disease control. Informed consent was received from the patient for the publication of this manuscript. Case presentation is followed by a concise review of the literature.

2. Case Report

A 22-year-old Caucasian female, nulligravida, presented to our institute (a tertiary referral center) complaining of a slowly growing painful mass at the right lateral neck. Past medical history included a resected desmoid tumor with free surgical margins from the same region six months ago in another center (Figure 1). No other comorbidities were reported. Her family history included mother with systemic lupus erythematosus. Physical examination revealed a hard, tender, palpable mass over the upper half of the right SCM, painful head rotation, and right upper extremity extension but no other sensory deficits or motion restrictions.

MRI revealed an enhancing mass at the cephalic third of the SCM, in close contact with the right IJV, with no signs of vessel infiltration (Figure 2). No pathologic cervical lymph nodes were detected by MRI and ultrasound tomography.

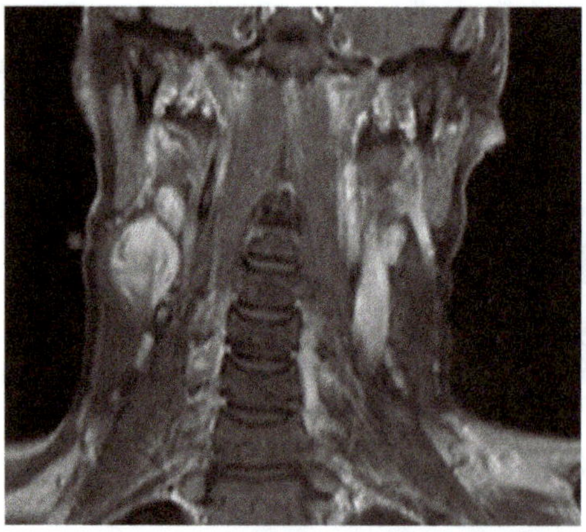

Figure 1: Coronal T1-weighted fast spin-echo (T1FSE) MRI depicting the tumor as an enhancing mass at the cephalic part of the right sternocleidomastoid muscle.

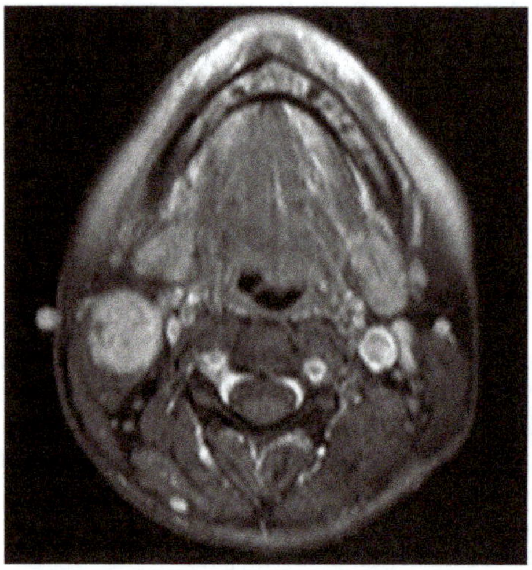

Figure 2: Axial T1-weighted fast spin-echo (T1FSE) MRI showing an enhancing mass indicative of local tumor recurrence following surgery.

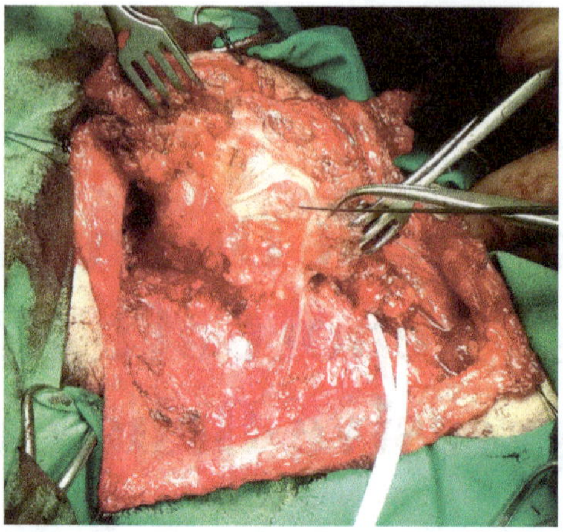

Figure 3: Surgical excision of the desmoid tumor.

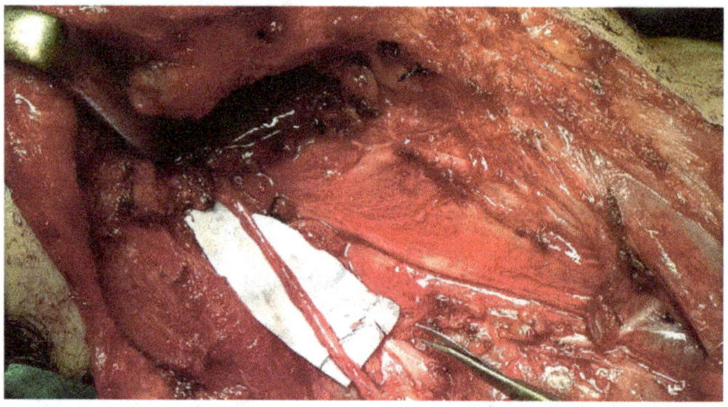

Figure 4: End-to-end anastomosis of the stumps of the spinal accessory nerve after macroscopic complete resection of the desmoid tumor.

Given her past medical history, imaging findings, and clinical presentation, the patient was scheduled two months later for surgical excision of the tumor recurrence under general anesthesia. Access to the surgical field was via an oblique right lateral neck incision. The neoplasm was found to originate from the upper portion of the SCM, extending to the parapharyngeal space, and infiltrating the SAN (Figure 3). A wide excision was performed, including the upper two-thirds of the SCM, the tumor extension to the prestyloid parapharyngeal space, the stylohyoid muscle, and part of the styloid process. The completely thrombosed ipsilateral IJV was ligated and excised. Intraoperatively, it was deemed impossible to dissect the SAN free from the neoplasm and so it had to be sacrificed. However, remaining length of the nerve was satisfactory, and a microsurgical end-to-end anastomosis was performed (Figure 4). A close suction drain was placed, and the wound was closed in layers. Patient recovery from the operating room was without any incidents.

The patient was discharged on the second postoperative day in good condition. The range of right upper extremity extension was limited, and the patient was referred for physiotherapy.

Microscopically, the tumor consisted of fascicles of uniform elongated fibroblast-like cells, surrounded and separated by abundant collagen, with no cell-to-cell contact. Neoplastic cells had sharply defined nuclei with one or more delicate nucleoli and poorly defined cell borders often merging with the extracellular collagen. Regenerative multinucleated skeletal muscle cells were found in the periphery of the lesion. Mitotic activity was typically low (2 mitoses per 10 HPFs) without atypical mitoses. Immunohistochemically, neoplastic cells stained vimentin (Figure 5(c)), smooth muscle actin (Figure 5(b)), and desmin (Figure 5(a)) and were negative for CD34. β-Catenin nuclear staining was also present (Figure 5(d)). The index of proliferation Ki-67 was 1-2%. Focally close excision margins were noted at the parapharyngeal border of the biopsy specimen.

On the 3-month postoperative follow-up, no clinical signs of tumor recurrence were noted, and the right upper extremity mobility was satisfactory, indicating successful anastomosis of the SAN. Unfortunately, on the 6-month follow-up, local pain and swelling indicated new tumor recurrence which was confirmed by MRI. The case of our patient was brought to the Oncology Board. Unanimously, it was agreed that a wait-and-see policy was not a sound option

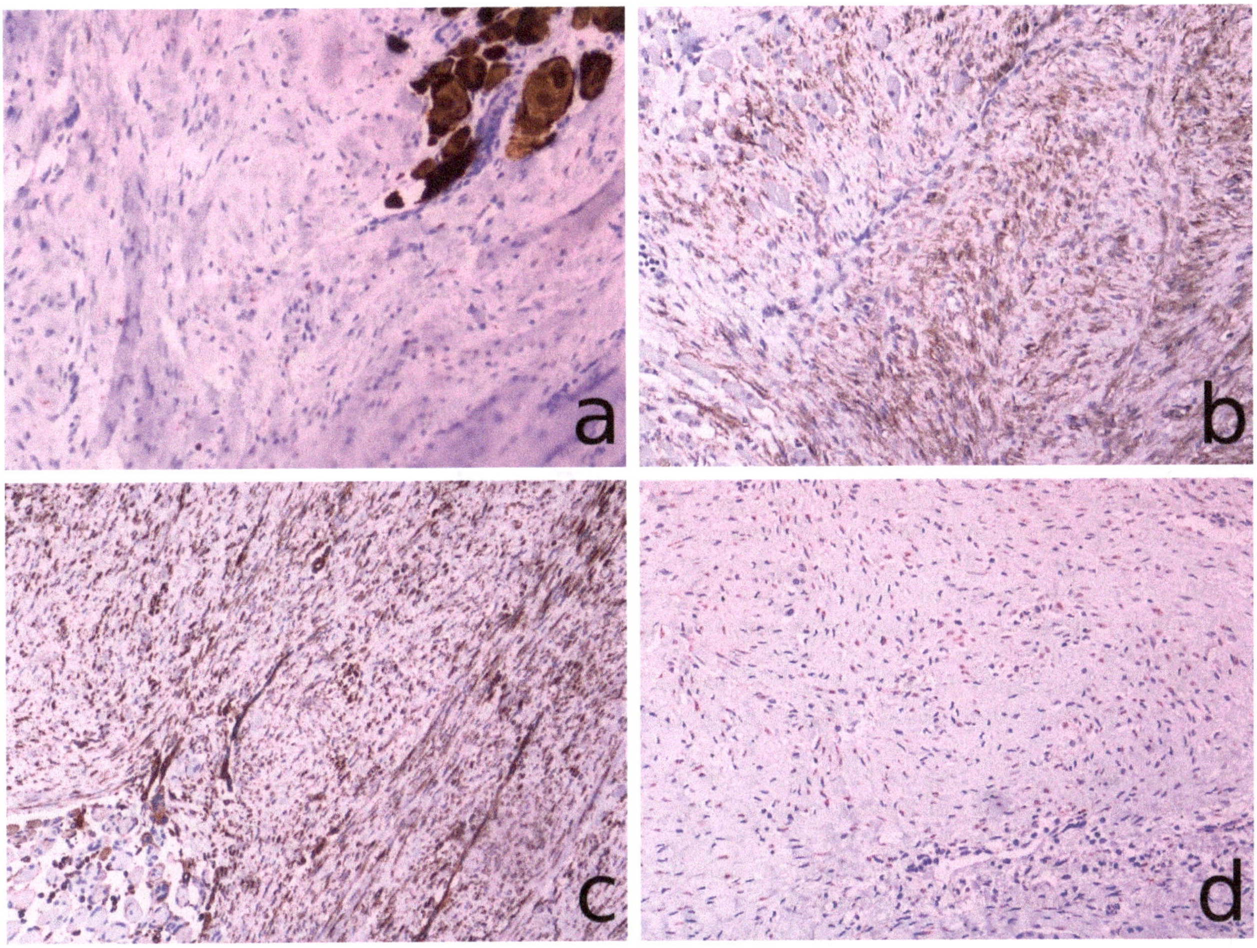

FIGURE 5: Immunohistochemical staining of the biopsy specimen: (a) desmin; (b) smooth muscle actin; (c) vimentin; (d) β-catenin.

and some kind of treatment should be administered since the tumor recurred within six months. Based on imaging findings, excellent performance status of the patient, and our experience as a tertiary referral center on head and neck surgery, excision of the new tumor recurrence was considered as the primary treatment modality. RT was also recommended, but given its long-term side-effects and the proximity of neural structures to the tumor bed, it was considered as an alternative option. Cytotoxic agents, tyrosine kinase inhibitors, and hormonal therapy were considered but discarded, given the reproductive age of our patient and the absence of contraindications for surgery or RT. The patient declined the option of further surgery but elected for RT and received 54 Gy of external beam RT over six weeks. Treatment was well tolerated. After the completion of RT, complete clinical remission of the disease was noted. No evidence of recurrence has been detected on clinical evaluation and imaging studies after twelve months of follow-up.

3. Discussion

According to the location of occurrence, desmoid tumors are classified into intra-abdominal, abdominal, and extra-abdominal types [2]. About 30% are extra-abdominal and only 10–25% of these develop in the head and neck area [2]. Tumor etiology is obscure although multiple mechanisms have been implicated. A history of prior trauma has been associated with their occurrence although their monoclonal nature does not support this hypothesis [3]. Observations on pattern of behavior during pregnancy, menopause, and contraceptive and tamoxifen administration suggest a sex hormone dependency. Cyclooxygenase-2 has been shown to modulate fibroblast proliferation on desmoid tumors [3]. Some cases of desmofibromatosis are associated with familial adenomatous polyposis in the hereditary Gardner syndrome, with a relative risk of about 850 times higher than that of the general population [3].

Desmoid tumors present as circumscribed, firm overgrowths of fibrous tissue arising from virtually any area with a connective tissue component, showing propensity to infiltrate surrounding tissues and occasionally encase blood vessels and nerves, without apparent deep invasion [4]. Histologically, the neoplasm is composed of mature spindle-form fibroblasts with a rich collagenous component, with a variable mitotic index but no evidence of cellular anaplasia or abnormal mitoses [4]. Diagnosis is almost always established by open or core needle biopsy since fine-needle aspiration cytology does not reliably yield diagnostic results [5, 6]. Computerized tomography and/or magnetic resonance imaging (MRI) are usually employed for tumor extension assessment and preoperative planning [5]. Patients with head and neck desmofibromatosis usually present with a nontender mass, in addition to sensory or motor deficits when nerve or muscular structures are involved [7]. Other symptoms, like dysphagia or hoarseness, may appear when the mass compresses the upper aerodigestive tract [7]. These neoplasms have zero metastatic potential, even though malignant transformation has been very rarely described [8]. Tumor growth speed is typically slow; however, rapid progression of the disease may be seen occasionally [6, 8]. Differential diagnosis should always include metastasis of unknown origin, as well as more unusual diseases such as neurofibroma, fibromatosis colli, congenital generalized or solitary fibromatosis, and diffuse infantile fibromatosis [8, 9].

No universally acceptable therapeutic protocols for extra-abdominal desmoid tumors have been introduced to date. Most information regarding this rare entity originates from retrospective studies and sporadic case reports. It should be noted that while the vast majority of patients are adults, it does not spare the pediatric population [10]. As such, vigilance is required and the disease should always be included in the differential diagnosis of a child with a lateral neck tumor.

Surgical excision of the disease has long been the mainstay of treatment. Tumors of the head and neck pose considerable challenges for the surgeon due to close proximity to vital structures. In addition, treatment-induced morbidity and unsatisfactory local control rates, along with spontaneous regression observed occasionally, have put aggressive surgical treatment into question. Finally, there are no established prognostic factors that can be employed for decision-making on treatment modality [11].

Significance of surgical margin status for this neoplasm is a matter of debate. When technically feasible, complete tumor resection with negative microscopic margins is the optimal treatment choice. The importance of microscopic positive margin status with regard to local recurrence rates is still unclear; the presence of microscopic disease has not been shown to affect long-term disease-free survival [12, 13]. Moreover, peripheral nerve involvement is not uncommon. Although it is usually feasible to preserve these structures during surgery [12], this was not possible in our case.

Further research is required to decrypt the molecular mechanisms underlying desmoid tumor genesis and progression. Acquiring such knowledge may lead to better patient selection, superior treatment, and optimal assessment of prognosis of each case. According to the current literature, CTNNB1 (41A, 45F, 45P), β-catenin, and APC locus gene mutations have been implicated with tumor pathogenesis and disease prognosis [14], but there is still no final verdict on the molecular determinants of desmofibromatosis.

Multiple conservative treatment modalities have been recommended and used in different settings. Radiotherapy has been applied primarily for inoperable or inaccessible disease. In addition, it has been used as adjuvant treatment in cases with positive surgical margins and a higher risk of local recurrence. Noncytotoxic regimens like nonsteroidal anti-inflammatory drugs (NSAIDs) and/or tamoxifen have been employed as first-line medical treatment. Cytotoxic agents including anthracycline-containing regimens, doxorubicin, vinblastine, methotrexate, and hydroxyurea have also been employed in cases where surgery and/or radiotherapy are contraindicated, producing variable but, in general, satisfactory results. Response rates to tyrosine kinase inhibitors (imatinib) administration have been shown to be subpar, and this choice should be reserved for cases that have failed other treatment options [3, 10, 14, 15]. Finally, in selected cases, a period of watchful waiting until clinically significant recurrence develops may be the indicated management strategy [3].

4. Conclusion

Desmofibromatosis of the head and neck has negligible mortality but high morbidity, due to high recurrence rates and unpredictable biological behavior and response to treatment. A high level of suspicion, appropriate patient counseling, and close follow-up are warranted in all cases [16].

Conflicts of Interest

The authors declare that there are no conflicts of interest regarding the publication of this article.

Authors' Contributions

Dionisios A. Klonaris was responsible for writing the manuscript and original draft preparation. Alexander D. Karatzanis was involved in conceptualization, methodology, supervision, and writing, reviewing, and editing the manuscript. Stylianos G. Velegrakis and Eleni D. Lagoudakis were responsible for writing and original draft preparation of the study. Emmanuel P. Prokopakis wrote, reviewed, and edited the manuscript. George A. Velegrakis was responsible for methodology and supervision.

References

[1] A. Z. Alherabi, O. A. Marglani, D. H. Bukhari, and T. A. Al-Khatib, "Desmoid tumor (fibromatosis) of the head and neck," *Saudi Medical Journal*, vol. 36, no. 1, pp. 101–103, 2015.

[2] C.-P. Wang, Y.-L. Chang, J.-Y. Ko, C.-H. Cheng, C.-F. Yeh, and P.-J. Lou, "Desmoid tumor of the head and neck," *Head & Neck*, vol. 28, no. 11, pp. 1008–1013, 2006.

[3] E. de Bree, O. Zoras, J. L. Hunt et al., "Desmoid tumors of the head and neck: a therapeutic challenge," *Head & Neck*, vol. 36, no. 10, pp. 1517–1526, 2014.

[4] J. K. Masson and E. H. Soule, "Desmoid tumors of the head and neck," *American Journal of Surgery*, vol. 112, no. 4, pp. 615–622, 1966.

[5] A. Hoos, J. J. Lewis, M. J. Urist et al., "Desmoid tumors of the head and neck--a clinical study of a rare entity," *Head & Neck*, vol. 22, no. 8, pp. 814–821, 2000.

[6] Z. A. Sobani, M. Junaid, and M. J. Khan, "Successful management of aggressive fibromatosis of the neck using wide

surgical excision: a case report," *Journal of Medical Case Reports*, vol. 5, no. 1, p. 244, 2011.

[7] M. C. Fasching, J. Saleh, and J. E. Woods, "Desmoid tumors of the head and neck," *American Journal of Surgery*, vol. 156, no. 4, pp. 327–331, 1988.

[8] R. Prabhu, A. Natarajan, R. Shenoy, and K. Vaidya, "Aggressive fibromatosis (desmoid tumour) of the head and neck: a benign neoplasm with high recurrence," *BMJ Case Reports*, vol. 2013, article bcr2013200156, 2013.

[9] A. Niv, N. Sion-Vard, M. Nash, A. Gatot, J. Peiser, and D. M. Fliss, "Desmoid tumor (aggressive fibromatosis) of the neck," *Indian Journal of Otolaryngology and Head & Neck Surgery*, vol. 52, no. 2, pp. 182–184, 2000.

[10] H. Miyashita, S. Asoda, T. Soma et al., "Desmoid-type fibromatosis of the head and neck in children: a case report and review of the literature," *Journal of Medical Case Reports*, vol. 10, no. 1, p. 173, 2016.

[11] M. Al-Jazrawe, M. Au, and B. Alman, "Optimal therapy for desmoid tumors: current options and challenges for the future," *Expert Review of Anticancer Therapy*, vol. 15, no. 12, pp. 1443–1458, 2015.

[12] M. G. Siqueira, P. L. Tavares, R. S. Martins et al., "Management of desmoid-type fibromatosis involving peripheral nerves," *Arquivos de Neuro-Psiquiatria*, vol. 70, no. 7, pp. 514–519, 2012.

[13] I. Koukoutsis, A. Pappas, G. Karanikas et al., "Desmoid tumor of the supraclavicular region: a case report," *Cases Journal*, vol. 2, no. 1, p. 7222, 2009.

[14] S. Bonvalot, A. Desai, S. Coppola et al., "The treatment of desmoid tumors: a stepwise clinical approach," *Annals of Oncology*, vol. 23, no. 10, pp. x158–x166, 2012.

[15] K. Dafford, D. Kim, A. Nelson, and D. Kline, "Extraabdominal desmoid tumors," *Neurosurgical Focus*, vol. 22, no. 6, p. E21, 2007.

[16] A. S. Lessow, P. Song, and A. Komisar, "Unusual fibromatosis of the head and neck," *Otolaryngology - Head and Neck Surgery*, vol. 130, no. 3, pp. 366–369, 2004.

25

Oropharyngeal CSF Leak Secondary to Anterior Cervical Discectomy and Fusion

Wyatt J. Weinheimer,[1] Justin G. Rowley,[2] Randal Otto,[1] John Floyd,[3] and Philip G. Chen[1]

[1]*Department of Otolaryngology Head Neck Surgery, University of Texas Health at San Antonio, 7703 Floyd Curl Dr, MC 7777, San Antonio, TX 78229, USA*
[2]*UT Long School of Medicine, University of Texas, Austin, TX 78712, USA*
[3]*Department of Neurosurgery, University of Texas Health at San Antonio, 7703 Floyd Curl Drive, MC 7843, San Antonio, TX 78229, USA*

Correspondence should be addressed to Philip G. Chen; chenpg@uthscsa.edu

Academic Editor: I. Todt

We present a case of an oropharyngeal cerebrospinal fluid (CSF) fistula in a patient that presented with headache, rhinorrhea, and pneumocephalus years after an anterior cervical discectomy and fusion. Imaging suggested a defect in the fovea ethmoidalis, but endoscopic surgery revealed the defect in the oropharynx. A second procedure was performed to remove the spinal hardware and repair the leak. This case is not only unique in the literature but also highlights the importance of maintaining a broad differential diagnosis to include rare complications and shows that despite dramatic improvements in imaging, locating CSF leaks still presents a challenge.

1. Introduction

Cerebrospinal fluid (CSF) leaks represent a pathological connection and communication between the subarachnoid space with another nonnative cavity. CSF leakage can result from innumerable processes: iatrogenic, trauma, tumors, or spontaneous disruption of a barrier. Patients often present when the CSF leaks are large enough to result in pneumocephalus or meningitis, a serious and life-threatening condition that can result in permanent neurologic deficits.

Identification of the site of the leak can pose a challenge. Multiple imaging modalities including high-resolution computed tomography (HRCT), CT cisternography/myelography, and magnetic resonance imaging can be and have been used. All have been shown to be useful, but the sensitivity and specificity varies greatly depending on size, location, etiology, and status of leak (active versus inactive) [1–4].

Anterior cervical discectomy and fusion (ACDF) procedures are very common and relatively safe. Although rare, patients undergoing ACDF surgeries can develop intraoperative CSF leaks through accidental dural breach during the procedure (0.2% to 1.8% of cases) with the vast majority of these being noted and repaired at the time of surgery [5, 6]. Development of a postoperative fistula is even less common (<0.2%) and usually presents as clear drainage externally from the surgical neck incision [6].

The purpose of this study is to discuss the workup and management of a patient that presented five years after ACDF with chronic dysphagia, acute headache, pneumocephalus, and signs of meningitis that was subsequently found to have a CSF-oropharyngeal fistula. Imaging suggested that the site of the CSF communication was the left fovea ethmoidalis. The correct anatomic location of the fistula, however, was not identified until a negative endoscopic exploration of the skull base led to identifying the oropharyngeal defect.

After a thorough literature review, we identified 3 case reports of post-ACFD fistula presenting as a neck mass and dysphagia [7–9] and one case of spinal hardware eroding into the esophagus and two cases of erosion into the pharynx [10–12]. To the best of our knowledge, there have been no cases reported of oropharyngeal mucosal erosion from ACDF hardware with resultant delayed CSF fistula.

2. Case Report

A 64-year-old male presented to the emergency room with a 2-week history of a severe, persistent headache. The patient's pertinent past medical and surgical history included obesity and an anterior cervical discectomy and fusion five years prior. A CT scan of the head followed by an MRI of the brain and spine revealed extensive pneumocephalus and concerns for meningitis. The MRI of the spine showed the ACDF hardware but did not reveal surrounding defects. The neurosurgery team was consulted, and the patient was admitted.

CT cisternogram/myelogram and high-resolution CT sinus were obtained. The cisternogram/myelogram was negative for leak at the skull base and cervical spine. CT imaging showed an air-fluid level within a left posterior ethmoid air cell with an apparent 2 mm adjacent osseous dehiscence along the fovea ethmoidalis, suspicious for the source of the CSF leak in this patient (Figure 1). The radiology report also commented that hardware from the anterior and posterior fusion between C3-C6 appeared intact without evidence of fistula or pseudomeningocele.

The otolaryngology/rhinology team was consulted due to the radiographic findings on the sinus CT. On further history and exam, the patient reported intermittent clear rhinorrhea and occasional salty tasting drainage. He denied any significant history of rhinosinusitis. Physical exam demonstrated an obese man who was uncomfortable. Holding the neck in flexion demonstrated clear fluid from the left nostril. The nasal endoscopy was normal. Based on clinical presentation and imaging, there was concern for a left skull defect.

The patient was taken to the operating room for identification and repair of the CSF leak. The neurosurgery team placed a lumbar drain and dilute fluorescein dye injected intrathecally. On nasal endoscopy, fluorescein dye was noted to be pooling in the nasopharynx throughout the case. A total sphenoethmoidectomy was performed, and the area of the potential defect was located and confirmed with intraoperative surgical navigation. Inspissated mucus was found at the area of mucosal thickening on CT (Figure 1) without evidence of fluorescein-dyed cerebrospinal fluid or bony dehiscence at the fovea ethmoidalis. The location was reconfirmed with surgical navigation. The right sinonasal cavity was evaluated without identification of any leak.

Subsequent endoscopic evaluation of the nasopharynx and oropharynx revealed significant pooling of fluorescein, but both openings to the eustachian tubes were normal. Close inspection of the mid-oropharynx, however, revealed a bulge in the posterior oropharynx, and a small, pinpoint fistula with actively leaking fluorescein-dyed CSF was found (Figure 2).

The CT scan of the neck region was reviewed to evaluate the cervical hardware (Figure 3), and the head and neck surgery team was asked to assist neurosurgery with repair of the fistula. An anterior neck approach to the cervical hardware was performed. The anterior cervical hardware was removed and revealed a profuse CSF leak in association with the hardware. The defect was repaired with DuraSeal followed by rotation of the right omohyoid muscle into the site of the defect between the prevertebral fascia and the oropharyngeal mucosa. The neck incision was closed in a layered fashion. The patient was transported to the neurosurgery intensive care unit with the lumbar drain in place. He remained in the ICU on bed rest with the lumbar drain open at 10 ml/hr for 5 days. The patient was then allowed to mobilize, and the lumbar drain was removed. His headaches resolved, and repeat imaging showed resolution of the pneumocephalus. He was discharged and has done well with no evidence of CSF leak. A repeat CT myelogram of the spine at 8 months showed no signs of persistent leak.

3. Discussion

This case illustrates two points. The first is that CSF leak localization can be challenging [13, 14]. The second is that this is a first known case of delayed CSF leak after ACDF with an oropharyngeal fistula.

As observed in this case, localizing a CSF leak can be difficult. Multiple imaging modalities are used to localize defects. High-resolution CT scan has the benefit of wide available and noninvasive to the patient. It is useful for evaluating the sinonasal and bony anatomy [1–3]. A systematic review by Oakley et al. found sensitivity and specificity for identification of a CSF leak was between 44–100% and 45–100%, respectively, with most studies at the upper end of this range [2]. It is considered the first-line imaging modality for CSF leak localization.

MRI is another common option. CSF is bright on T2-weighted imaging and can be seen passing through a defect. While also noninvasive, it is more expensive than CT scanning. The sensitivity and specificity ranges from 56–94% and 57–100% [1–4].

CT cisternography/myelography combines intrathecal contrast injection followed by CT scanning to identify a fistula. Studies report relatively lower accuracy compared to other options [2]. This lower accuracy and the invasive nature make it less attractive as a first-line imagining modality.

Other options include MRI cisternography and single proton emission CT. Some studies suggest improved sensitivity and specificity with these modalities, but they are not widely available and are further associated with higher cost. Additionally, MR cisternography is invasive and requires intrathecal injection [2, 4]. Using a combination of modalities (i.e., HRCT and MRI) has also shown to improve the accuracy [1, 2].

Despite the use of multiple imaging modalities preoperatively in our patient, only operative exploration with the use of intrathecal fluorescein positively located the fistula. Intrathecal fluorescein is suggested to be safe at diluted doses with the benefit of localizing defects [15, 16].

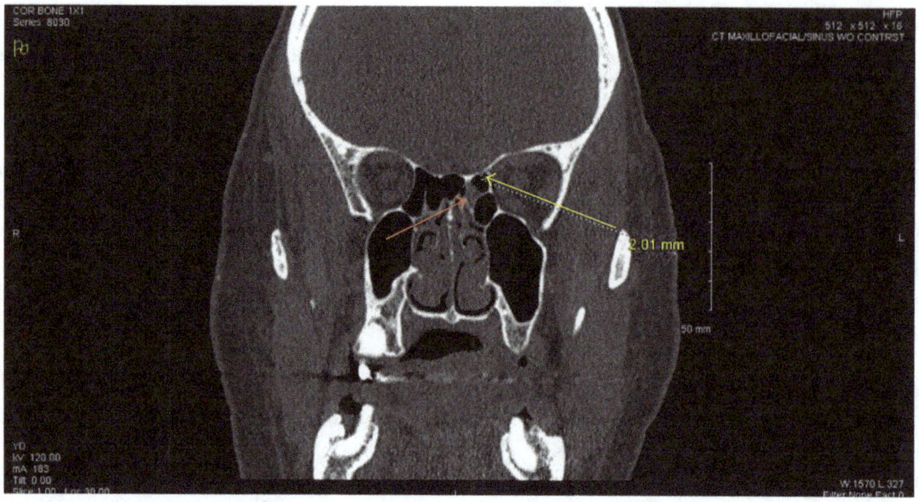

FIGURE 1: High-resolution CT showing area suspicious for a small skull base defect (yellow arrow) and adjacent opacification in the posterior ethmoid sinus (red arrow).

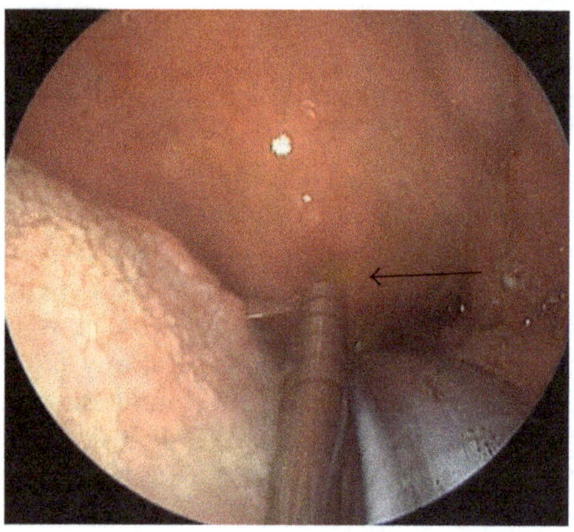

FIGURE 2: Endoscopic identification of fluorescein-dyed CSF in the oropharynx.

Intrathecal fluorescein is, however, invasive in nature, and some studies have failed to show a significant benefit [17].

The best localization technique would be one that is widely available, relatively low in cost, noninvasive, and highly accurate. This case highlights the fact that such a technique does not currently exist. Also, a thorough literature search reveals that most published reports on CSF leak identification are retrospective series with relatively small patient populations. Additional research is needed to determine the best approach to CSF leak localization.

After a thorough literature review, we identified 3 case reports of post-ACFD fistula presenting as a neck mass and dysphagia [7–9] and one case of spinal hardware eroding into the esophagus resulting in CSF leak and pneumocephalus [10]. These cases were uncommon, but even these all occurred within one month of surgery. The case we present is interesting because of its location in the oropharynx, but even more so due to the delayed nature. This highlights that CSF leaks can occur even five years after ACDF.

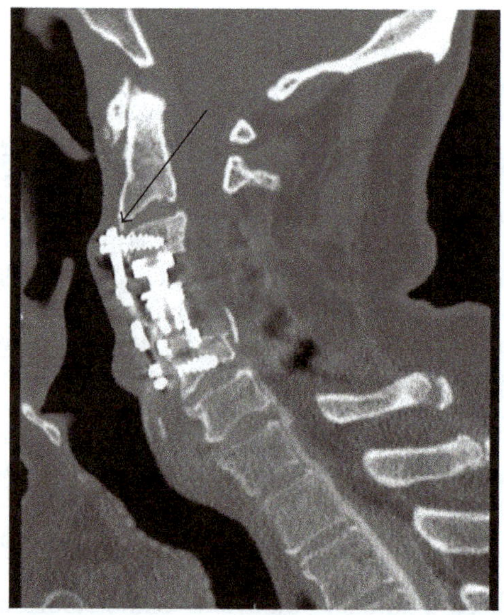

FIGURE 3: CT neck showing cervical hardware with thinning of the oropharyngeal mucosa. CT myelogram was negative for leak in this region.

4. Conclusion

CSF leak after ACDF is an uncommon complication in the postoperative period, and it is a rare fistula to develop years after the procedure.

Despite using several imaging modalities to identify the CSF leak location, none of these identified the site of fistula in our patient. This case highlights the need for research to identify the best approach for defect localization that is accurate, cost effective, and minimally invasive.

Conflicts of Interest

The authors have no conflicts of interest or financial disclosures.

References

[1] P. G. Shetty, M. M. Shroff, D. V. Sahani, and M. V. Kirtane, "Evaluation of high-resolution CT and MR cisternography in the diagnosis of cerebrospinal fluid fistula," *American Journal of Neuroradiology*, vol. 19, no. 4, pp. 633–639, 1998.

[2] G. M. Oakley, J. A. Alt, R. J. Schlosser, R. J. Harvey, and R. R. Orlandi, "Diagnosis of cerebrospinal fluid rhinorrhea: an evidence-based review with recommendations," *International Forum of Allergy and Rhinology*, vol. 6, no. 1, pp. 8–16, 2015.

[3] J. D. Zuckerman and J. M. DelGaudio, "Utility of preoperative high-resolution CT and intraoperative image guidance in identification of cerebrospinal fluid leaks for endoscopic repair," *American Journal of Rhinology*, vol. 22, no. 2, pp. 151–154, 2008.

[4] K. Ohwaki, E. Yano, T. Shinohara et al., "Spinal cerebrospinal fluid leaks detected by radionuclide cisternography and magnetic resonance imaging in patients suspected of intracranial hypotension," *Advances in Medical Sciences*, vol. 59, no. 2, pp. 196–199, 2014.

[5] P. Syre, L.-E. Bohman, G. Baltuch, P. Le Roux, and W. C. Welch, "Cerebrospinal fluid leaks and their management after anterior cervical discectomy and fusion," *Spine*, vol. 39, no. 16, pp. E936–E943, 2014.

[6] H. Bertalnaffy and H. R. Eggert, "Complications of anterior cervical spine discectomy without fusion in 450 consecutive patients," *Acta Neurochirurgica*, vol. 99, no. 1-2, pp. 41–50, 1989.

[7] M. R. Schaberg, J. I. Altman, S. M. Shapshay, and P. Woo, "Cerebrospinal fluid leak after anterior cervical disc fusion: an unusual cause of dysphagia and neck mass," *Laryngoscope*, vol. 117, no. 11, pp. 1899–1901, 2007.

[8] K. N. Fountas, E. Z. Kapsalaki, and K. W. Johnston, "Cerebrospinal fluid fistula secondary to dural tear in anterior cervical discectomy and fusion," *Spine*, vol. 30, no. 10, pp. E277–E280, 2005.

[9] S. B. Nair, L. M. Flood, and F. Nath, "An unusual complication of Cloward's procedure presenting to the otolaryngologist," *Journal of Laryngology and Otology*, vol. 112, no. 11, 1998.

[10] R. C. Goodwin, C. E. Boone, J. Pendleton et al., "Pneumocephalus leading to the diagnosis of cerebrospinal fluid leak and esophageal perforation after cervical spine surgery," *Journal of Clinical Neuroscience*, vol. 26, pp. 141-142, 2016.

[11] S. A. Quadri, J. Capua, V. Ramakrishnan et al., "A rare case of pharyngeal perforation and expectoration of an entire anterior cervical fixation construct," *Journal of Neurosurgery: Spine*, vol. 26, no. 5, pp. 560–566, 2017.

[12] Y.-C. Kuo and M. S. Levine, "Erosion of anterior cervical plate into pharynx with pharyngotracheal Fistula," *Dysphagia*, vol. 25, no. 4, pp. 334–337, 2010.

[13] C. Martín-Martín, G. Martínez-Capoccioni, R. Serramito-García, and F. Espinosa-Restrepo, "Surgical challenge: endoscopic repair of cerebrospinal fluid leak," *BMC Research Notes*, vol. 5, no. 1, p. 459, 2012.

[14] J. Daele, Y. Goffart, and S. Machiels, "Traumatic, iatrogenic, and spontaneous cerebrospinal fluid (CSF) leak: endoscopic repair," *B-ENT*, vol. 7, no. 17, pp. 47–60, 2011.

[15] R. Keerl, R. K. Weber, W. Draf, A. Wienke, and S. D. Schaefer, "Use of sodium fluorescein solution for detection of cerebrospinal fluid fistulas: an analysis of 420 administrations and reported complications in Europe and the United States," *Laryngoscope*, vol. 114, no. 2, pp. 266–272, 2004.

[16] J. I. Moseley, C. A. Carton, and W. E. Stern, "Spectrum of complications in the use of intrathecal fluorescein," *Journal of Neurosurgery*, vol. 48, no. 5, pp. 765–767, 1978.

[17] R. Seth, K. Rajasekaran, M. S. Benninger, and P. S. Batra, "The utility of intrathecal fluorescein in cerebrospinal fluid leak repair," *Otolaryngology Head and Neck Surgery*, vol. 143, no. 5, pp. 626–632, 2010.

26

Head and Neck Myxoma Presenting as Isolated Laryngeal Polyp

Smriti Panda,[1] **Rajeev Kumar**,[1] **Vikram Raj Gopinath**,[2] **and Prem Sagar**[1]

[1]*Department of Otorhinolaryngology and Head and Neck Surgery, All India Institute of Medical Sciences, New Delhi, India*
[2]*Department of Pathology, All India Institute of Medical Sciences, New Delhi, India*

Correspondence should be addressed to Rajeev Kumar; rajeev9843@yahoo.co.in

Academic Editor: Kamal Morshed

Myxoma is a benign tumour with a propensity for local infiltration and recurrence. Laryngeal myxoma presents as a submucosal polyp. Being an uncommon tumour and mimicking vocal cord polyp, only anecdotal evidence is available in the literature. The literature was reviewed from 1986 onwards using the keywords "myxoma" and "larynx." The databases used were PubMed, Google Scholar, Scopus, and Web of Science. Along with this, we also report our case of vocal fold myxoma. We found a total of 19 studies reporting laryngeal myxoma. Laryngeal myxoma typically affects males in the 6th decade with a history of smoking. Unlike myxomas originating outside the larynx, recurrence is not widely described, and microlaryngeal surgery will usually suffice. Laryngeal myxomas should definitely be kept in the list of differential diagnosis when dealing with a benign-looking vocal fold lesion.

1. Introduction

Myxomas are a rare benign myxoid neoplasm of mesenchymal origin. They are a heterogeneous group of soft tissue neoplasms with a variable degree of invasiveness, ranging from benign to highly aggressive forms [1]. Although benign, they are known to be locally infiltrative in nature with a tendency to recur if not excised with margins [2]. Myxomas of head and neck region are rare tumours with the larynx being a less commonly affected site. Clinical presentation of laryngeal myxomas is very much similar to common benign mucosal fold disorders like laryngeal polyp or cyst. Clinically, laryngeal myxomas are indistinguishable from a laryngeal polyp. They are diagnosed on histology supplemented with immunohistochemistry.

2. Case Report

A 53-year-old male presented with hoarseness of 12-year duration. He gave no history of breathing or swallowing difficulty. On enquiring further, he had complaints related to gastric acid reflux. He was a smoker but had quit smoking 6 months back. He is a politician with a history of voice abuse. On flexible fibreoptic evaluation, there was a 0.5 cm polypoidal, cystic mass pedicled on the medial free edge of the middle 1/3 of the right true vocal fold. There was no abnormality of vocal fold mobility. Rest of the ENT examination was normal.

Based on a history of long-standing hoarseness, voice abuse, and presence of a solitary polypoidal lesion over the true vocal fold, a preoperative diagnosis of a laryngeal polyp was made. No preoperative radiology was taken due to the unambiguous nature of the clinical findings. The patient was taken up for microlaryngeal surgery (MLS), and the lesion was excised with cold instruments. Postoperative period was uneventful with patient reporting near-normal voice during first follow-up after one week. Surprisingly, the postoperative histology showed features consistent with laryngeal myxoma.

On histological examination, our case showed a polypoidal tumour lined by hyperplastic stratified squamous epithelium (Figure 1(a)). A subepithelial unencapsulated lesion was noted. The latter was paucicellular formed by small, bland, spindle to stellate cells having indistinct cytoplasmic margins and hyperchromatic nuclei (Figure 1(b)). No significant atypia or mitotic activity or any necrosis was noted (Figure 1(c)). These cells were embedded within an abundant myxoid matrix. Immunohistochemically (IHC),

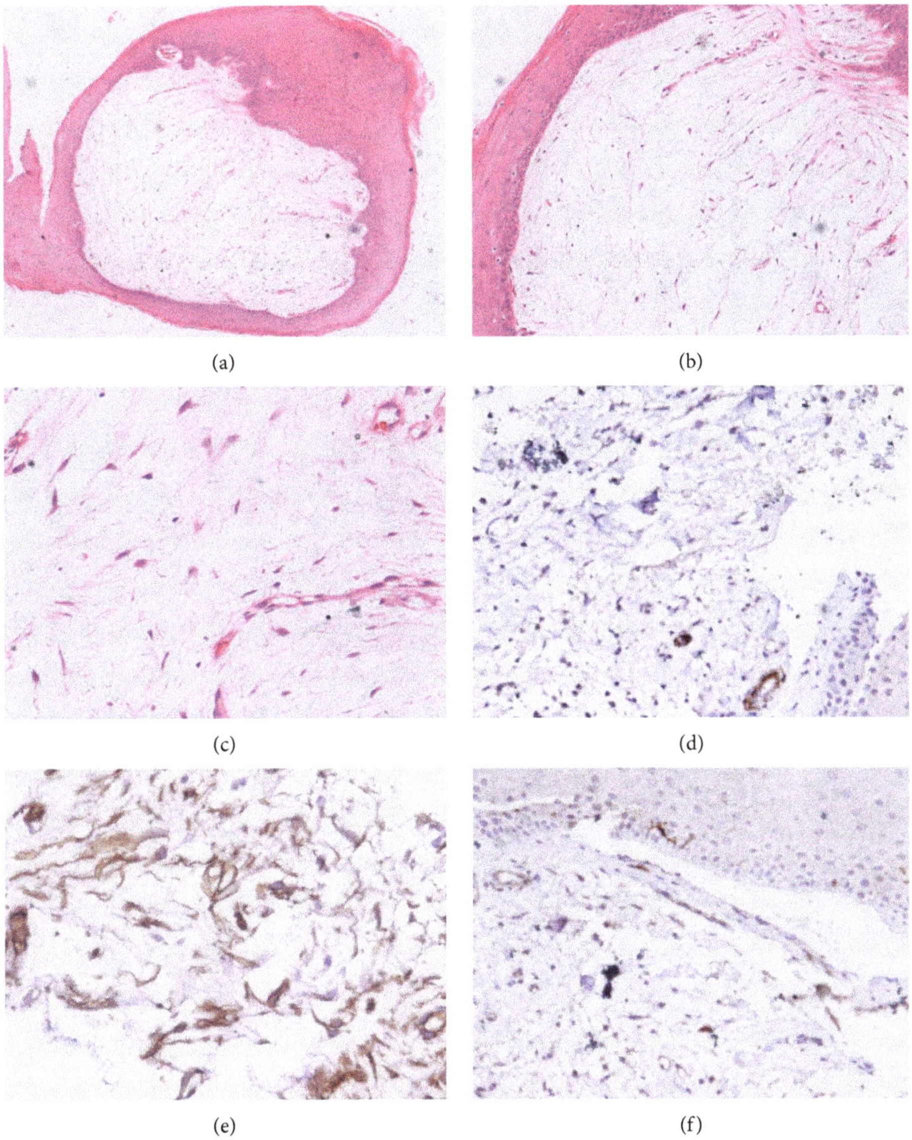

FIGURE 1: Histopathology. (a–c) A polypoidal lesion lined by hyperplastic stratified squamous epithelium. Subepithelium shows a paucicellular mesenchymal tumour comprising small, bland, spindle, or stellate-shaped cells with small and hyperchromatic nuclei and inconspicuous cytoplasm dispersed in an abundant myxoid stroma. Cellular pleomorphism, mitotic figures, and necrosis are absent. (e–f) Results of immunohistochemistry with CD34, SMA, and S-100. The tumour cells are immunonegative for CD34, smooth muscle actin (SMA), and S100 ((a) HE 40x, (b) HE 100x, (c) HE 200x, (d) CD34 200x, (e) SMA 200x, and (f) S100 200x).

the cells were negative for CD34, smooth muscle actin (SMA), and S100 (Figures 1(d)–1(f)). Thus, a final diagnosis of laryngeal myxoma was rendered. The absence of stromal vasculature, hemorrhage, hemosiderin-laden macrophages, and hyalinization of basement membrane helped to differentiate it from a vocal fold polyp [3].

3. Discussion

We did a comprehensive review of all the anecdotal cases of laryngeal myxoma reported in the literature so far which is summarized in Table 1 [3–20] after searching across PubMed, Google Scholar, Scopus, and Web of Science using the terms "Myxoma" and "laryngeal." All articles reporting laryngeal myxoma specifying tumour location and histological feature were included.

Larynx as a site for head and neck myxoma is extremely rare. Our comprehensive literature search revealed 19 cases of laryngeal myxoma till date (Table 1). Male preponderance (M : F of 5 : 1) with a history of smoking is seen in a majority of cases reported. Our case also had both of these characteristics. Mean age at presentation was 52.16 years (range 36 to 77 years). Hoarseness was the most common presenting symptom signifying a predilection for the glottis, as seen in our case also. Dysphagia was reported in the studies by Baruah et al. and Chen et al. due to the involvement of the epiglottis [15, 20]. All authors documented the presence of a submucosal polypoidal mass ranging in size from 0.4 cm to 6.5 cm. Microlaryngeal surgery

Table 1: Systematic review of all cases of laryngeal myxoma.

Author (year)	Number of cases	Age/sex	Presentation	Addiction	Association	Site	Size	Approach	Follow-up	Histology	Need for tracheostomy
Tang et al. (2015) [4]	1	ND	Dysphonia	ND	—	Glottis	ND	Two approaches	?Recurrence		—
Ritchie et al. (2015) [3]	1	77/M	Hoarseness 6 months	Smoker	Reinke's edema	Glottis	<1 cm	MLS	3 months, NED	Stellate cell, spindle cell, and mucinous matrix. CD 34−, S100+, and SMA+	—
Singh et al. (2014) [5]	1	65/M	Hoarseness 4 months and dyspnoea 1 week	ND	—	Glottis	17 × 12 mm	MLS	8 months, NED	-do- No IHC	Tracheostomy
Shah et al. (2014) [6]	1	50/M	Hoarseness 2 months	ND	—	Glottis	—	MLS	No f/u	-do- No IHC	—
Garca et al. (2013) [7]	1	61/M	Hoarseness 3 months	Smoker	—	Glottis	0.5 × 0.5 cm	MLS	No f/u	-do- CD 34−, S100−, desmin−, and SMA−	—
Kanlıada et al. (2012) [8]	1	42/f	Hoarseness 3 months	—	—	Glottis	4 mm	MLS	12 months, NED	-do- No IHC	—
Nakamura et al. (2008) [9]	1	74/f	Hoarseness	Alcohol	—	Glottis	4 mm	MLS	NED	-do- No IHC	—
Song et al. (2008) [10]	1	36/M	Hoarseness 2 months	—	—	Glottis	7 mm × 5 mm	MLS	4 months, NED	-do- No IHC	—
Ali et al. (2008) [11]	1	48/F	Hoarseness childhood	Smoker	Reinke's edema	Glottis	—	MLS	—	-do- CD34+, S100−, and SMA−, Ki-67+	—
Leu et al. (2007) [12]	1	53/m	Hoarseness 2 years	—	—	Glottis	5 mm	MLS	—	-do- No IHC	—
Kim et al. (2007) [13]	2	62/m	Hoarseness 5 years	Smoker	—	Glottis	1.5 × 0.8 × 0.4 cm	MLS	8 years, NED	-do- No IHC	—
		52/M	Hoarseness and dyspnoea 3 weeks	Smoker	—	Glottis	2 × 0.4 × 0.4 cm	MLS	3 years, 6 months, NED	-do- NED	—
Idrees et al. (2005) [14]	1	46/M	—	Smoker	—	Glottis	8 mm	MLS	—	-do- No IHC	—
Baruah et al. (2001) [15]	1	57/M	Hoarseness	—	—	AEF/epiglottis	6.5 × 5.0 × 1 cm	MLS	ND	-do- No IHC	—
Kim et al. (1997) [16]	1	62/M	Dyspnoea 3 days	Smoker, alcoholic	Reinke's edema	Glottis, obstructing airway	2.5 × 2.5 × 1.5 cm	MLS	—	-do- No IHC	Tracheostomy
Tsunoda et al. (1997) [17]	1	57/m	Hoarseness	Alcoholic	—	Glottis	7 × 7 × 7 mm	MLS	NED	No IHC	—
Hadley et al. (1994) [18]	1	64/M	Hoarseness 4 years	Alcoholic, smoker	—	Glottis	1 × 0.6 × 0.2 cm	MLS	18 months, NED	No IHC	—
Sena et al. (1991) [19]	1	70/M	Hoarseness	Alcoholic, smoker	—	AEF	0.5 × 0.5 × 2.5 cm	Transcervical	12 months, NED	No IHC	—
Chen and Ballecer (1986) [20]	1	37/M	Dysphonia and dysphagia	—	—	Epiglottis	5.6 × 4.3 × 2.4 cm	MLS	12 months, NED	No IHC	—
Present study (2016)	1	53/M	Hoarseness 12 years	Smoker	—	Glottis	0.5 cm	MLS	4 months, NED	Immunonegative for CD34, SMA, and S100	—

and excision by cold instruments was the preferred approach with one reported recurrence which responded to subtotal excision [4]. Tracheostomy was required preoperatively in two glottic myxomas due to airway compromise which was sorted after complete excision [5, 16]. Sena et al. utilized a transcervical route in his case where the primary one was located in the aryepiglottic fold [19].

Although we did not find any systemic association, at least three studies have revealed an association with Reinke's edema [3, 11, 16]. Possibility of Reinke's edema being a precursor lesion or sharing the same etiopathogenesis with myxoma needs to be studied in detail.

Demographically, laryngeal myxomas differ from other head and neck myxomas. A comprehensive review on head and neck myxoma by Andrews et al. [2] shows a female preponderance, with age group 18–67 years being affected. This study also quoted involvement of the paediatric age group. Laryngeal myxoma, on the contrary, seems to be a disease of males in the 5th–6th decade with a history of smoking.

Various theories for its etiopathogenesis have been put forth. Due to the abundance of mucinous matrix and glycosaminoglycans, fibroblast immaturity has been cited as a factor [21]. Another theory traces its origin to odontogenic primordial mesenchyme [3]. The latter probably explains the most common location for a myxoma in head and neck, that is, maxilla. Immature fibroblasts could be responsible for the occurrence in the larynx and also the association seen with Reinke's edema. Myxomas have been reported in mucopolysaccharidosis, Carney complex, and Mazabraud syndrome [3]. Mazabraud syndrome belongs to the spectrum of fibrous dysplasias where intramuscular myxomas have been described [22]. Carney complex is an autosomal dominant disorder characterized by cardiac myxomas, cutaneous hyperpigmentation, and multiple endocrinopathies in the form of raised ACTH and growth hormone. PRKAR1 alpha is the tumour suppressor gene implicated in this syndrome.

Histopathology forms the mainstay for diagnosing this entity. The usual clinical appearance is that of a benign vocal fold lesion like an intracordal cyst, polyp, or a nodule. It is the presence of myxoid stroma and abundance of stellate cells and spindle cells that help in clinching the diagnosis. There is no general consensus regarding myxoma-specific immunohistochemistry markers. All studies (Table 1) have reported submucosal involvement, a predominance of stellate cells and spindle cells against the background of a mucinous matrix. Immunohistochemistry markers were available in three studies with no consensus regarding the significance of positivity of markers like CD34, SMA, S100, desmin, and Ki-67.

Head and neck myxomas are known for locally infiltrative nature and tendency to recur if not excised radically [2]. However, literature review suggested that microlaryngeal surgery performed from the point of view of a vocal fold polyp or cyst will generally suffice as it is evident by only one recurrence reported so far and long disease free intervals in other patients.

4. Conclusion

Laryngeal myxomas should definitely be kept in the list of differential diagnosis when dealing with a benign looking vocal fold lesion. Patients need to be kept on close follow-up if excision has been suboptimal due to the absence of capsule and locally infiltrative nature.

Conflicts of Interest

The authors declare that they have no conflicts of interest.

References

[1] A. D. Baheti, S. H. Tirumani, M. H. Rosenthal et al., "Myxoid soft-tissue neoplasms: comprehensive update of the taxonomy and MRI features," *American Journal of Roentgenology*, vol. 204, no. 2, pp. 374–385, 2015.

[2] T. Andrews, S. E. Kountakis, and A. A. J. MaiHard, "Myxomas of the head and neck," *American Journal of Otolaryngology*, vol. 21, no. 3, pp. 184–189, 2000.

[3] A. Ritchie, J. Youngerman, J. E. Fantasia, L. B. Kahn, and R. S. Cocker, "Laryngeal myxoma: a case report and review of the literature," *Head and Neck Pathology*, vol. 8, no. 2, pp. 204–208, 2014.

[4] C. G. Tang, D. L. Monin, B. Puligandla, and R. M. Cruz, "Glottic myxoma presenting as chronic dysphonia: a case report and review of the literature," *Ear, Nose, & Throat Journal*, vol. 94, no. 1, pp. E30–E33, 2015.

[5] B. R. Singh, A. Pandey, and A. M. Thakral, "Laryngeal myxoma: emergency management," *Indian Journal of Clinical Practice*, vol. 24, no. 11, pp. 1027–1032, 2014.

[6] S. U. Shah, S. Verma, S. Hamid, M. H. Kirmani, M. Sangoo, and A. Wani, "Laryngeal myxoma: a rare case report," *International Journal of Clinical and Surgical Advances*, vol. 2, no. 2, pp. 35–38, 2014.

[7] M. F. Garca, H. Cankaya, M. Turan, and M. Kosem, "Laryngeal myxoma resembling a laryngeal polyp: case report," *Van Tip Dergisi*, vol. 20, no. 2, pp. 100–102, 2013.

[8] D. Kanlıada, B. Başaran, O. Mete, and K. Değer, "Laryngeal myxoma mimicking intracordal cyst," *Turkish Archives of Otolaryngology*, vol. 50, no. 2, pp. 26-27, 2012.

[9] A. Nakamura, H. Iguchi, M. Kusuki, H. Yamane, M. Matsuda, and S. Osako, "Laryngeal myxoma," *Acta Oto-Laryngologica*, vol. 128, no. 1, pp. 110–112, 2008.

[10] Y. S. Song, H. S. Jang, K. W. Min, W. N. S. M. Jang, Y. J. Jun, and S. S. Paik, "Myxoma of the larynx presenting as a nodule," *Korean Journal of Pathology*, vol. 42, pp. 306-307, 2008.

[11] S. Ali, G. MacDougall, and W. Wallace, "Myxoma-rare laryngeal presentation," *Internet Journal of Otorhinolaryngology*, vol. 11, no. 1, 2008.

[12] G. Leu, A. M. Klein, A. T. Deyrup, and M. M. Johns III, "Pathology quiz case 1. Laryngeal myxoma," *Archives of Otolaryngology-Head & Neck Surgery*, vol. 133, no. 1, pp. 94-96, 2007.

[13] D. H. Kim, J. W. Eom, T. H. Han, and M. S. Kang, "Two cases of laryngeal myxoma," *Korean Journal of Otorhinolaryngology*, vol. 50, pp. 275–277, 2007.

[14] M. T. Idrees, R. Hessler, D. Terris, C. Mixson, and B. Y. Wang, "Unusual polypoid laryngeal myxoma," *Mount Sinai Journal of Medicine*, vol. 72, no. 4, pp. 282–284, 2005.

[15] P. Baruah, D. N. Jha, A. K. Karak, and R. Kumar, "Laryngeal myxoma," *Journal of Laryngology & Otology*, vol. 115, no. 3, pp. 231-232, 2001.

[16] K. M. Kim, S. C. Kim, H. J. Jeong, and J. H. Kie, "Myxoma: life threatening benign non epithelial tumour of the larynx," *Yonsei Medical Journal*, vol. 38, no. 3, pp. 187–189, 1997.

[17] K. Tsunoda, K. Nosaka, M. Housui, E. Murano, M. Ishikawa, and Y. Imamura, "A rare case of laryngeal myxoma," *Journal of Laryngology & Otology*, vol. 111, no. 3, pp. 271–273, 1997.
[18] J. Hadley, Q. Gardiner, M. Dikes, and M. Boyle, "Myxoma of larynx: a case report and a review of literature," *Journal of Laryngology & Otology*, vol. 108, no. 9, pp. 811-812, 1994.
[19] T. Sena, M. S. Brady, A. G. Huvos, and R. H. Spiro, "Laryngeal myxoma," *Archives of Otolaryngology–Head and Neck Surgery*, vol. 117, no. 4, pp. 430–432, 1991.
[20] K. T. Chen and R. A. Ballecer, "Laryngeal myxoma," *American Journal of Otolaryngology*, vol. 7, no. 1, pp. 58-59, 1986.
[21] Z. Tataryn, J. Tracy, CT. J. Wu, C. B. Heilman, and R. O. Wein, "Intramuscular myxoma of the cervical paraspinal musculature: case report and review of the literature," *American Journal of Otolaryngology–Head and Neck Medicine and Surgery*, vol. 36, no. 2, pp. 273–276, 2015.
[22] D. Dreizin, C. Glen, and J. Jose, "Mazabraud Syndrome," *American Journal of Orthopedics*, vol. 41, no. 7, pp. 332–335, 2012.

27

Parapharyngeal Abscesses Caused by Group G Streptococcus

Shori Tajima, Takashi Anzai, Rina Matsuoka, Hiroko Okada, Takuma Ide, Mitsuhisa Fujimaki, Shota Kaya, Shin Ito, and Katsuhisa Ikeda

Department of Otorhinolaryngology, Juntendo University Faculty of Medicine, Tokyo, Japan

Correspondence should be addressed to Takashi Anzai; tanzai@juntendo.ac.jp

Academic Editor: Hidenori Yokoi

Deep neck abscess is a life-threatening infection that causes laryngeal edema and upper airway occlusion. The predominant bacterial species involved in this disorder is group A streptococcus. Group G streptococcus (GGS) constitutes the normal commensal flora of the human upper airway. Although rarely, it can cause pharyngitis, tonsillitis, and peritonsillar abscess. Here, we report a case of a woman with parapharyngeal abscess caused by GGS. A 56-year-old woman presented to the emergency department with complaints of sore throat and cervical swelling, and a diagnosis of parapharyngeal abscess was established. She had upper airway occlusion, requiring urgent tracheostomy. Endoscopic incision and drainage of the abscess using a specially designed, rigid curved laryngoscope was successfully performed. Since a rigid curved laryngoscope creates a wide viewing field and working space, it was useful for incision and drainage of the parapharyngeal abscess.

1. Introduction

Deep neck abscess, including parapharyngeal and retropharyngeal abscesses, is a life-threatening infection that can cause laryngeal edema and upper airway occlusion. Several case reports showed that group G streptococcus (GGS) bacteria are normal commensal flora of the human upper airway that can cause severe pharyngitis, tonsillitis, and, rarely, peritonsillar abscess [1–3]. Here, we present a case of parapharyngeal abscess with upper airway occlusion caused by GGS. We successfully performed endoscopic surgery for incision and drainage of the abscess using a rigid curved laryngoscope that is a specially designed laryngoscope developed by Satou (Satou's Curved Laryngo-Pharyngo Scope®; Nagashima Medical Instruments Company, Tokyo, Japan).

1.1. Case Presentation. A 56-year-old woman presented to our emergency department with complaints of sore throat and cervical swelling. Her medical history included hypertension, habitual smoking, and occasional alcohol consumption. She developed a sore throat and visited a local clinic 3 days before presenting to our emergency department.

She was diagnosed with tonsillitis. Group A antigen test was negative, and she was administered amoxicillin 750 mg/day. However, 2 days later, she developed dyspnea, dysphagia, and neck stiffness. On arrival at our hospital, she had a severe sore throat and muffled voice and was drooling. Laryngeal fiberscopy revealed swelling of the caudal oropharyngeal mucosa on the right side and a severely swollen epiglottis and arytenoid region that caused upper airway occlusion. Her SpO_2 was 97% on 2 L oxygen, and her body temperature was 37.4°C. Blood test results suggested strong inflammation (white blood cell count, 15.3 × 109/L; C-reactive protein, 27.6 mg/L).

We established a diagnosis of parapharyngeal abscess. Because of a high risk of suffocation, we first performed tracheostomy with the patient under local anesthesia. Enhanced computed tomography after tracheostomy revealed hypodense lesions at the left lateral and posterior pharyngeal walls (Figure 1). Incision and drainage of the abscess was performed with the patient under general anesthesia using a rigid curved laryngoscope.

Peritonsillitis containing mucus and pus from the posterior pillar was observed (Figure 2(a)). We incised and opened a part of the swollen posterior pillar and lateral and

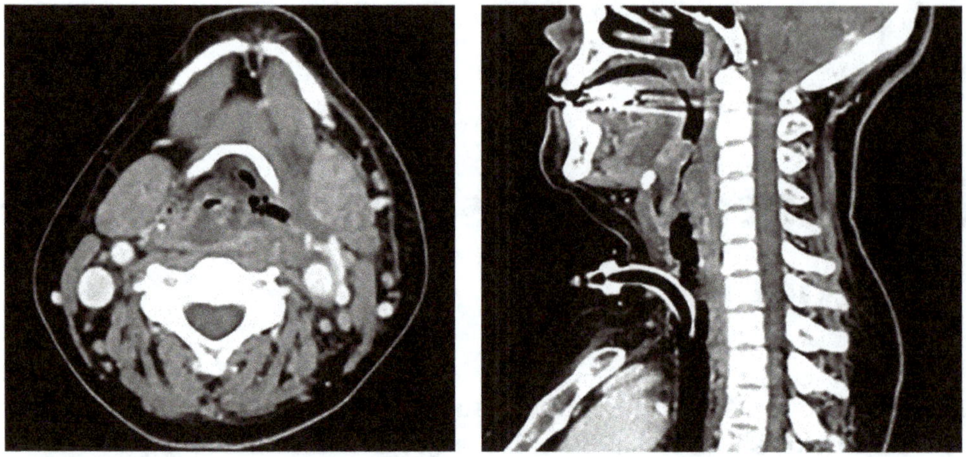

(a) (b)

FIGURE 1: Enhanced CT findings (after tracheostomy). Enhanced CT scan revealed a large mass involving the left parapharyngeal and retropharyngeal space, causing significant airway narrowing.

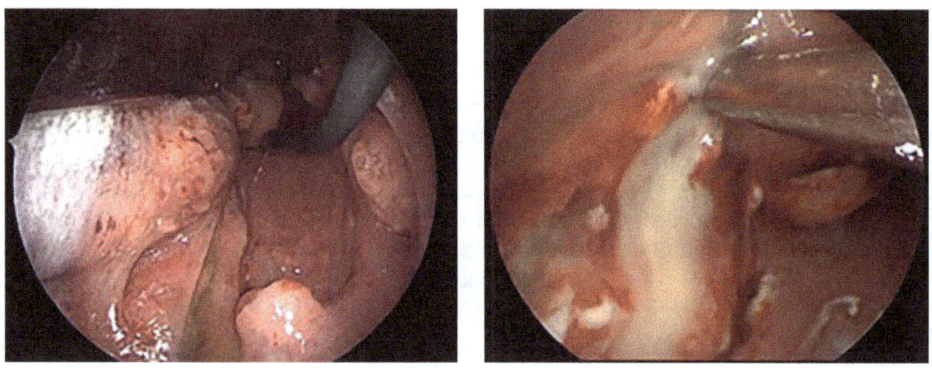

(a) (b)

FIGURE 2: Intraoperative findings. (a) There was peritonsillitis containing mucus and pus from the posterior pillar on the right side. (b) Incision at the left lateral and posterior pharyngeal walls. A large amount of pus flowed out from the peritonsillar and lateral pharyngeal wall.

posterior pharyngeal walls, draining pus from these regions (Figure 2(b)). The operation was completed without any adverse events.

The patient was administered 3 g/d meropenem as empiric therapy. On postoperative day 4, culture for aerobes and anaerobes revealed GGS and *Parvimonas micra*, respectively. Therefore, the antibiotics were changed to 4 g/d piperacillin and 1.2 g/d clindamycin. The recovery course was uneventful.

2. Discussion

GAS is a major microbial pathogen causing pharyngitis, peritonsillar abscess, and deep neck infection. In our case, GGS and *Parvimonas micra* were isolated from the pus. It is often the case that mixed aerobic and anaerobic bacteria can be identified through pus culturing. Tsai et al. reported that polymicrobial growth was observed in 57.39% of pus cultures [4]. Empirical antibiotics targeting both aerobes and anaerobes would be appropriate. However, considering GGS's aggressive characteristic like GAS, GGS appeared to be an important pathogen of the parapharyngeal and concomitant peritonsillar abscesses that could cause potentially fatal upper airway occlusion. GGS is frequently present in the human pharynx and tonsils. Group C and G streptococci are two antigenic variants of the same organism, *Streptococcus dysgalactiae* subspecies *equisimilis* (SDSE). Genomic sequence homology analysis of GGS revealed that GGS was closest in sequence to GAS, with 72% similarity [5]. Virulence profile analysis of SDSE revealed that its genetic basis of disease propensity is shared with GAS, including the antiphagocytic M protein, streptolysin O, streptolysin S, streptokinase, and one or more pyrogenic exotoxins [6]. The burden of SDSE infection is comparable to that caused by invasive GAS infection [7]. We reviewed the bacteriology of the peritonsillar abscess from previous studies searching the PubMed database. There were 9 studies from 2014 to 2018. Two studies were excluded as the detailed *Streptococcus* sp. was not mentioned. As shown in Table 1, GGS or GCS has a prevalence of less than 5% [8–14]. Notably, GGS was

Table 1: Previous studies involved in bacteriology of peritonsillar abscess.

Investigator	Country	Year	Number of samples, *n*	GGS or GCS, *n* (%)
J. Wiksten et al. [8]	Finland	2010-2011	149	2 (1.3)
Vaikjarv et al. [9]	Estonia	2011-2012	22	1 (4.5)
Tachibana et al. [10]	Japan	2008–2013	100	1 (1.0)
Lepelletier et al. [11]	French	2009–2012	412	11 (2.6)
Plum et al. [12]	USA	2002–2012	69	1 (1.4)
Mazur et al. [13]	Poland	2003–2013	45	1 (2.2)
Gavriel et al. [14]	Israel	1996–2003	132	1 (0.76)

GGS, group G streptococcus; GCS, group C streptococcus.

not detected using the rapid antigen test because of the lack of group A antigen, which is the target of these tests. Current pharyngitis guidelines focus only on group A streptococci and only recommend antibiotics. However, as we demonstrated, GGS also causes life-threatening diseases, such as a deep neck abscess. It is important for the primary care physician to consider carefully negative results.

During surgery, it is important to visualize the abscess lesion and create a sufficient working space. The intraoral approach using a self-retaining mouth gag with ipsilateral tonsillectomy can be used to access diseases in the parapharyngeal space [15]. However, a Davis gag can be used to visualize oropharyngeal structures around the oral cavity and tonsils but cannot be used to visualize the caudal oropharynx. Therefore, physicians should perform invasive surgery to remove the ipsilateral tonsil and approach the parapharyngeal space. We describe a novel method using a rigid curved laryngoscope for incision and drainage of a parapharyngeal abscess. This instrument was designed for laryngopharyngeal surgery under endoscopic vision [16, 17] (Figure 3). Recent case reports have described successful removal of a fish bone in the hypopharynx and drainage of retropharyngeal abscesses using a rigid curved laryngoscope [18, 19], which is useful for hypopharyngeal and oropharyngeal surgery. The blade is inserted into the pharynx and lifted forward. The oropharynx is well visualized. After exposing the whole oropharynx, the handle is attached to a holder fixed to the operating table. Because of a crooked line path, we used devices such as malleable high-frequency knives (KD-600®; Olympus, Tokyo, Japan) and malleable forceps (Laryngo FIT®; Karl Storz, Tuttlingen, Germany). In our procedure, the rigid curved laryngoscope exposed the whole oropharynx including the caudal oropharynx. A conventional straight laryngoscope can be used to visualize the caudal oropharynx; however, it provides only a small visual and working space. This curved instrument can provide a wide working space that permits easy and complete incision and drainage while avoiding neck incision or tonsillectomy; therefore, it is useful for incision and drainage of a parapharyngeal abscess.

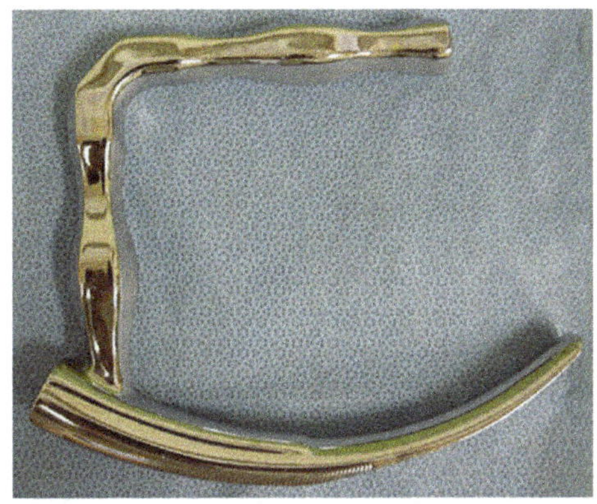

Figure 3: A rigid curved laryngosocpe. This curved rigid laryngoscope can enable visualization of the whole oropharynx.

3. Conclusion

GGS is an important pathogen of deep neck abscesses. A rigid curved laryngoscope enables a wide viewing field and working space; therefore, it is useful for incision and drainage of a parapharyngeal abscess.

Conflicts of Interest

The authors declare that there are no conflicts of interest associated with this manuscript.

Authors' Contributions

ST, TA, and KI prepared and edited this manuscript. RM, HO, TI, MF SK, and SI contributed to the collection of data. TA and KI gave final approval for this version of the manuscript. All authors read and approved the final manuscript.

References

[1] N. Gupta, J. Lovvorn, and R. M. Centor, "Peritonsilar abscess requiring intensive care unit admission caused by group C and G Streptococcus: a case report," *Cases Journal*, vol. 2, no. 1, p. 6808, 2009.

[2] M. Shah, R. M. Centor, and M. Jennings, "Severe acute pharyngitis caused by group C streptococcus," *Journal of General Internal Medicine*, vol. 22, no. 2, pp. 272–274, 2007.

[3] H. Faden, "Group C and G streptococcal disease among children," *Pediatric Infectious Disease Journal*, vol. 24, no. 11, pp. 1014-1015, 2005.

[4] Y. W. Tsai, Y. H. Liu, and H. H. Su, "Bacteriology of peritonsillar abscess: the changing trend and predisposing factors," *Brazilian Journal of Otorhinolaryngology*, 2017.
[5] Y. Shimomura, K. Okumura, S. Y. Murayama et al., "Complete genome sequencing and analysis of a Lancefield group G streptococcus dysgalactiae subsp. equisimilis strain causing streptococcal toxic shock syndrome (STSS)," *BMC Genomics*, vol. 12, no. 1, p. 17, 2011.
[6] M. R. Davies, D. J. McMillan, R. G. Beiko et al., "Virulence profiling of streptococcus dysgalactiae subspecies equisimilis isolated from infected humans reveals 2 distinct genetic lineages that do not segregate with their phenotypes or propensity to cause diseases," *Clinical Infectious Diseases*, vol. 44, no. 11, pp. 1442–1454, 2007.
[7] L. N. Broyles, C. Van Beneden, B. Beall et al., "Population-based study of invasive disease due to beta-hemolytic streptococci of groups other than A and B," *Clinical Infectious Diseases*, vol. 48, no. 6, pp. 706–712, 2009.
[8] J. Wiksten, E. Kaltiainen, A. Pitkaranta, and K. Blomgren, "Renewal of peritonsillar abscess: impact of the bacterial species of the infection and clinical features of the patient-a prospective comparative aetiological study," *Clinical Otolaryngology*, vol. 42, no. 6, pp. 1358–1362, 2017.
[9] R. Vaikjarv, P. Kasenomm, L. Jaanimae et al., "Microbiology of peritonsillar abscess in the South Estonian population," *Microbial Ecology in Health & Disease*, vol. 27, p. 27787, 2016.
[10] T. Tachibana, Y. Orita, S. Takao et al., "The role of bacteriological studies in the management of peritonsillar abscess," *Auris Nasus Larynx*, vol. 43, no. 6, pp. 648–653, 2016.
[11] D. Lepelletier, V. Pinaud, P. Le Conte et al., "Peritonsillar abscess (PTA): clinical characteristics, microbiology, drug exposures and outcomes of a large multicenter cohort survey of 412 patients hospitalized in 13 French university hospitals," *European Journal of Clinical Microbiology & Infectious Diseases*, vol. 35, no. 5, pp. 867–873, 2016.
[12] A. W. Plum, A. J. Mortelliti, and R. E. Walsh, "Microbial flora and antibiotic resistance in peritonsillar abscesses in upstate New York," *Annals of Otology, Rhinology & Laryngology*, vol. 124, no. 11, pp. 875–880, 2015.
[13] E. Mazur, E. Czerwinska, I. Korona-Glowniak, A. Grochowalska, and M. Koziol-Montewka, "Epidemiology, clinical history and microbiology of peritonsillar abscess," *European Journal of Clinical Microbiology & Infectious Diseases*, vol. 34, no. 3, pp. 549–554, 2015.
[14] H. Gavriel, Y. Golan, T. Lazarovitch, and E. Eviatar, "Bacteriology of peritonsillar abscess in patients over 40 years—a neglected age group," *European Archives of Oto-Rhino-Laryngology*, vol. 272, no. 4, pp. 981–984, 2015.
[15] Y. Okumura, H. Hidaka, N. Noguchi, and Y. Katori, "Intraoral drainage under surgical microscopy with tonsillectomy for parapharyngeal abscesses," *Journal of Laryngology & Otology*, vol. 129, no. 6, pp. 595–597, 2015.
[16] Y. Satou, T. Omori, and M. Tagawa, "Treatment of superficial carcinoma in the hypopharynx," *Nippon Jibiinkoka Gakkai Kaiho*, vol. 109, no. 7, pp. 581–586, 2006.
[17] I. Tateya, M. Muto, S. Morita et al., "Endoscopic laryngopharyngeal surgery for superficial laryngo-pharyngeal cancer," *Surgical Endoscopy*, vol. 30, no. 1, pp. 323–329, 2016.
[18] H. Sakaida, K. Chiyonobu, H. Ishinaga, and K. Takeuchi, "Use of a rigid curved laryngoscope for removal of a fish bone in the hypopharynx," *Case Reports in Otolaryngology*, vol. 2016, Article ID 9689521, 3 pages, 2016.
[19] K. Watanabe, D. Yamauchi, Y. Takanashi, H. Hidaka, and Y. Katori, "Novel application of a rigid curved laryngopharyngoscope for examination and treatment of hypopharyngeal lesions," *Auris Nasus Larynx*, vol. 45, no. 2, pp. 367–370, 2018.

28

Chronological Progression of an Enlarged Styloid Process: A Case Report of Eagle Syndrome

Daisuke Maki, Kenji Okami, Koji Ebisumoto, and Akihiro Sakai

Department of Otolaryngology, Head and Neck Surgery, Tokai University, Kanagawa, Japan

Correspondence should be addressed to Daisuke Maki; d.maki@tokai.ac.jp

Academic Editor: Richard T. Miyamoto

Eagle syndrome is characterized by an elongated styloid process. However, the time frame over which the styloid process becomes elongated and extends is unknown. How the condition worsens over time is also unclear. To date, there has been no report describing the chronologic change that occurs in the styloid process in Eagle syndrome. We describe a 53-year-old patient with Eagle syndrome in whom the styloid process enlarged progressively over time and the elongated styloid process fused with the hyoid bone. The styloid process was resected via a transcervical approach, and the patient's subjective symptoms improved. This is the first report showing how the styloid process can enlarge over a few years in a patient with Eagle syndrome. Surgical resection via a transcervical approach is an appropriate treatment for a patient in whom the styloid process has become excessively enlarged and elongated.

1. Introduction

Eagle syndrome (an elongated styloid process) causes a range of symptoms because of physical irritation by mastication and swallowing and nerve compression by the deformed styloid process [1]. Although many case reports have been published, complete connection of the styloid process to the hyoid bone is rare, and no study has described the natural history of the enlarging course of the elongated styloid process. Herein, we report the case of a patient with a massively enlarged styloid process in whom sequential changes were observed by chance.

2. Case Presentation

A 53-year-old man presented to our institution with a 3-year history of pain in the left throat and trismus caused by pain. Magnetic resonance imaging in the Department of Neurology revealed an abnormal shadow above the hyoid bone. The patient was referred to the Department of Otorhinolaryngology, where no abnormal signs other than trismus were found. Computed tomography (CT) revealed that the left styloid process was connected to the hyoid bone, had a total length of 70 mm, and was approximately 10 mm thick along almost its entire length (Figures 1(a) and 2). Five years earlier, the patient had been transferred to our emergency clinic with a facial injury, and cervical CT images taken also revealed elongation of the styloid process. At that time, the styloid process had been approximately 5–7 mm thick, and its enlargement in the subsequent 5 years was evident (Figure 1(b)).

The patient was diagnosed with Eagle syndrome and treated initially with analgesics. However, the treatment with analgesics had not improved his pain, so he underwent transcervical resection of the styloid process under general anesthesia. A horizontal skin incision was made in the upper part of the neck, and the submandibular gland was removed to ensure a wide surgical field (Figure 3). The styloid process was firmly connected to the hyoid bone on the dorsal side of the hypoglossal nerve, and a 40 mm portion was resected from the attachment to the hyoid bone. No invasion of the surrounding tissue was found intraoperatively, and it was easy to separate and resect the bone. Pathologic examination revealed that the lesion consisted of bony tissue with a bone marrow component and a cartilaginous component in contact with the trabecular bone. There were no signs of active inflammation or malignancy. The symptoms such as pain and trismus

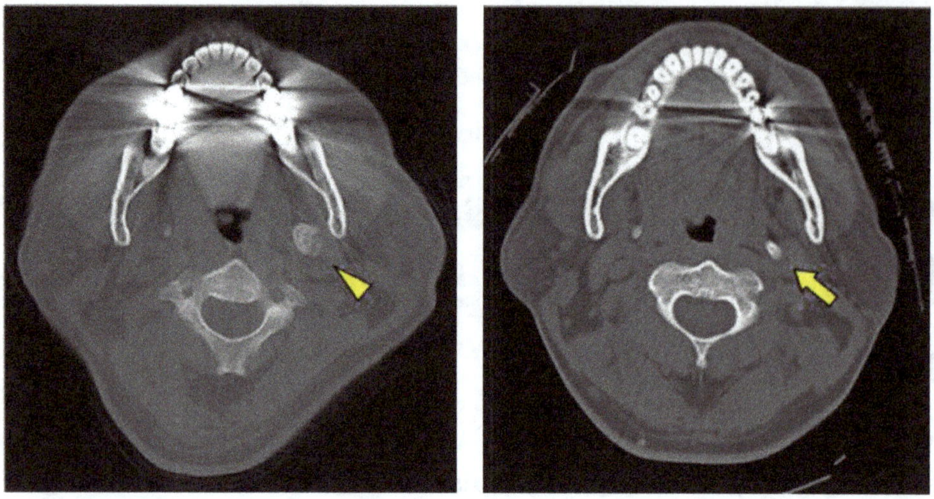

(a) (b)

FIGURE 1: (a) Preoperative computed tomographic image showing enlargement of the left styloid process to approximately 10 mm thick (arrowhead). (a) A computed tomographic image taken 5 years earlier showing enlargement of the styloid process to around 5–7 mm thick (arrow) when the patient was examined for a facial injury.

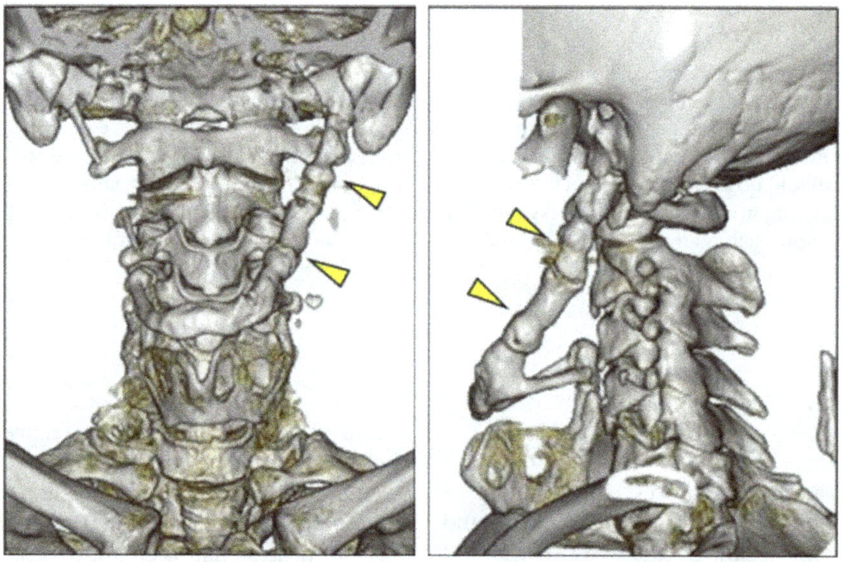

FIGURE 2: Three-dimensional reconstruction of a computed tomographic image taken preoperatively showing that the left styloid process was fused completely to the hyoid bone and had a total length of 70 mm (arrowheads). It was approximately 10 mm thick along almost its entire length.

disappeared completely. Preoperatively, the patient scored pain on opening his mouth and pain on swallowing as 8 on a visual analog scale, and both scores improved to 0 postoperatively. The patient had no recurrence of subjective symptoms at the most recent follow-up 19 months postoperatively. Postoperative CT revealed that a good portion of the left styloid process was resected (Figure 4). The stylohyoid ligament on the right side was partially calcified and requires ongoing observation in the future.

3. Discussion

Eagle syndrome causes a wide range of symptoms because of elongation of the styloid process and calcification of the stylohyoid ligament [1]. Some of these symptoms are attributable to direct physical irritation, while others are caused by compression of branches of the glossopharyngeal and vagal nerves. Symptoms include laryngopharyngeal pain, pain on swallowing, dysphagia, earache, trismus, pain when turning the neck, and facial pain. Eagle syndrome may also cause internal carotid artery dissection [2, 3]. Although the cause of Eagle syndrome is unknown, abnormal bone metabolism and developmental anomalies are thought to be involved [4]. The styloid process is normally 25–30 mm in length, but according to Eagle et al., the styloid process measures ≥25 mm in approximately 4% of adults, and approximately 4% of these individuals will exhibit symptoms [1, 2]. Patients with this syndrome may be treated

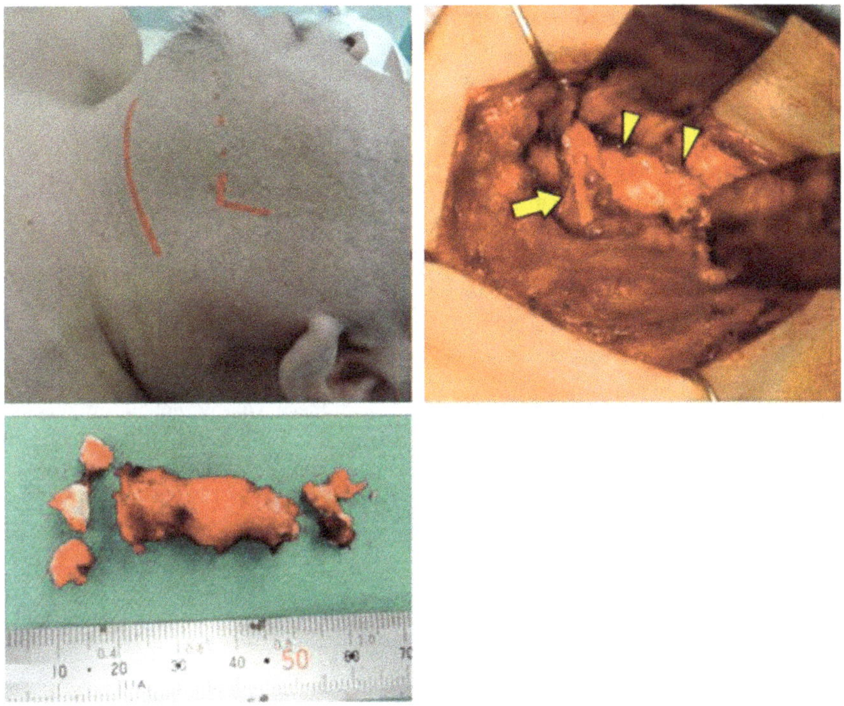

FIGURE 3: Intraoperative findings and the resected styloid process. The styloid process was resected via a transcervical approach. The submandibular gland was removed to ensure a clear field of view. The styloid process (arrowheads) was observed to be continuous with the hyoid bone on the dorsal side of the hypoglossal nerve (arrow), and a 40 mm portion was resected from the site of attachment to the hyoid bone.

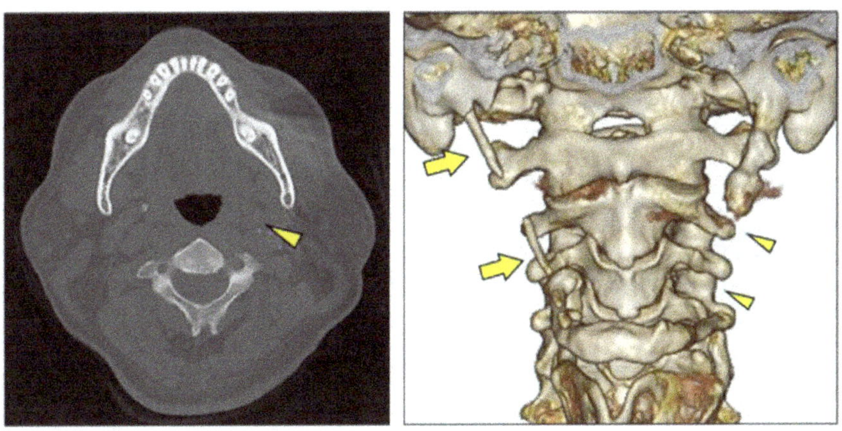

FIGURE 4: Postoperative computed tomographic image and three-dimensional reconstruction. A good portion of the left styloid process was resected (arrowheads). The styloid process on the right side was also elongated, and the stylohyoid ligament was partially calcified (arrows). Ongoing observation is required.

conservatively or surgically. No study has demonstrated the long-term efficacy of conservative therapy, such as oral analgesics or a nerve blocking agent. Surgery is recommended as a curative treatment and may be performed via a transoral approach or a transcervical approach [5]. The oral approach involves first removing the palatine tonsil and making an incision in the pharyngeal constrictor muscle to resect the hyoid process lateral to it. This approach has the advantages of a shorter operating time, a shorter period of hospitalization, and not requiring a skin incision. The transcervical approach involves resecting the hyoid process from below the mandible via a skin incision in the neck. This approach provides a broad field of view ensuring clear visibility of the anatomic structures and enabling resection of a large portion of the hyoid process; however, it has the disadvantages of a longer period of hospitalization, a longer operating time, and leaving a scar on the neck [6]. Although there have been almost no studies comparing the post-operative courses after these two procedures, a comparative report of a small number of patients found no major difference in visual analog scale scores for subjective symptoms [5].

Patients such as the one reported here in whom the styloid process was thick and completely continuous with the hyoid bone are rare, with only three previous cases reported [7–9]. The patient's course, including treatment, was unknown in one patient, but surgery was performed via the external cervical approach in the other two patients. This procedure is recommended for patients with a long and large styloid process because the oral approach does not provide an adequate field of view.

To the best of our knowledge, no previous case report of Eagle syndrome has described the enlarging course of the elongated styloid process. The present case was unusual in that the styloid process could be seen to have approximately doubled in thickness over a 5-year period. The styloid process does not usually enlarge over time; however, the contralateral styloid process extended in this case and the stylohyoid ligament became calcified. Therefore, it was thought that this patient had some unusual features. He had been punched in the face 5 years earlier and suffered a traumatic cervical syndrome. There is a report suggesting that inflammation can cause elongation of the styloid process [10]. The injury-related inflammation might have caused the elongation in this case. Although the patient consented to surgery only on the left side, careful follow-up of the right side is needed.

Although the etiology of the development of Eagle syndrome has been considered for a long time, the exact cause is not known. As in our present case, a styloid process may become excessively elongated. If elongation of the styloid process is discovered by chance, it should be explained to the patient that the elongation may worsen and that subjective symptoms may occur.

Acknowledgments

The authors would like to thank coworkers in their department for useful discussions.

References

[1] W. W. Eagle, "Elongated styloid process; further observations and a new syndrome," *Archives of Otolaryngology-Head and Neck Surgery*, vol. 47, no. 5, pp. 630–640, 1948.

[2] W. W. Eagle, "Symptomatic elongated styloid process; report of two cases of styloid process-carotid artery syndrome with operation," *Archives of Otolaryngology-Head and Neck Surgery*, vol. 49, no. 5, pp. 490–503, 1949.

[3] M. Zuber, J. F. Meder, and J. L. Mas, "Carotid artery dissection due to elongated styloid process," *Neurology*, vol. 53, no. 8, pp. 1886–1887, 1999.

[4] D. J. Fusco, S. Asteraki, and R. F. Spetzler, "Eagle syndrome: embryology, anatomy, and clinical management," *Acta Neurochirurgica*, vol. 154, no. 7, pp. 1119–1126, 2012.

[5] T. Müderris, S. Bercin, E. Sevil, S. Beton, and M. Kırıs, "Surgical management of elongated styloid process: intraoral or transcervical?" *European Archives of Oto-Rhino-Laryngology*, vol. 271, no. 6, pp. 1709–1713, 2014.

[6] J. H. Shin, S. R. Herrera, P. Eboli, S. Aydin, E. H. Eskandar, and K. V. Slavin, "Entrapment of the glossopharyngeal nerve in patients with Eagle syndrome: surgical technique and outcomes in a series of 5 patients," *Journal of Neurosurgery*, vol. 111, no. 6, pp. 1226–1230, 2009.

[7] L. E. Langstaff, T. Abed, and J. Philpott, "Massively enlarged styloid process presenting as a submandibular mass," *BMJ Case Reports*, vol. 2012, p. bcr-2012-007392, 2012.

[8] S. Kouki and M. Guerfel, "Eagle's syndrome presenting as a cervical mass," *BMJ Case Reports*, vol. 2013, p. bcr2013200312, 2013.

[9] Y. Fujita, H. Chisoku, G. Shimizu, I. Kato, T. Imai, and Y. Yura, "A case of elongated styloid process reaching the hyoid bone," *Japanese Journal of Oral and Maxillofacial Surgery*, vol. 59, no. 10, pp. 663–666, 2013.

[10] L. M. Ghosh and S. P. Dubey, "The syndrome of elongated styloid process," *Auris Nasus Larynx*, vol. 26, no. 2, pp. 169–175, 1999.

29

Intranasal Lobular Capillary Hemangioma with Multiple Sites of Origin during Pregnancy

Lama S. Alalula,[1] **Abdullah S. Arafat**,[2] **Riyadh A. Alhedaithy**,[2] **and Mohammed Elkrim**[2]

[1]*College of Medicine–King Saud bin Abdulaziz University for Health Sciences, Riyadh 11426, Saudi Arabia*
[2]*Division of Otolaryngology–Head and Neck Surgery, Department of Surgery, King Abdulaziz Medical City, National Guard Health Affairs, Riyadh, Saudi Arabia*

Correspondence should be addressed to Abdullah S. Arafat; arafat.as@outlook.sa

Academic Editor: Andrea Gallo

In the present case report, we describe a 33-year-old pregnant woman in the third trimester with a history of recurrent epistaxis leading to frequent visits to the emergency department. Each episode of epistaxis was managed by anterior nasal packing. During endoscopic examination, a left nasal mass was seen. She was admitted and managed conservatively until she delivered her baby without complication. After delivery, a CT scan was taken, which showed an enhancing mass in the middle and lower meatus of the nasal cavity with no bony erosions. For symptomatic relief and tissue diagnosis, endoscopic surgical removal was advised. An intraoperative examination revealed a red, smooth, and well-circumscribed mass occupying the left nasal cavity and originating from the medial surface of the inferior turbinate and the inferior surface of the posterior part of the middle turbinate. A complete en bloc resection of the mass was performed endoscopically. The mass was sent for histologic analysis, which confirmed the diagnosis of lobular capillary hemangioma. Eventually, upon follow-up at two weeks, one month, three months, and six months postsurgery, no evidence of recurrence was detected.

1. Introduction

Hemangiomas are benign vascular lesions commonly found on the skin and oral mucosa, with the nasal cavity being a rare site of involvement [1, 2]. They are classified according to their histopathological features. Lobular capillary hemangiomas (LCHs) visualized with a microscope contain numerous lobulated and dilated capillaries [1, 3]. Many names have been given to LCHs, including pyogenic granuloma and capillary granuloma, which indicate that its pathophysiology is still unknown [1, 4]. Studies have shown LCHs development to be associated with hormonal factors and local traumatic events to the skin or mucosa [1–5]. The anterior septum is the most frequently affected site, with epistaxis and nasal obstruction being predominating symptoms [1–5]. Proper investigations, including those that employ imaging techniques such as nasal endoscopy, are essential to differentiate LCHs from other dangerous entities, such as inflammatory or neoplastic lesions [1–5]. Despite the availability of multiple treatment options, surgical excision is the most effective form of management [1, 2]. In this case report, we describe a 33-year-old female patient in late pregnancy with a history of recurrent episodes of epistaxis and multiple visits to the emergency department. She was also found to have LCH with unusual and multiple sites of origin in the lateral wall of the nasal cavity.

2. Case Presentation

In June 2017, a 33-year-old gravida 3, para 2 female in her third trimester presented (ED) with active left nasal bleeding to the emergency department at King Abdulaziz Medical City in Riyadh, Saudi Arabia. The patient's vitals were stable upon presentation and she denied any history of trauma or nose picking. Additionally, she complained of a one-month history of persistent left-sided nasal obstruction. The patient was free of medical diagnoses and had no personal or family history of bleeding disorders or any other conditions.

Anterior nasal packing was applied, and bleeding stopped two hours later. Her hemoglobin level was 9.9 mg/dL. Normal saline nasal irrigation was prescribed, and first aid instructions were given. Nasal packs were removed, and the patient was advised to come back if bleeding recurred. Ten days later, the patient returned to the ED with another episode of epistaxis that was managed conservatively. At that time, her hemoglobin levels were 9.4 mg/dL. She was discharged and advised to follow up with otorhinolaryngology. On the same day, she arrived at the ED for a second time with epistaxis of moderate severity. Again, minimal anterior nasal packing was applied, and the patient was sent home. On the next day, she returned to the ED for the third time in 48 hours with active bleeding from her left nostril. Her hemoglobin level at this point measured 8.7 mg/dL. During a bed side examination, the right nasal cavity appeared clear. However, the left nasal cavity evidenced a large clot with moderate bleeding. A nasal endoscopy was performed, which revealed a large, red, smooth, and rounded mass in the left nasal cavity that was actively bleeding upon any application of pressure. The bleeding stopped with properly sized anterior nasal packing, and the patient was rehydrated with intravenous fluids. Obstetrics and Gynecology and Otorhinolaryngology (ORL) teams were consulted. Since the patient was in her 38th week of pregnancy, a decision was made to retain the nasal pack for 48 hours more and admit her for spontaneous delivery, after which she would be reassessed. Two days later, the patient delivered, and both the mother and the baby were in good health. The day after delivering, the patient was taken to the ORL clinic for reassessment. The nasal pack was removed, after which the patient proceeded to actively bleed. Endoscopic assessment illustrated no changes to the nasal mass. Her hemoglobin dropped to 7.8 mg/dL. A blood transfusion was recommended, but the patient refused one. On the same day, a contrasted CT scan of the paranasal sinuses was scheduled, which revealed a heterogeneously enhanced soft tissue mass involving the middle and lower meatus of the left nasal cavity measuring 3.2 × 2.2 × 1.5 cm with normal adjacent bony structures (Figure 1). Two treatment options were discussed with the patient. The first was to wait for spontaneous regression of the mass following hormonal withdrawal after delivery. The second was to undergo complete surgical excision for quick symptomatic relief and tissue diagnosis, which the patient agreed to. The surgery was explained to the patient and informed, written consent was obtained. During intraoperative examination using a telescope, a large, well-circumscribed, red, smooth mass occupying the left nasal cavity and originating from the medial surface of the inferior turbinate and the inferior surface of the posterior part of the middle turbinate was visualized without any attachment to the nasal septum (Figure 2). The mass was initially injected with lidocaine and epinephrine (1 : 100,000) and then excised completely from its site of origin via bipolar diathermy which resulted in no significant bleeding (Figure 3). Gross histopathological analysis revealed a polypoidal tissue mass measuring 3.0 × 1.5 × 1.0 cm with a smooth and glistening surface (Figure 4). Microscopically, the mass was composed of numerous capillaries, likely associated with edema, and inflamed stroma with no malignant cells noted. Based on this, a diagnosis of LCH was made (Figure 5). Postoperatively, left-sided nasal obstruction markedly improved. The patient was stable and recovered well with no additional episodes of epistaxis or requirement for blood transfusion. She was consequently discharged on the same day in good condition. The patient was completely asymptomatic during follow-up appointments in our clinic at two weeks, one month, three months, and six months postoperatively, with healthy mucosa and no evidence of mass recurrence during endoscopic nasal examination (Figure 6).

3. Discussion

Lobular capillary hemangioma is a rare, rapidly growing, benign tumor featuring vascular malformation [1, 5]. It was first described by Poncet and Dor in 1897 as botryomycosis hominis based on the assumption that it arose secondary to a fungal infection [6]. Because it has since been shown to be neither infectious nor granulomatous, the term pyogenic granuloma is now considered a misnomer [2, 3]. Based on its histopathological features, the name LCH was assigned to these tumors by Miller [7]. Grossly, it appears as a polypoidal mass with an ulcerated surface that is covered with fibrin and blood [7]. Microscopically, it is further characterized by an association with numerous capillary sized blood vessels featuring edematous and inflamed stroma [2–4, 7]. LCH can be either pedunculated, meaning that it has a stalk that attaches the mass to its site of origin, or it can be sessile, meaning that the mass is fixed to its base without any peduncles [8]. Mills et al. reviewed 639 vascular lesions found in the oral cavity and upper respiratory tract [7]. Of those lesions, 73 had characteristics of LCH. Among those cases, the most commonly affected site was the lip, followed by the nose, oral mucosa, and tongue. Another study by Ash and Old reviewed 3000 nasal polyps, 23 of which were found to be sinonasal hemangiomas [9]. When found in the nasal cavity, the most common site for these tumors to present is on the anterior nasal septum, followed by the nasal vestibule, inferior turbinate, middle turbinate, and uncinate process, as Puxeddu et al. concluded in a retrospective study of 40 patients [4, 10]. In pregnancy, the prevalence of these tumors ranges from 0.5% to 5% [10]. Table 1 summarizes five different cases of pregnant women in whom LCHs originated from dissimilar sites and were of different sizes [11–15]. LCH affects both genders beyond the age of 40 years equally. Despite this, there is a predominance of females who are affected by LCH in the third decade while males are more often affected if less than 18 years old [16]. At present, no underlying mechanisms for the development of LCH have been demonstrated. Nevertheless, the most prevalent risk factors for LCH development include local trauma to the skin and mucus membranes, as is seen with nose picking, as well as hormonal imbalances, as occur in pregnancy and in women who use oral contraceptives or are postmenopausal [16]. Furthermore, LCH often presents with recurrent unilateral epistaxis, nasal obstruction, and discharge, and proper examination and imaging studies are essential to exclude other causes of a similar intranasal mass,

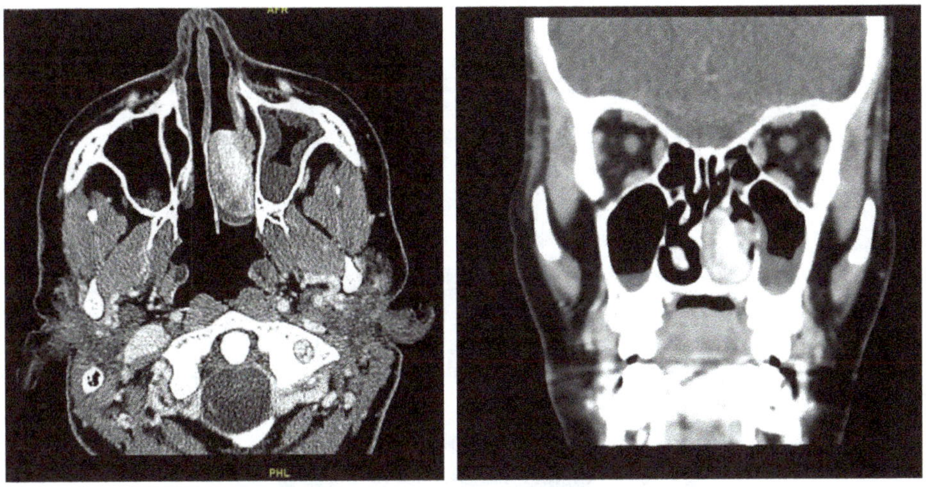

Figure 1: Axial and coronal sinus CT scans with contrast showing a heterogeneously enhanced mass involving the middle and lower meatus of the left nasal cavity with normal adjacent bony structures. In its maximum dimensions, the mass measured $3.2 \times 2.2 \times 1.5$ cm.

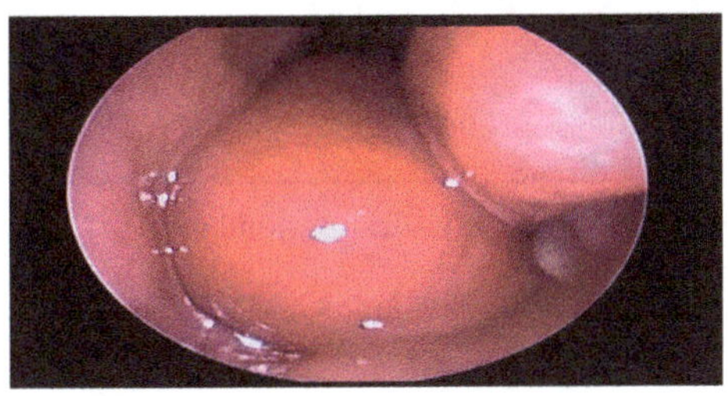

Figure 2: A preoperative endoscopic examination revealed a mass occupying the left nasal cavity.

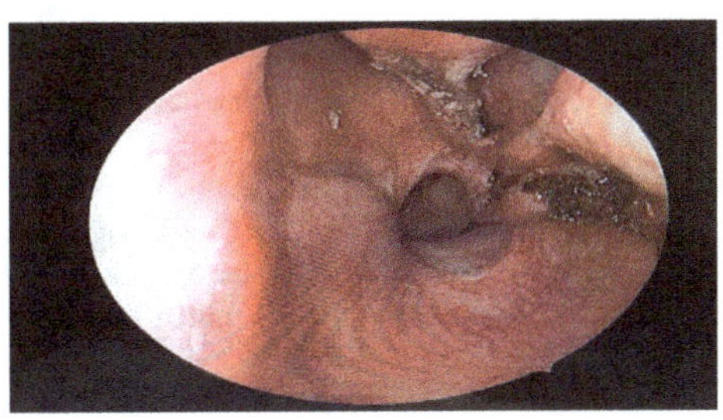

Figure 3: An intraoperative endoscopic examination after complete excision of a left nasal cavity mass revealed two sites of origin in the lateral nasal wall: the medial surface of the inferior turbinate and the inferior surface of the posterior part of the middle turbinate.

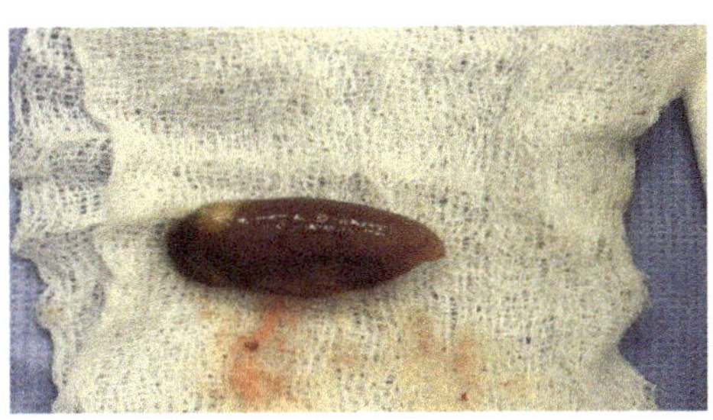

Figure 4: Gross appearance of the mass after excision, which had a smooth and glistening surface.

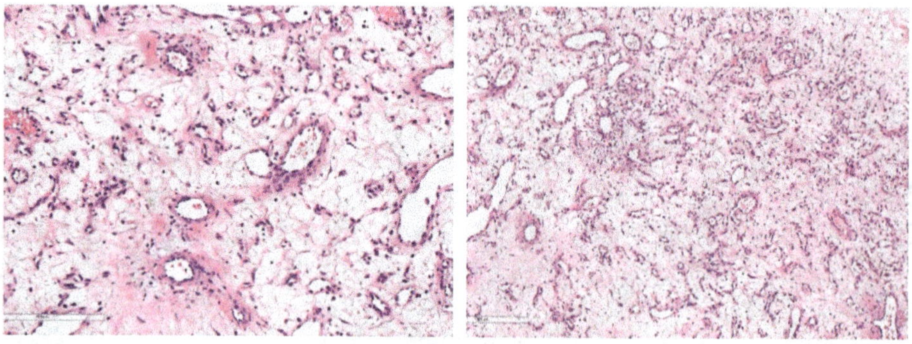

FIGURE 5: Microscopic examination of the tumor revealed lobulated and dilated capillaries with edematous stroma, confirming the diagnosis of lobular capillary hemangioma.

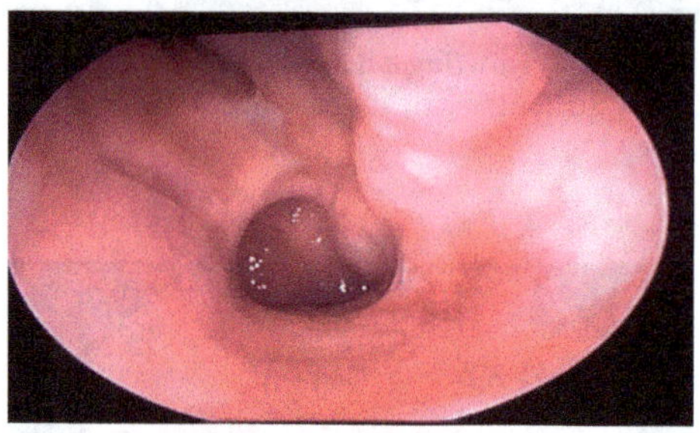

FIGURE 6: A 3-month postoperative examination via endoscopy indicating good mucosal healing at the site of procedure with no evidence of recurrence.

TABLE 1: A summary of the case presented in this report and other lobular capillary hemangioma cases found in the literature.

Case	Age	Trimester	Symptoms	Size	Site	Treatment
Our patient	33	Third	Epistaxis and nasal obstruction	3.2 × 2.2 × 1.5 cm	The medial surface of the inferior turbinate and the inferior surface of the posterior part of the middle turbinate	Postpartum excision under general anesthesia
1	35	Third	Epistaxis and nasal obstruction	1 × 1 cm and a pedicle with a base of 0.5 cm	Anterior part of the septum in the right nasal cavity	Antepartum excision under local anesthesia
2	33	Third	Nasal obstruction	2 × 1.5 cm	Lateral nasal wall in the nasal valve area of the left nasal cavity	Postpartum excision under local anesthesia
3	34	Third	Epistaxis and a rapidly growing mass	25 × 32 × 16 mm	Attached to the nasal septum	Antepartum excision under general anesthesia
4	34	After delivery	Epistaxis and nasal obstruction	4 × 5 cm	Inferior turbinate in the left nasal cavity	Preoperative embolization and postpartum excision under general anesthesia
5	30	Third	Epistaxis and nasal obstruction	4.0 × 2.8 × 2.0 cm	Right nasal vestibule	Postpartum excision under general anesthesia

inflammation, or neoplastic lesions [1]. The lobular arrangement of nasal capillaries differentiates LCH from granulation tissue in which there is a parallel capillary arrangement. Telangiectasia should be excluded if the patient has a family history of hereditary hemorrhagic telangiectasia and angiofibroma should be considered in the differential diagnosis if the patient is a male adolescent [1]. Typically, LCH presents as a well-circumscribed mass with marked enhancement and an absence of calcification on CT scans [17]. In the literature, different modalities have been utilized to treat LCH, such as intranasal steroids and harmonic scalpel, though endoscopic surgical resection remains the treatment of choice [5].

4. Conclusion

Based on the case study presented here, lobular capillary hemangioma (LCH) should be suspected if a pregnant woman has an intranasal mass causing nasal obstruction and recurrent epistaxis. In the patient described here, pregnancy was a risk factor that might have contributed to the development of LCH. However, further studies are needed to demonstrate the cause-effect relationship between pregnancy and LCH. Furthermore, the mass originated from the inferior and middle turbinate, which are uncommon sites of involvement. Finally, this patient underwent endoscopic surgical excision, which is the treatment of choice most supported by the literature, and was given a histologic diagnosis of LCH.

Conflicts of Interest

The authors declare that there are no conflicts of interest regarding the publication of this article.

Acknowledgments

We would like to thank the radiology department and Dr. Abdullatif Khan from the pathology department at King Abdulaziz Medical City, Riyadh, Saudi Arabia.

References

[1] A. Ragab, S. Rabiea, T. Alchammaa, and M. Ghobashy, "Lobular capillary hemangioma of the lateral nasal wall," *Anveshana Ayurveda Medical Journal*, vol. 13, no. 4, 2015.

[2] P. Kamath, V. Shenoy, and A. Mukundan, "Lobular capillary hemangioma of the nasal septum—a case report," *Egyptian Journal of Ear, Nose, Throat and Allied Sciences*, vol. 15, no. 3, pp. 255–257, 2014.

[3] P. Patil, S. Singla, R. Mane, and K. Jagdeesh, "Nasal lobular capillary hemangioma," *Journal of Clinical Imaging Science*, vol. 3, no. 1, p. 40, 2013.

[4] T. H. Chi, C. H. Yuan, and S. T. Chien, "Lobular capillary hemangioma of the nasal cavity: a retrospective study of 15 cases in Taiwan," *Balkan Medical Journal*, vol. 33, no. 1, pp. 69–71, 2014.

[5] S. K. Jha, D. Roy, A. Pal, and S. Jha, "Lobular capillary hemangioma of nose: case report and literature review," *Otolaryngology Online Journal*, vol. 5, no. 1, 2015.

[6] A. Poncet and L. Dor, "Botyromycose Humaine," *Revue de Chirurgie (Paris)*, vol. 18, p. 996, 1897.

[7] S. E. Mills, P. H. Cooper, and R. E. Fechner, "Lobular capillary hemangioma: the underlying lesion of pyogenic granuloma. a study of 73 cases from the oral and nasal mucous membranes," *American Journal of Surgical Pathology*, vol. 4, no. 5, pp. 470–479, 1980.

[8] A. Albossiouny, "Case series: lobular capillary hemangioma of the nasal cavity in pregnancy," *Medical Journal of Cairo University*, vol. 78, no. 1, pp. 237–240, 2010.

[9] J. E. Ash and J. W. Old, "Hemangiomas of the nasal septum," *Transactions American Academy of Ophthalmology and Otolaryngology*, vol. 54, pp. 350–356, 1950.

[10] R. Puxeddu, M. Berlucchi, G. P. Ledda, G. Parodo, D. Farina, and P. Nicolai, "Lobular capillary hemangioma of the nasal cavity: a retrospective study on 40 patients," *American Journal of Rhinology*, vol. 20, no. 4, pp. 480–484, 2006.

[11] Y. Noorizan and H. Salina, "Nasal septal hemangioma in pregnancy," *Medical Journal of Malaysia*, vol. 65, no. 1, pp. 70-71, 2010.

[12] H. Kurtaran, N. ARK, T. Yilmaz, A. Ayrim, and D. Aktas, "Lobular capillary hemangioma of the nasal valve area which appears during pregnancy," *New Journal of Medicine*, vol. 26, pp. 120-121, 2009.

[13] R. E. Oakes, S. J. Frampton, and P. M. Scott, "Granuloma gravidarum: management," *Journal of Obstetrics and Gynaecology*, vol. 32, no. 8, p. 805, 2012.

[14] S. Choudhary, C. MacKinnon, G. Morriessey, and S. Tan, "A case of giant nasal pyogenic granuloma gravidarum," *International Journal of Oral & Maxillofacial Surgery*, vol. 27, pp. 327–333, 1998.

[15] I. Hsu, L. Liao, P. Lou, and J. Shih, "Pyogenic granuloma of the nasal cavity: an unusual complication of pregnancy," *Taiwanese Journal of Obstetrics and Gynecology*, vol. 44, no. 1, 2005.

[16] M. G. Koo, S. H. Lee, and S. E. Han, "Pyogenic granuloma: a retrospective analysis of cases treated over a 10-year," *Archives of Craniofacial Surgery*, vol. 18, no. 1, pp. 16–20, 2017.

[17] J. H. Kim, S. W. Park, and S. C. Kim, "Computed tomography and magnetic resonance imaging findings of nasal cavity hemangiomas according to histological type," *Korean Journal of Radiology*, vol. 16, no. 3, pp. 566–574, 2015.

30

A Case of Septicemia due to Nonocclusive Mesenteric Ischemia Occurring in Induction Chemotherapy

Hideki Tanaka, Kiyoaki Tsukahara, Isaku Okamoto, Rio Kojima, Kazuhiro Hirasawa, and Hiroki Sato

Department of Otorhinolaryngology, Head and Neck Surgery, Tokyo Medical University, Tokyo, Japan

Correspondence should be addressed to Hideki Tanaka; hide.cola31@gmail.com

Academic Editor: Dinesh K. Chhetri

In nonocclusive mesenteric ischemia (NOMI), mesenteric ischemia and intestinal necrosis occur despite the absence of organic blockage in mesenteric blood vessels. As abdominal pain is often absent and few characteristic findings are seen in blood biochemistry, imaging diagnosis or other examinations, discovery is often delayed. With a mortality rate of 56–79%, NOMI is a very serious disease. However, few reports have described this pathology in association with chemotherapy regimens such as those used for malignant head and neck tumors. We encountered a case of NOMI during induction therapy combining cisplatin, docetaxel, and 5-fluorouracil. The patient was a 74-year-old man receiving chemotherapy for T2N2bM0 stage IVA oropharyngeal carcinoma. Febrile neutropenia appeared on treatment day 8. An antibacterial agent and a granulocyte colony-stimulating factor were administered, but septic shock developed and he was transferred to the intensive care unit. Abdominal distension was present and contrast-enhanced computed tomography of the abdomen suggested NOMI. Emergency surgery on day 9 resected the necrotized small intestine and created a single-hole ileostomy. The patient subsequently recovered with 2 weeks of continuous hemodiafiltration and other intensive therapies. Otolaryngological surgeons seldom encounter intestinal diseases, which are thus easily overlooked. The present case report may help in achieving early diagnosis.

1. Introduction

Induction chemotherapy combining the 3 agents of cisplatin (CDDP), docetaxel (DOC), and 5-fluorouracil (5-FU) is standard treatment in head and neck cancer. This triple-therapy is also referred to as TPF (Taxotere, Platinol, and fluorouracil). As TPF is a powerful therapy, adverse events are frequent, and sometimes fatal.

Nonocclusive mesenteric ischemia (NOMI) is an intestinal blood flow disorder without blockage of the main trunk of the mesenteric artery. NOMI has few specific clinical symptoms and findings on medical examinations. As diagnosis is often delayed and irreversible intestinal necrosis results, NOMI is a serious disease. This pathology has a wide range of causes, and chemotherapy has been reported as one. However, no previous reports have described NOMI occurring as a complication of chemotherapy in head and neck cancer [1–4]. We report herein a case of NOMI due to induction chemotherapy with TPF for oropharyngeal carcinoma.

2. Case Details

The patient was a 74-year-old man who was examined for the major complaint of swelling in the right neck. His medical history included pneumonia and sensorineural hearing loss, but no family history of note was elicited. He had smoked 40 cigarettes a day until 32 years old. He had first noted swelling of the right neck 5 years earlier, and had been referred to our department in April 2016 after noticing a growing tendency. Pharyngolaryngeal endoscopy had revealed swelling of the lateral wall on the right side of the oropharynx. On cervico-thoracic contrast-enhanced computerized tomography (CT), a mass with a maximum diameter of 24 mm was noted in the lateral wall of the right oropharynx, but no infiltration into the parapharyngeal space or epiglottis was seen. Swelling was also observed in the right upper and middle deep neck lymph nodes and the right node of Rouviere. In blood biochemistry, a squamous cell carcinoma-related antigen was elevated to 2.8 ng/mL. Biopsy of the right oropharynx lateral wall revealed p40-and p16-positive squamous cell carcinoma. The diagnosis was T2N2bM0 stage IVA oropharyngeal carcinoma of the right lateral wall. The treatment plan was to manage the disease through induction chemotherapy with TPF. As induction chemotherapy, CDDP and DOC were both administered at 60 mg/m^2 on day 1 and 5-FU at 600 mg/m^2 from day 1 to day 5. Daily urine volume was ≥3,000 mL. Although bodyweight decreased day by day from day 4, compared to before the start of chemotherapy, no deterioration in patient condition had been seen; so, we kept the patient under observation with particular attention to vital signs. On day 8, neutrophil count had dropped to 2250/μL and blood pressure fell to 70/50 mmHg. However, as no fever was evident, febrile neutropenia was ruled out. As fluid balance continued to be negative each day, we conducted fluid replacement for extracellular fluids to prevent dehydration. The diarrhea that appeared was considered to be drug-induced colitis due to 5-FU, and symptomatic treatment was initiated. On day 9, he showed a fever of 38.0°C, and neutrophil count had decreased to 212/μL. Febrile neutropenia was diagnosed, and administration of cefepime (CFPM), an antibacterial agent, and a granulocyte colony-stimulating factor (G-CSF) agent was commenced. However, 3 h later, the patient lost consciousness and blood pressure fell to 50/40 mmHg. Septic shock was diagnosed, and he was transferred to the Intensive Care Unit (ICU). Treatment of the septic shock according to early goal-directed therapy was combined with continuous hemodiafiltration and polymyxin B-immobilized fiber column hemoperfusion. As nausea and marked abdominal distension were present, contrast-enhanced CT of the abdomen was conducted (Figures 1 and 2). While a decrease in contrast effect was observed in the small intestine wall, no prominent thrombosis of the mesenteric artery or veins was observed, so NOMI was considered. In consultation with our gastrointestinal surgery department, conservative therapy was considered problematic, and the decision was made to conduct emergency surgery. Partial resection of the small intestine was performed and an ileostomy was created. Numerous ischemic locations were seen in the small intestine, and about 1 m of the intestine was resected (Figure 3). No intestinal perforation or intraperitoneal contamination was observed. Postoperative pathological examination showed necrosis in the intestinal wall but no organic blockage or blood clots in the mesenteric artery.

On day 2 after surgery, the shock abated. On day 12, the patient was returned to the general ward from the ICU. Contrast-enhanced CT of the neck on postoperative day 15 showed partial response of the oropharyngeal carcinoma. As additional chemotherapy was considered problematic, treatment with cetuximab was conducted in combination with radiotherapy. Both the primary cancer and neck lymph node lesions subsequently disappeared. After half a year, the ileostomy was closed off. In the 9 months following the completion of treatment, no recurrence or metastasis was observed.

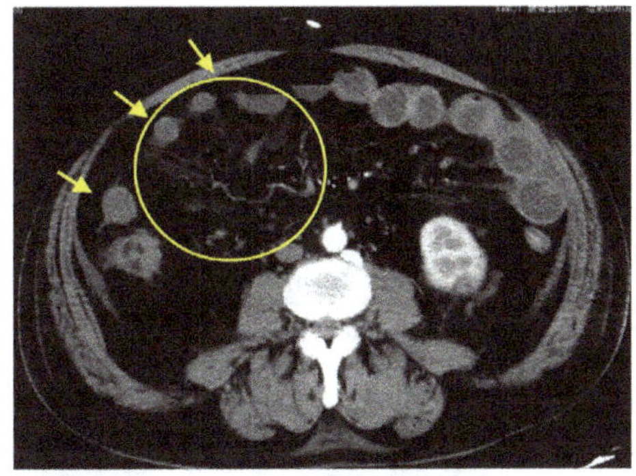

Figure 1: Axial-section contrast-enhanced CT of the abdomen performed in the ICU. Poor contrast effects can be seen in the small intestine (arrows). Disruption of peripheral blood vessels of the superior mesenteric artery is apparent (circled).

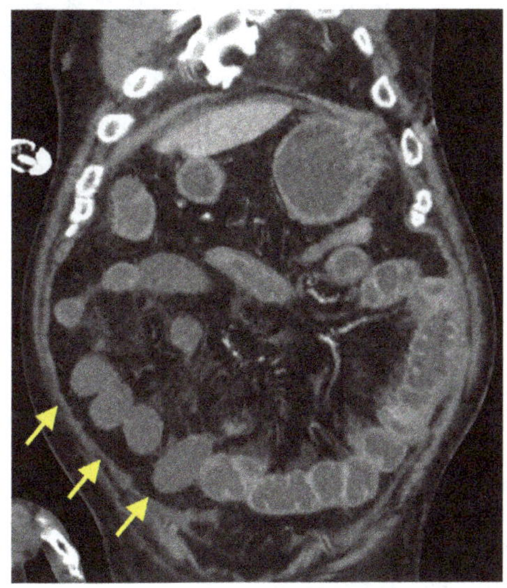

Figure 2: Coronal-section contrast-enhanced CT of the abdomen performed in the ICU. Poor contrast effects can be seen in the small intestine (arrows).

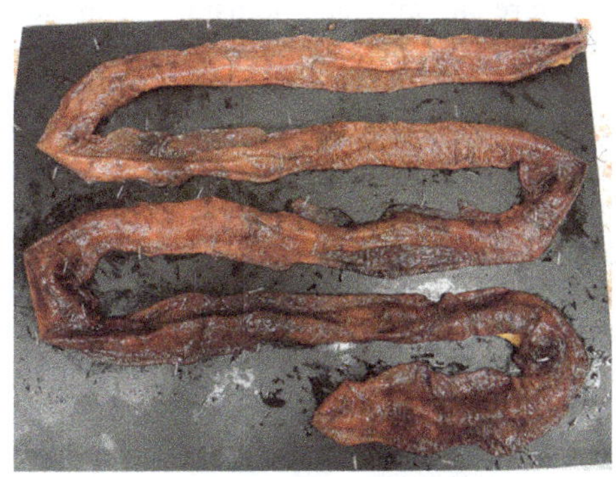

Figure 3: Resected small intestine. Multiple ischemic locations are seen, for around 200 cm from the ligament of Treitz to about 10 cm from the terminal ileum.

3. Discussion

NOMI is a disease of the mesenteric blood vessels without organic blockage that causes mesenteric ischemia and intestinal necrosis. This pathology is the cause of 15–27% of intestinal ischemia and shows a high mortality rate of 56–79% [5, 6]. However, patients frequently show few

TABLE 1: Previously reported case of NOMI during chemotherapy.

Author	Age/sex	Cancer region	Chemotherapy regimen	Year reported
Pearson et al. [3]	53/female	Metastatic liver cancer	CDDP, ADM, MMC	2008
Awano et al. [1]	80/female	Lung Adenocarcinoma	gefitinib	2013
Matsuzawa et al. [4]	74/female	Melanoma	DTIC, ACNU, VCR, ß-interferon	2015
Yamane et al. [2]	68/male	Small cell lung cancer	CDDP, ETP	2015
Present case	74/male	Oropharynx cancer	CDDP, 5-FU, DOC	2017

CDDP: cisplatin; ADM: adriamycin; MMC: mitomycin C; CBDCA: carboplatin; DTIC: dacarbazine; ACNU: nimustine; VCR: vincristine; ETP: etoposide; DOC: docetaxel.

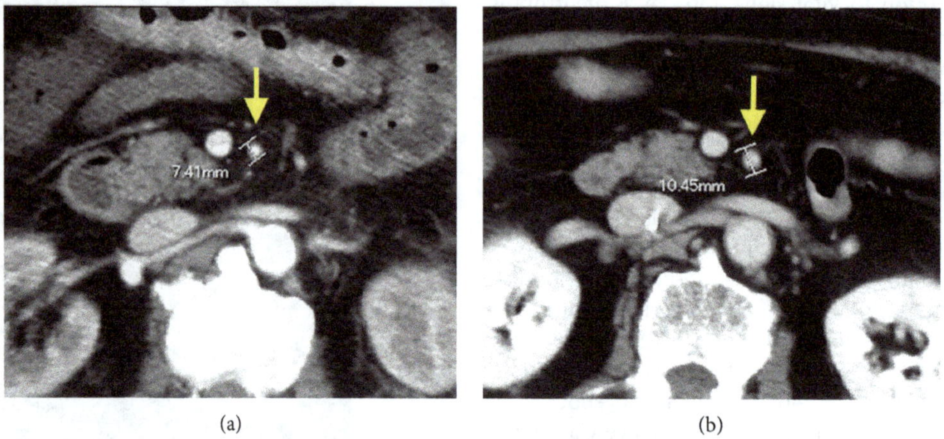

FIGURE 4: Coronal-section contrast-enhanced CT of the abdomen. (a) Before surgery. (b) 3 months after surgery. The diameter of the superior mesenteric artery is 7.41 mm before surgery and 10.45 mm at 3 months after surgery (arrows).

findings from blood biochemistry or imaging examinations. One reason for the high mortality rate is delayed discovery because of the lack of characteristic findings. Abdominal distension and abdominal pain were observed in the present case, but abdominal pain is not seen in 20–30% of cases [7–9].

The major features in the pathology of NOMI are an extreme drop and unevenness in intestinal blood flow. Another cause is peripheral vascular spasm due to exaggerated responses in sympathetic nerves and fluid factors, such as vasopressin and angiotensin, accompanying decreases in cardiac output and circulating plasma volume [10]. The three major risks are thus congestive heart failure, digitalis intoxication, and hemagglutination. Other causes include sympathomimetic drugs, diuretics, dialysis, and septic shock. However, chemotherapy has not been reported as a risk factor for NOMI.

A search of PubMed for NOMI and chemotherapy found only 4 cases of NOMI due to chemotherapy (Table 1). However, the sites of the primary cancer and regimens varied. Various adverse events occur with chemotherapy and may cause NOMI as a secondary effect. In the present case, daily decreases in bodyweight were seen from day 4 of administering TPF, and hemoconcentration, one of the risk factors for NOMI, occurred. Also, as septic shock resulted from febrile neutropenia, impaired blood flow in the intestinal mucosa was considered to have been exacerbated.

Drug-induced colitis may occur as an adverse event of the 5-FU used in TPF therapy. Symptoms are diarrhea and nausea in mild cases and hemorrhagic colitis and necrotizing enterocolitis in serious cases, resembling NOMI. However, major differences exist between these pathologies regarding treatment and prognosis. In 5-FU-induced colitis, 1.8% of all diarrhea that occurs may be fatal [11]. Furthermore, NOMI may be hidden among patients diagnosed with 5-FU-induced colitis.

With the NOMI diagnosis algorithm used in the United States, selective angiography has been suggested as the number-one diagnostic modality. However, when NOMI is discovered, systemic conditions are frequently unstable. The rate of conducting selective angiography is thus reportedly low [12]. Diagnostic criteria for mesenteric vascular spasm are proximal stenosis of the superior mesenteric artery and main branch, abnormal images of mesenteric branches, arcade spasm of the mesenteric artery, and poor contrast on internal images of the blood vessels in the mesenteric wall.

The appearance of multidetector row CT (MDCT) in recent years has improved the visualization of veins. MDCT allows angiography diagnostic criteria-related findings to be evaluated [13]. With MDCT, it is also possible to diagnose loss of blood flow contrast effect in the intestinal wall and thinning of the intestinal wall due to decreased mesenteric blood flow. Intestinal ischemia is regional in nature, from the small intestine to the colon, and is distributed unevenly. Regarding the present case, the presence of an extensive poor contrast effect in the intestinal wall and vascular disruption in the superior mesenteric artery periphery on MDCT led to the diagnosis of NOMI. Compared with the results of CT 3 months after surgery, the superior mesenteric artery appeared narrowed on CT before surgery (Figure 4). However, angiography should be performed in accordance with the American standards where possible. Regrettably, due to the emergency nature of the intervention and in-hospital circumstances, we were unable to perform angiography.

Thinking that the present case represented 5-FU-induced colitis, the patient had initially been put under observation, with only fluid replenishment and symptomatic treatment. If we had performed MDCT at that time, the disease state may not have become as serious. The drug 5-FU and its derivatives are a major part of treatment in head and neck cancer, and inclusion of NOMI among the differential diagnoses of colitis is therefore important.

Treatment of NOMI can be divided into surgical and nonsurgical methods. For the latter, continuous intra-arterial infusion of vasodilators, such as papaverine hydrochloride, is useful. Peritoneal irritation symptoms are often an indicator for surgery. However, in many cases, physical findings cannot be relied upon in elderly patients and those in a poor state of consciousness. Nakao et al. actively performed surgery without angiography for 17 patients with NOMI complicated by shock, and found that colectomy was necessary in 14 patients (82%) [14].

If an irreversible ischemic state is determined to have developed in the large intestine, as in the present case, surgery is absolutely necessary. In our patient, prompt diagnosis and surgical intervention enabled early infection control, and the early discovery of NOMI potentially saved his life. The emphasis should thus be on early diagnosis of NOMI by means of contrast-enhanced MDCT and teamwork in therapy involving intensive care specialists and gastroenterological surgeons.

4. Conclusion

We encountered a rare case of NOMI occurring during induction chemotherapy for head and neck cancer. Otolaryngology department surgeons such as ourselves seldom encounter intestinal diseases and may overlook them. For NOMI in particular, characteristic clinical findings are few, and differentiation from 5-FU-induced colitis is difficult. However, contrast-enhanced MDCT is useful for distinguishing between these pathologies. The unstable hemodynamics in chemotherapy may cause NOMI. The association between chemotherapy and NOMI should be verified in a larger population.

References

[1] N. Awano, K. Kondoh, T. Andoh, S. Ikushima, T. Kumasaka, and T. Takemura, "Three cases of lung carcinoma complicated by gastrointestinal necrosis and perforation," *Haigan*, vol. 53, no. 6, pp. 809–814, 2013.

[2] H. Yamane, N. Fukuda, K. Nishino et al., "Non-occlusive mesenteric ischemia after splenic metastasectomy for small-cell lung cancer," *Internal Medicine*, vol. 54, no. 7, pp. 743–747, 2015.

[3] A. C. Pearson, S. Steinberg, M. H. Shah, and M. Bloomston, "The complicated management of patient following trans-arterial chemoembolization for metastatic carcinoid," *World Journal of Surgical Oncology*, vol. 6, no. 1, p. 125, 2008.

[4] M. Matsuzawa, K. Harada, N. Hosomura et al., "Non-occlusive mesenteric ischemia after chemotherapy for metastatic melanoma," *Journal of Dermatology*, vol. 42, no. 1, pp. 105-106, 2015.

[5] Y. Mishima, "Acute mesenteric ischemia," *Japanese Journal of Surgery*, vol. 18, no. 6, pp. 615–619, 1988.

[6] S. J. Boley, S. Sprayregan, S. S. Siegelman, and F. J. Veith, "Initial results from an aggressiveroentgenologial and surgicall approach to acute mesenteric ischemia," *Surgery*, vol. 82, pp. 848–855, 1977.

[7] L. G. Britt and R. C. Cheek, "Nonocclusive mesenteric cascular disease: clinical and experimental observantions," *Annals of Surgery*, vol. 169, no. 5, pp. 704–711, 1969.

[8] S. Klotz, T. Vestring, J. Rotker, C. Schmidt, H. H. Scheld, and C. Schmid, "Diagnosis and treatment of nonocclusive mensenteric ischema after open heart surgery," *Annals of Thoracic Surgery*, vol. 72, no. 5, pp. 1583–1586, 2001.

[9] M. Trompeter, T. Brazda, C. T. Remy et al., "Non-occlusive mesenteric ischemia: etiology, diagnosis, and intervenetional therapy," *European Radiology*, vol. 12, no. 5, pp. 1179–1187, 2002.

[10] T. Yamaguchi, "Experimental studies on the etiology of gas in the portal venous system," *Japanese Journal of Gastroenterological Surgery*, vol. 13, no. 11, pp. 1260–1270, 1980.

[11] H. Ogi, Y. Yoshitake, T. Tanaka, M. Yoneda, M. Maki, and M. Shinohara, "A case of serious drug-induced enteritis that developed during chemoradiotherapy with S-1 in a patient with oral cancer," *Japanese Journal of Oral and Maxillofacial Surgery*, vol. 62, no. 7, pp. 352–357, 2016.

[12] T. J. Howard, L. A. Plaskon, E. A. Wiebke, M. G. Wilcox, and J. A. Madura, "Nonocclusive mesenteric ischemia remains a diagnostic dilemma," *American Journal of Surgery*, vol. 171, no. 4, pp. 405–458, 1996.

[13] R. Woodhams, H. Nishimaki, K. Fujii et al., "Usefulness of multidetector-row CT(MDCT) for the diagnosis of non-occlusive mesenteric ischemia (NOMI): assessment of morphology and diameter of the superior mesenteric artery (SMA) on multi-planar reconstructed (MPR) images," *European Journal of Radiology*, vol. 76, no. 1, pp. 96–102, 2010.

[14] S. Nakao, H. Watanabe, Y. Takahashi, H. Yamamoto, and T. Matsuoka, "Effectiveness of emergency laparotomy for diagnosis and treatment of severe non-occlusive mesenteric ischemia (NOMI)," *Journal of Abdominal Emergency Medicine*, vol. 31, no. 7, pp. 1021–1027, 2011.

Primary Atypical Meningioma of the Nasal Cavity

Leison Maharjan, Yogesh Neupane, and Bibhu Pradhan

Department of ENT-HNS, Institute of Medicine (IOM), Kathmandu, Nepal

Correspondence should be addressed to Leison Maharjan; leison.maharjan@gmail.com

Academic Editor: Rong-San Jiang

Background. Meningioma is a central nervous system tumor that typically arises in proximity to meninges. Extracranial primary atypical meningioma of sinonasal tract is a rare one. *Methods.* We discuss the clinical, radiological, and histological presentation of an elderly female with primary atypical meningioma of the nasal cavity, which was excised via endoscopic endonasal approach. *Results.* There was no recurrence even up to 20 months of follow-up after endoscopic excision. *Conclusion.* Extracranial primary atypical meningioma should be kept in mind as one of the differential diagnoses of nasal mass. Histopathological diagnosis along with immunohistochemistry should be used for definitive diagnosis.

1. Introduction

Meningioma is a central nervous system tumor that typically arises in proximity to meninges. Rarely in less than 2% of the cases, meningiomas appear extracranially, especially in head and neck regions, sinonasal tract, ear, temporal bone, and scalp [1]. Histopathological and immunohistochemistry examination is usually diagnostic. WHO (World Health Organization) has classified meningioma into 3 grades: benign, atypical, and anaplastic [2]. Some studies have shown 30% of meningiomas to be atypical [3].

Here, we are presenting a case of primary atypical nasal meningioma.

2. Case Report

A 63-year-old female presented to our outpatient department with complaints of right-sided nasal obstruction and intermittent epistaxis for 6 months. Her nasal obstruction was insidious in onset, gradually progressive, and for the last 3 months, there was complete obstruction. Epistaxis was intermittent, 1 episode in a month, spontaneous, and 250–500 ml in amount in each episode. There was no history of any systemic diseases.

Examination of the nasal cavity revealed pinkish fleshy mass occupying the entire right nasal cavity that bled easily on touch. CECT (contrast-enhanced computed tomography) of the nose and paranasal sinuses (Figure 1) showed heterogeneously enhancing mass in the right nasal cavity, likely centered in middle turbinate with extension into the right ethmoid sinus superiorly and choana and sphenoid sinus posteriorly with erosion of the adjacent bone. There was destruction of the nasal septum along with extension of the mass to the contralateral nasal cavity, features suggestive of inverted papilloma.

To confirm the diagnosis, biopsy of the mass was taken. Histopathological examination (Figure 2) revealed unencapsulated tumor composed of tumor cells arranged in lobules, nests, and sheets with focal whorling pattern in subepithelium. The tumor cells were epithelioid to spindle-shaped with monomorphic round nuclei, moderate amount of eosinophilic cytoplasm, and indistinct cell borders. The chromatin was fine with occasional intranuclear inclusions and many prominent nucleoli. Some areas also showed spindling with oval nucleus arranged in short fascicles. Mitotic figures were present: 4 per 10 high-power field. Neither necrosis nor pigmentation was seen. Features were suggestive of a WHO grade II atypical transitional meningioma. Due to

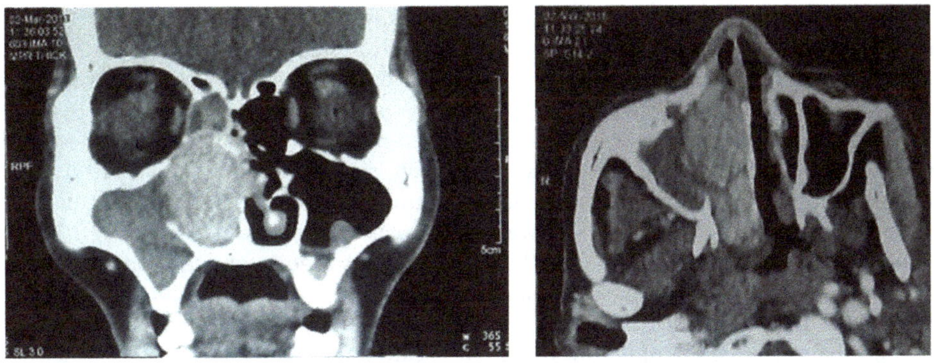

(a) (b)

Figure 1: CECT nose and PNS (coronal and axial cut) showing heterogeneously enhancing mass in the right nasal cavity, likely centered in the middle turbinate with extension into the right ethmoid sinus superiorly, floor of nasal cavity inferiorly, choana and sphenoid sinus posteriorly with the erosion of the adjacent bone, and destruction of the nasal septum with extension of the mass to the contralateral side.

prominent nuclei and S100 positivity, HMB-45 was done which was negative, thus ruling out malignant melanoma.

Initially, preoperative internal maxillary artery embolization was planned, but catheterization could not be performed due to tortuosity of the right common iliac artery. She underwent endoscopic excision of the mass. Preoperatively, there was a pinkish, vascular, and friable mass occupying the right nasal cavity, extending anteriorly up to the anterior end of the right middle turbinate and posteriorly occupying the choana along with extension towards the left side (Figure 3). Superiorly, the mass was attached to the roof of ethmoid and inferiorly to the floor of the right nasal cavity. No destruction of septum was seen as suggested by CECT. There was no recurrence even after 20 months of follow-up.

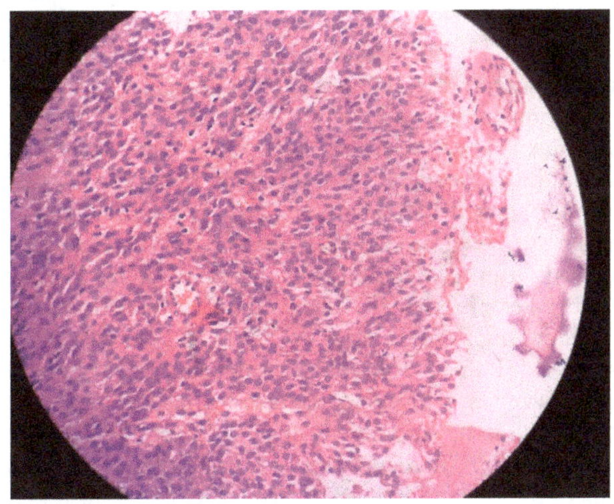

Figure 2: Histopathological examination suggestive of a WHO grade II atypical transitional meningioma (H&E stain).

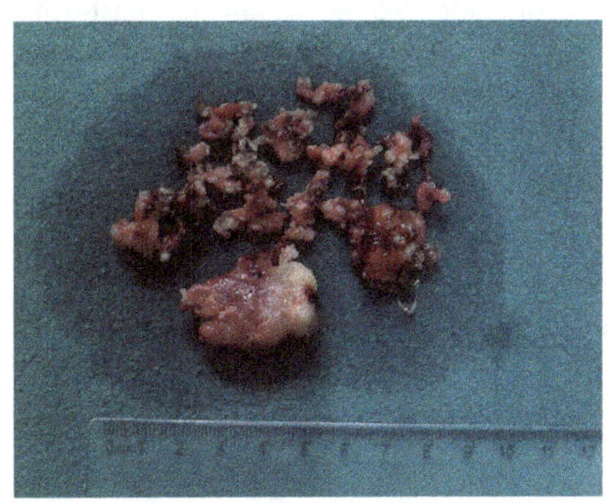

Figure 3: Meningioma after endoscopic excision.

3. Discussions

Meningiomas are nonglial tumors of the central nervous system, representing 24–30% of all intracranial neoplasms. They arise from the arachnoid cap cells (meningocytes) that are derived from the neural crest. These tumors have a predilection for females and have bimodal age distribution with first peak at the second decade of life and second peak during fifth through seventh decades [1, 4]. They have been reported to occur extracranially in only 1-2% of cases, and 20% of extracranial meningiomas are secondary extensions of intracranial tumors [5]. Primary extracranial meningiomas without direct communication with the intracranial region are rare. Histologically, primary extracranial meningiomas are identical to intracranial counterparts.

There are different mechanisms contributing to the development of the extracranial meningiomas. During embryogenesis, when arachnoidal cells that are present in the sheaths of nerves or vessels emerge through the skull foramina, the then displaced Pacchionian bodies are detached, pinched off, or entrapped in an extracranial location. It can also occur following a traumatic event or cerebral hypertension that displaces the arachnoid islets, originated from undifferentiated or multipotent mesenchymal cells, such as fibroblasts, Schwann cells, or a combination of these, perhaps explaining the diverse pathologic spectrum found in meningiomas [1, 6, 7].

Bassiouni et al. have classified primary extradural meningiomas into four types: Type I (epidural), tumor located between the dura mater and the inner calvarial table; Type II (calvarial or diploic), located between the outer and the inner calvarial table; Type III (extracranial), located outside the outer calvarial table; and Type IV (mixed), tumor extending from the dura to extracalvarial space [8].

They have been reported to occur in the sinonasal tract, cranial bones, middle ear, scalp, and soft tissues of the face and neck, and parotid gland. An analysis of 146 cases of primary extracranial meningiomas showed that the majority of them originated from the skin and scalp ($n = 59$) followed by middle ear ($n = 26$) and sinonasal tract ($n = 25$). Other rare locations in the head and neck are the temporal bone, mandible, nasopharynx, parotid gland, orbit, and neck [9].

Symptoms depend on the anatomic site of involvement. Meningiomas involving the sinonasal tract may mimic sinusitis with patients presenting with the nasal obstruction, anosmia, facial pain, nasal discharge, and epistaxis [5, 10]. Some authors describe that an average duration of extracranial sinonasal meningioma is 31.1 months. Nasal endoscopy usually shows a firm reddish pink to grey mass in the nasal cavity which could be globular or lobulated but well circumscribed with displacement and without infiltration into the surrounding tissues [1]. Radiological findings are usually nonspecific and include clouding or opacification of the sinuses, bony sclerosis, and focal destruction of the surrounding sinusoidal or nasal cavity bony tissues [11].

In the current WHO edition (2007), grade I meningiomas (benign) are recognized by their histologic subtype and lack of anaplastic features. Grade II meningiomas (atypical) are defined by one or more of the following four criteria: (1) chordoid or clear cell histologic subtype, (2) 4 to 19 mitoses per ten high-power field (HPFs), (3) brain infiltration, and (4) 3 or more of the following five histologic features: small cell change, increased cellularity, prominent nucleoli, sheet-like growth, or necrosis. Grade III meningiomas (anaplastic/malignant) are defined by rhabdoid or papillary subtypes, a histological picture of frank malignancy resembling that of carcinomas, melanomas, or high-grade sarcomas, or 20 or more mitoses per 10 HPFs [2]. A report of an atypical primary meningioma of nasal septum undergoing malignant transformation with distant metastasis into scalp and anterior chest wall can be found in literature [12].

In a study done in 163 cases, the most common histopathological subtype in primary extracranial meningiomas of head was meningothelial meningioma (53.4%) followed by transitional type (12.3%), psammomatous type (11.7%), and fibrous type (6.7%). Meanwhile microcystic, metaplastic, secretory, and regressive types were rare consisiting of 2.4% [4].

The differential diagnosis of sinonasal tract meningiomas includes mucocele, olfactory neuroblastoma, carcinoma, hemangioma, sarcoma, and angiofibroma [1, 10]. Histopathology and immunohistochemistry are confirmatory. Meningiomas are strongly immunoreactive to vimentin, EMA (epithelial membrane antigen), and pancytokeratin. Besides these, some meningiomas also show positive reactions to CK7, S100 protein, CAM 5.2, synaptophysin, CK20, GFAP, Ki-67 index (>1%), CD34, SMA, PCNA, progesterone receptor, and estrogen receptor [1, 9].

Studies have shown that the growth of the tumor is slow; hence, surgical extirpation without the necessity of adjuvant therapy is the treatment of choice, but complete excision is not always possible due to complex anatomy of nasal cavity and paranasal sinuses [1, 9]. Complete extirpation of these masses may be accomplished by endoscopic, open, or a combination of both approaches. Radiation therapy has been suggested to improve survival in meningiomas of central nervous system, but its role in extracranial meningiomas has not been studied yet. In our case, endoscopic surgery was done, and microdebrider along with monopolar cautery was used to excise the tumor in piecemeal due to vascular nature of the mass. In cases with high-risk tumor locations, stereotactic surgery has shown improved results. Studies have found that tumors ranging from 1 to 8 cm with an average of 3.5 cm usually infiltrate bone of the sinus or nasal cavity and an intact surface epithelium without ulceration or penetration [1].

In our case, there was no recurrence on subsequent follow-up of 20 months. Usually, recurrence occurs at the same anatomic site as the primary lesion, and depending on the time interval, it may be distinguished from the residual disease. A study analyzing the relationships between tumor sites and recurrence and death in 170 cases has found statistically significant difference among recurrence and type of removal. They found 9.7%, 14.3%, and 66.7% recurrence rates in total, subtotal, and partial removal cases, respectively. Further, they found death rates of 5.4% and 28.6% in total and subtotal removal cases, respectively. Recurrence was found to be 8% in benign meningioma, 11.1% in atypical, and 57.1% in malignant type [4]. Additional surgery, if clinically feasible, is advisable as radiation therapy does not always result in a clinical response.

A 5-year disease-free survival rate was found to be 66.9% to 82.1%, and 10-year disease-free survival rate was found to be 54.6% to 78.6% [1, 9]. Death rate of malignant (57.1%) is highest compared to atypical (11.1%) and benign (2.3%) [4].

4. Conclusions

Primary sinonasal atypical meningioma is a rare condition. It should be considered as one of the differential diagnoses of a nasal mass. Histopathological diagnosis along with immunohistochemistry should be used for definitive diagnosis. Excision can be done by endoscopic endonasal approach.

Acknowledgments

The authors are thankful to Dr. Pramila Vaidhya, Department of Pathology, Institute of Medicine (IOM), for providing them the histopathology slide of the case.

References

[1] L. D. R. Thompson and K. A. Gyure, "Extracranial sinonasal tract meningiomas: a clinicopathologic study of 30 cases with a review of the literature," *American Journal of Surgical Pathology*, vol. 24, no. 5, pp. 640–650, 2000.

[2] D. N. Louis, H. Ohgaki, O. D. Wiestler et al., "The 2007 WHO classification of tumours of the central nervous system," *Acta Neuropathologica*, vol. 114, no. 2, pp. 97–109, 2007.

[3] T. Backer-Grøndahl, B. H. Moen, and S. H. Torp, "The histopathological spectrum of human meningiomas," *International Journal of Clinical and Experimental Pathology*, vol. 5, no. 3, pp. 231–242, 2012.

[4] Y. Liu, H. Wang, H. Shao, and C. Wang, "Primary extradural meningiomas in head: a report of 19 cases and review of literature," *International Journal of Clinical and Experimental Pathology*, vol. 8, no. 5, pp. 5624–5632, 2015.

[5] C. D. Friedman, P. D. Costantino, B. Teitelbaum, R. E. Berktold, and G. A. Sisson, "Primary extracranial meningiomas of the head and neck," *Laryngoscope*, vol. 100, no. 1, pp. 41–48, 1990.

[6] C. Y. Chang, S. W. Cheung, and R. K. Jackler, "Meningiomas presenting in the temporal bone: the pathways of spread from an intracranial site of origin," *Otolaryngology-Head and Neck Surgery*, vol. 119, no. 6, pp. 658–664, 1998.

[7] J. G. Batsakis, "Pathology consultation. Extracranial meningiomas," *Annals of Otology, Rhinology & Laryngology*, vol. 93, no. 3, pp. 282-283, 1984.

[8] H. Bassiouni, S. Asgari, U. Hübschen, H. J. König, and D. Stolke, "Dural involvement in primary extradural meningiomas of the cranial vault," *Journal of Neurosurgery*, vol. 105, no. 1, pp. 51–59, 2006.

[9] E. J. Rushing, J. P. Bouffard, S. McCall et al., "Primary extracranial meningiomas: an analysis of 146 cases," *Head and Neck Pathology*, vol. 3, no. 2, pp. 116–130, 2009.

[10] R. E. Swain, T. T. Kingdom, J. M. Del Gaudio, S. Muller, and W. J. Grist, "Meningiomas of the paranasal sinuses," *American Journal of Rhinology*, vol. 15, no. 1, pp. 27–30, 2001.

[11] K. F. Lee, J. H. Suh, Y. E. Lee, and R. G. Berry, "Meningioma of the paranasal sinuses," *Neuroradiology*, vol. 17, no. 3, pp. 165–171, 1979.

[12] B. J. Baek, J. M. Shin, C. K. Lee, J. H. Lee, and K. H. Lee, "Atypical primary meningioma in the nasal septum with malignant transformation and distant metastasis," *BMC Cancer*, vol. 12, no. 1, p. 275, 2012.

32

Non-Hodgkin's Lymphoma of the Middle Ear Presenting as Mastoiditis

Marwan Alqunaee,[1] Abdullah Aldaihani,[2] and Mohammed AlHajery[3]

[1] Otorhinolaryngology, Head and Neck Surgery Resident, Kuwait Institute of Medical Specialization, Kuwait City, Kuwait
[2] Department of Surgery, Adan Hospital, Hadiya, Kuwait
[3] Department of ENT, Zain and Al Sabah Hospitals, Kuwait City, Kuwait

Correspondence should be addressed to Marwan Alqunaee; marwanalqunaee@gmail.com

Academic Editor: Rong-San Jiang

Lymphoma originating from the middle ear is rare. The diagnosis of lymphoma as with other cancers of the temporal bone is often made late, and this has a negative implication on the treatment and prognosis of the condition. The delay of diagnosis is mainly due to the similar presentation shared with other benign conditions of the middle ear. We present a case of a 62-year-old man who was treated as a case of chronic otitis media for a period of time before presenting with advanced symptoms; a final diagnosis of lymphoma of the middle ear was given. Other similar cases in the literature are discussed and reviewed. Severe and persistent symptoms of the middle ear should raise red flags and warrant detailed investigations.

1. Introduction

Lymphoma is a cancer of the reticuloendothelial system; it has two subtypes, Hodgkin's lymphoma and non-Hodgkin's lymphoma. Furthermore, lymphomas constitute 10% of all head and neck tumors; 60% of these are non-Hodgkin's lymphoma and the other 40% are Hodgkin's lymphoma.

Diffuse large cell B lymphoma is the largest subunit of non-Hodgkin's lymphoma, and it is characterized by extranodal involvement. The most common sites of extranodal involvement are the stomach and the gastrointestinal tract; however, lymphoma can present in any type of tissues. The bony involvement comprises 1-2% of malignant lymphomas and 3–5% of extranodal lymphomas; involvement of temporal bone is extremely rare with only few reported cases in the literature [1–3].

2. Case

A 62-year-old man presented to the otolaryngology clinic with a House-Brackmann grade 4 left lower motor facial nerve palsy with a 10-day history of left postauricular pain. This was preceded by 6 months of intermittent purulent discharge from the left ear for which he received multiple antibiotic courses. On examination, the patient was vitally stable; however, he was febrile. The left postauricular area was mildly tender on palpation and the overlying skin was normal. Otoscopic examination of the left ear was only significant for an erythematous and retracted tympanic membrane. The rest of the examination of the right ear along with a full head and neck exam was unremarkable. White blood count was elevated with 13900 (76% neutrophils, 16.2% lymphocytes, and 8.3% monocytes).

The patient was admitted to the hospital and had an initial diagnosis of mastoiditis with facial nerve paralysis. He was started on intravenous antibiotics. High-resolution computed tomography (HRCT) and magnetic resonance imaging were performed (Figures 1–4).

Due to the severe complication of the facial nerve palsy a decision was made for surgical intervention; cortical mastoidectomy with facial nerve decompression and left middle ear exploration was performed. Granulation tissue in the mastoid air cells and the middle ear were encountered

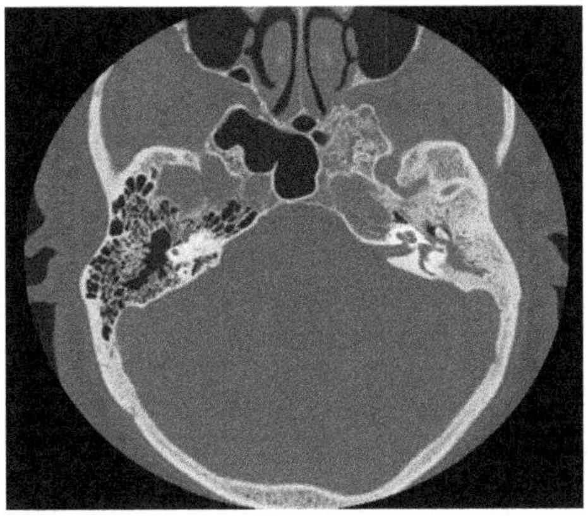

FIGURE 1: High-resolution CT scan (axial cut) of the temporal bone. Total opacification of the left-sided hypo- and mesotympanum by a soft tissue density. Mastoid air cells totally opacified with resorption of septae and partially sclerosed bone. Partial dehiscence of the mastoid portion of the facial nerve canal. The left tympanic membrane is thickened and retracted inwards. The left middle ear ossicles and scutum are intact. Normal aeration of the external auditory canals with intact bony and cartilaginous boundaries. The right middle ear cavity is normally aerated with intact ossicles. The right mastoid air cells are unremarkable.

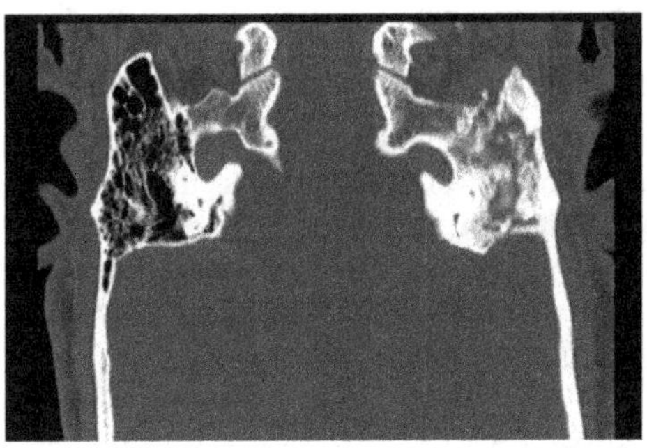

FIGURE 2: High-resolution CT scan (coronal cut) of the temporal bone. Total opacification of the left-sided hypo- and mesotympanum by a soft tissue density. Mastoid air cells totally opacified with resorption of septae and partially sclerosed bone. Partial dehiscence of the mastoid portion of the facial nerve canal. The left tympanic membrane is thickened and retracted inwards. The left middle ear ossicles and scutum are intact. Normal aeration of the external auditory canals with intact bony and cartilaginous boundaries. The right middle ear cavity is normally aerated with intact ossicles. The right mastoid air cells are unremarkable.

and removed. Biopsies were also taken and sent for histopathology.

The histopathological assessment of the tissue revealed diffuse proliferation of large monomorphic atypical lymphoid cells admixed with few medium-sized cells (centroblastic and prominent immunoblastic lymphoid cells) (Figure 5).

The cells showed scant to moderate amphophilic cytoplasm, vesicular nuclei, or focal irregular chromatin clumping with prominent 1-2 nucleoli.

Frequent mitoses and few tumor giant cells were regarded along with subendothelial infiltrate and occasional pseudorosette (Figures 6 and 7).

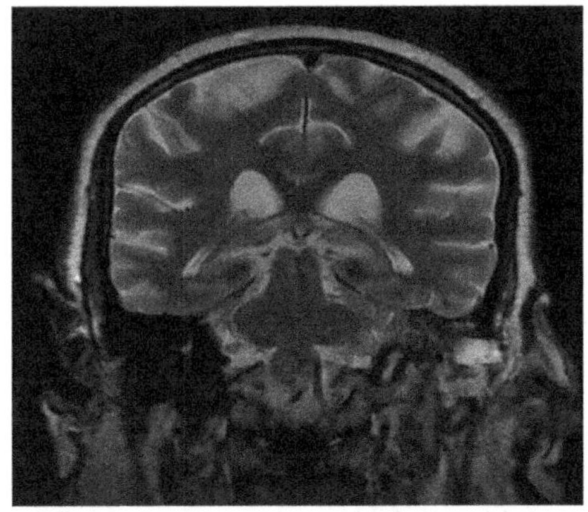

FIGURE 3: MRI of cerebellopontine angles and posterior fossa (coronal cut). Opacification of the left mastoid air cells and middle ear cavity with soft tissue signal which elicits low signal in T1WI and high signal in T2WI with restricted diffusion in DWI. There is homogeneous enhancement following IV contrast administration. No evidence of adjacent intracranial abscess formation or sinus thrombosis. The region of brain stem and cerebellar hemispheres are normal. No focal lesions are seen. Both the VII and VIII cranial nerves show normal course and signal intensity. No intra- or extra-canalicular enhancing lesion is seen.

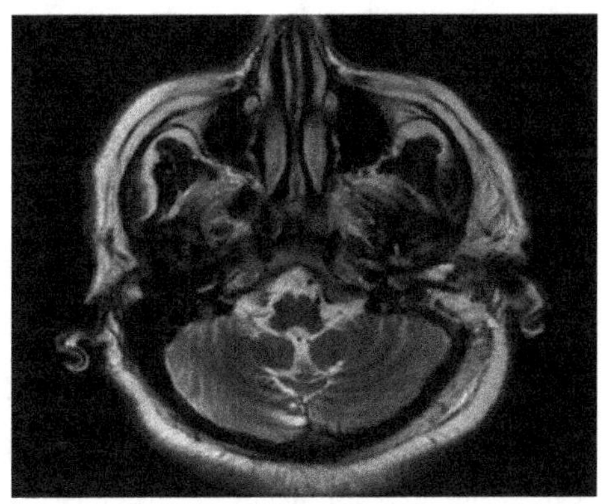

FIGURE 4: MRI of cerebellopontine angles and posterior fossa (axial cut). Opacification of the left mastoid air cells and middle ear cavity with soft tissue signal which elicits low signal in T1WI and high signal in T2WI with restricted diffusion in DWI. There is homogeneous enhancement following IV contrast administration. No evidence of adjacent intracranial abscess formation or sinus thrombosis. The region of brain stem and cerebellar hemispheres are normal. No focal lesions are seen. Both the VII and VIII cranial nerves show normal course and signal intensity. No intra- or extra-canalicular enhancing lesion is seen.

The proliferative fraction as detected by Ki67 immunostaining is very high (80–90% positivity) (Figure 8).

The patient was then transferred to the oncology unit for staging and further management. There was no distant spread and the patient was treated with courses of chemotherapy. At the most recent follow-up his ear symptoms of otalgia and persistent discharge have resolved; however, he still showed a House-Brackmann grade 3 left lower motor neuron facial palsy.

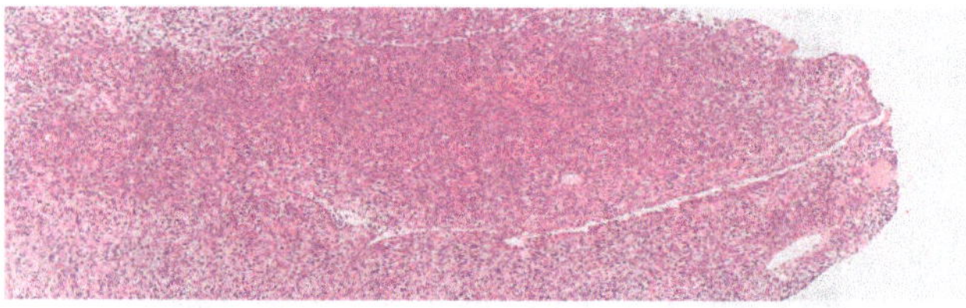

FIGURE 5: Microphotograph shows diffuse infiltration of large neoplastic lymphoid cells. HEx100x.

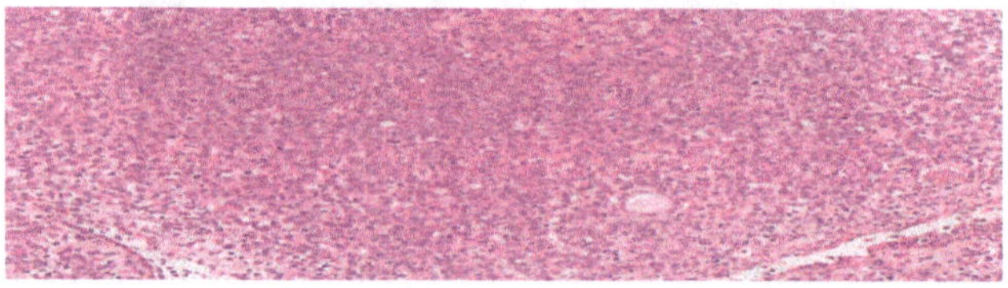

FIGURE 6: Microphotograph shows atypical large lymphoid cells with prominent 1-2 nucleoli, subendothelial infiltration, frequent mitoses, and a pseudorosette. HEx200x.

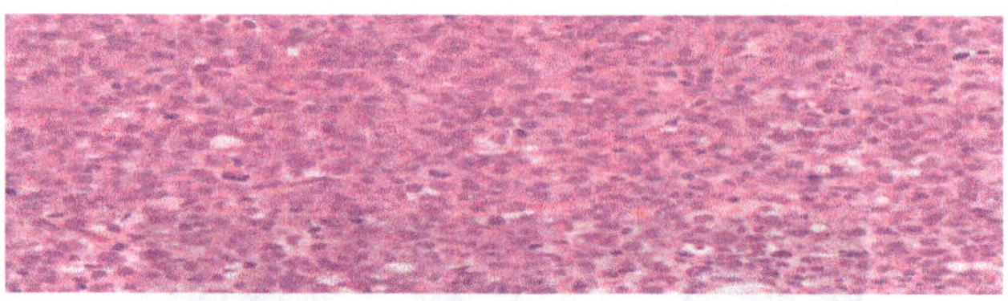

FIGURE 7: High-power view of transformed lymphoid cells and mitoses. HEx400x.

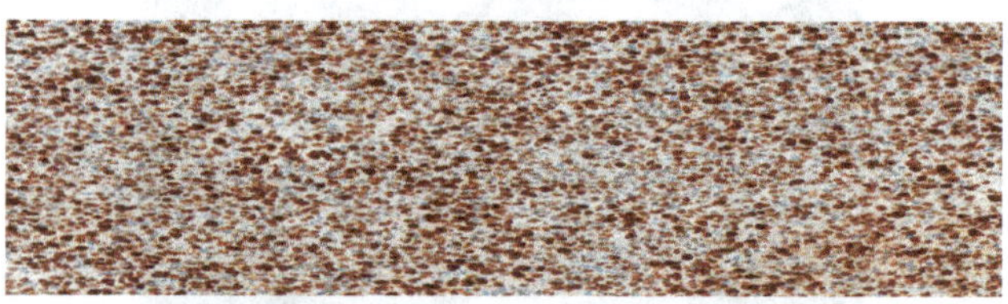

FIGURE 8: Ki67 by immunohistochemistry shows high proliferation index (80–90%). 200x.

3. Discussion

Carcinoma of the temporal bone is rare, and most of the pathological diagnosis in such cases turns out to be squamous cell carcinoma. In addition, adenoid cystic carcinoma, adenocarcinoma, and basal cell carcinomas along with metastasis are also reported. Other malignant tumors that can occur in the temporal bone are melanoma, rhabdomyosarcoma, chondrosarcoma, and lymphoma [4].

Lymphoma of the middle ear can arise from the mucosa of the mastoid antrum, tympanum, or the tympanic orifice of the eustachian tube. In addition to that it can arise primarily from the temporal bone, as in our case, which is in the mastoid part of the temporal bone.

Diagnosis of cancer in the middle ear and the mastoid process is seldom made early; this can contribute to the unique anatomy of middle ear and the fact that many benign pathologies such as otitis media and its complications share similar clinical presentations; most commonly reported symptoms include otorrhea, otalgia, aural fullness, tinnitus, and hearing loss [5].

Severe hearing loss, facial nerve weakness, and vestibular dysfunction are advanced sequel of middle ear pathology that should raise red flags for a more sinister cause. In addition to malignancy, autoimmune conditions such as granulomatosis with polyangiitis and sarcoidosis and immunodeficiency conditions should also be considered in the differential diagnosis of cases of refractory chronic otitis media with facial nerve palsy. Delay in management of such cases usually occurs due to a low index of suspicion of the treating physician.

Saito et al. presented a similar case in a 58-year-old woman who presented with headache and auditory disturbances in addition to otitis media; further investigations revealed that the patient has transverse sinus thrombosis. Surgery was performed 6 years after initial presentation, when only the diagnosis of lymphoma was made. The patient then recovered fully after a course of chemotherapy. They have also reviewed the literature and found 10 cases of lymphoma arising around the middle ear; the most common presentations were facial nerve palsy and otorrhea which is consistent with the presentation of our case [6].

Roberts et al. have presented a case of a 78-year-old woman with large B-cell lymphoma of the middle ear presenting as chronic otomastoiditis. However, in their case there was no involvement of any of the cranial nerves, and emphasis was made on the early detection of temporal bone malignancy through neurotological examination and imaging as early diagnosis and aggressive chemotherapeutic treatment for primary lymphoma of the middle ear lymphoma are crucial for a good outcome [7].

Our case presented similarly to other cases in the literature; however, earlier detection within the period where he had persistent symptoms refractory to medical treatment may have prevented the advanced complication of facial nerve palsy and increased his chances of cure.

4. Conclusion

Lymphoma in the temporal bone is very rare; it may manifest with symptoms that are similar to other common benign middle ear pathologies. In severe and persistent symptoms a malignant cause should be put into consideration; this ensures early detection and thus management of the condition.

Conflicts of Interest

The authors have no conflicts of interest to declare.

References

[1] L. Airaghi, I. Greco, M. Carrabba et al., "Unusual presentation of large B cell lymphoma: a case report and review of literature," *Clinical and Laboratory Haematology*, vol. 28, no. 5, pp. 338–342, 2006.

[2] S. Ogawa, I. Tawara, S. Ueno et al., "De novo CD5-positive diffuse large B-cell lymphoma of the temporal bone presenting

with an external auditory canal tumor," *Internal Medicine*, vol. 45, no. 11, pp. 733–737, 2006.
[3] S. Vaid, J. Jadhav, A. Chandorkar, and N. Vaid, "Bilateral non-Hodgkin's lymphoma of the temporal bone: a rare and unusual presentation," *Case Reports in Otolaryngology*, vol. 2016, Article ID 2641876, 5 pages, 2016.
[4] N. M. Agarwal, V. C. Popat, C. Traviad, and A. Srivastava, "Clinical and histopathological study of mass in ear: a study of fifty cases," *Indian Journal of Otolaryngology and Head & Neck Surgery*, vol. 65, no. S3, pp. 520–525, 2013.
[5] D. Hinton, "Cancer of the mastoid and the middle ear," *Journal of the National Medical Association*, vol. 66, no. 2, pp. 125–128, 1974.
[6] A. Saito, W. Jia, T. Sasaki et al., "B-cell malignant lymphoma presenting as otitis media and mastoiditis associated with sinus thrombosis," *Case Reports in Neurology*, vol. 6, no. 2, pp. 161–165, 2014.
[7] J. M. Roberts, J. Fastenberg, E. Redd, and D. Foyt, "Primary diffuse large B-cell lymphoma presenting as chronic otomastoiditis," *Journal of Otology & Rhinology*, vol. 1, no. 3, 2012.

33

Oncocytoma of the Parotid Gland with Facial Nerve Paralysis

Seijiro Hamada,[1] **Keishi Fujiwara**,[1] **Hiromitsu Hatakeyama,**[1,2] **and Akihiro Homma**[1]

[1]*Department of Otolaryngology Head and Neck Surgery, Faculty of Medicine and Graduate School of Medicine, Hokkaido University, N15W7, Kita-Ku, Sapporo 0608638, Japan*
[2]*Department of Otolaryngology Head and Neck Surgery, Yokohama City University Medical Center, 4-57 Urafune-cho, Minami-ku, Yokohama 2320024, Japan*

Correspondence should be addressed to Keishi Fujiwara; boron700@med.hokudai.ac.jp

Academic Editor: M. Tayyar Kalcioglu

Parotid gland tumor with facial nerve paralysis is strongly suggestive of a malignant tumor. However, several case reports have documented benign tumors of the parotid gland with facial nerve paralysis. Here, we report a case of oncocytoma of the parotid gland with facial nerve paralysis. A 61-year-old male presented with pain in his right parotid gland. Physical examination demonstrated the presence of a right parotid gland tumor and ipsilateral facial nerve paralysis of House–Brackmann (HB) grade III. Due to the facial nerve paralysis, a malignant tumor of the parotid gland was suspected and right parotidectomy was performed. Oncocytoma was confirmed histopathologically. The facial nerve paralysis was resolved 2 months after surgery. During the follow-up period (one and a half years), no recurrence was observed. As the tumor showed a distinctive dumbbell shape and increased somewhat due to inflammation (i.e., infection), the facial nerve was pinched by the enlarged tumor. Ischemia and strangulation of the nerve were considered to be the cause of the facial nerve paralysis associated with the benign tumor in this case.

1. Introduction

Parotid tumor with facial nerve paralysis is generally considered as a criterion for malignancy. However, several case reports have documented benign tumors of the parotid gland with facial nerve paralysis, with almost all of these cases diagnosed as Warthin's tumor [1–5] or pleomorphic adenoma [6, 7]. Oncocytomas are rare benign tumors that comprise about 0.1 to 1.5% of all salivary gland tumors [8].

We herein describe the case of a 61-year-old male who suffered from right parotid oncocytoma with facial nerve paralysis.

2. Case Presentation

A 61-year-old male had been aware of a right parotid mass for about 10 years; however, he did not seek treatment as the mass was painless. On experiencing serious right parotid pain, he visited our affiliated hospital. Physical examination revealed a painful mass in his right parotid gland of approximately 30 mm in diameter and ipsilateral facial nerve palsy of House–Brackmann (HB) grade III. Laboratory findings showed a leukocyte count of 12,190/μL and C-reactive protein (CRP) of 0.18 mg/dL. Computed tomography (CT) revealed an enhanced irregularly shaped mass in the right parotid gland (Figure 1(a)). T1-weighted SE MR imaging of the mass showed lower intensity than that of the native parotid tissue (Figure 2(a)). T2-weighted SE MR imaging also showed intermediate signal intensity and partial hyperintensity (Figure 2(b)). At this stage, a malignant neoplasm of the parotid gland was suspected.

Nine days after the appearance of symptoms, he was referred to our hospital. On physical examination, the mass was found to be still present but the pain had eased. In addition, the facial nerve palsy showed some improvement to HB grade II. Ultrasound examination revealed an inhomogeneous, lobulated mass (approximately 30×25 mm) in the right parotid gland. CT showed that the tumor had become smaller than at the time of the previous scan in our affiliated hospital (Figure 1(b)). We tried ultrasound-guided fine needle aspiration cytology (FNAC) twice, with an initial finding of necrotic material and a subsequent finding of a large number of histiocytes and acinar cells and a small number of eosinophilic cells with no atypical findings observed. However, no definitive diagnosis was provided.

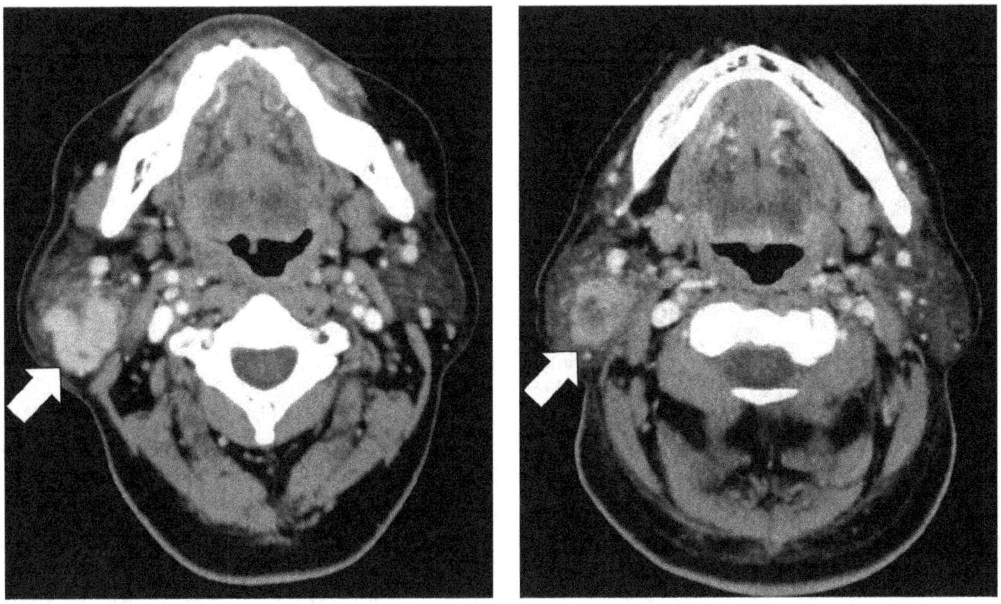

(a) (b)

FIGURE 1: Postcontrast computed tomography (CT) findings. The right parotid gland tumor in scans obtained in our hospital (b) is smaller than that in scans obtained in our affiliated hospital (a).

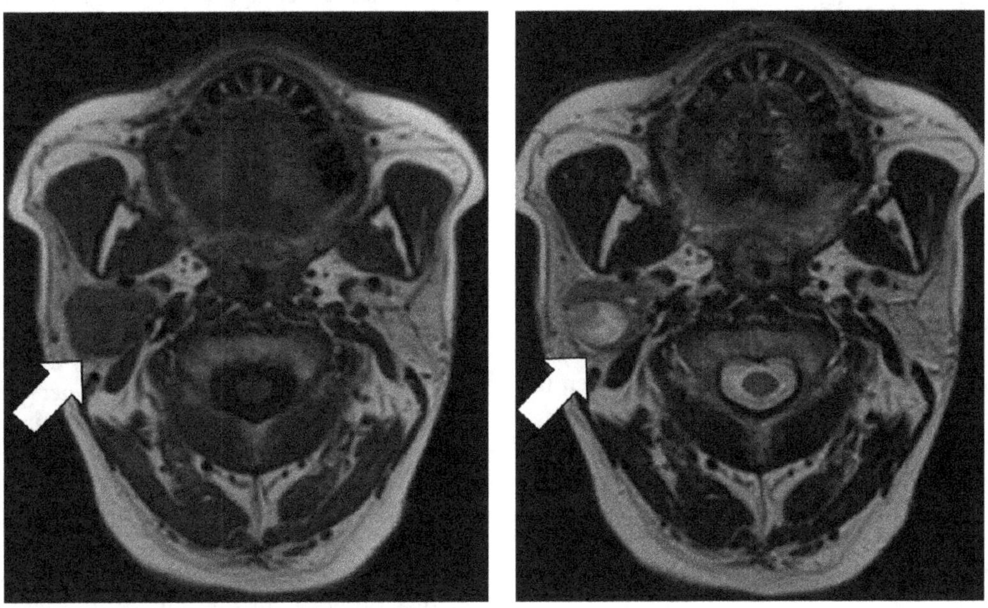

(a) (b)

FIGURE 2: MR imaging findings. (a) A T1-weighted image showing the tumor to have lower intensity than that of the native parotid tissue. (b) A T2-weighted image showing the tumor to have an intermediate signal intensity and partial hyperintensity.

We suspected a malignant tumor because of the associated facial nerve paralysis and parotid pain. On the contrary, we considered the possibility of a benign tumor with inflammation due to the reduction in tumor size and pain. We planned a total parotidectomy including exeresis and reconstruction of the facial nerve. However, we also made preparations to preserve the facial nerve should a benign tumor be suggested during the surgery.

The patient underwent surgery at 31 days after the appearance of symptoms. A modified Blair incision was made, and a dumbbell-shaped parotid tumor, extending from the superficial to the deep lobe of the parotid gland, was identified. The buccal and marginal mandibular branches of facial nerve were pinched by the tumor (Figure 3). The nerve branches were in contact with the tumor, but not involved. The temporal and zygomatic branches were present on the tumor capsule. A portion of the tumor was cut off and used for frozen section diagnosis (FSD). It was found to consist of solid and cystic components. The solid component was

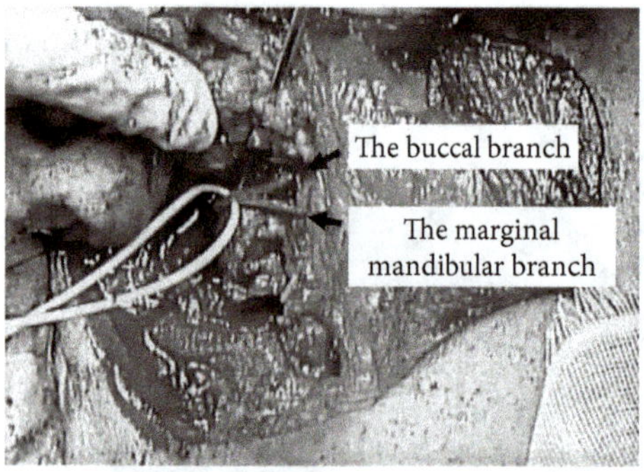

Figure 3: Intraoperative view of the facial nerve. The buccal branch and marginal mandibular branch can be seen to be compressed by the tumor.

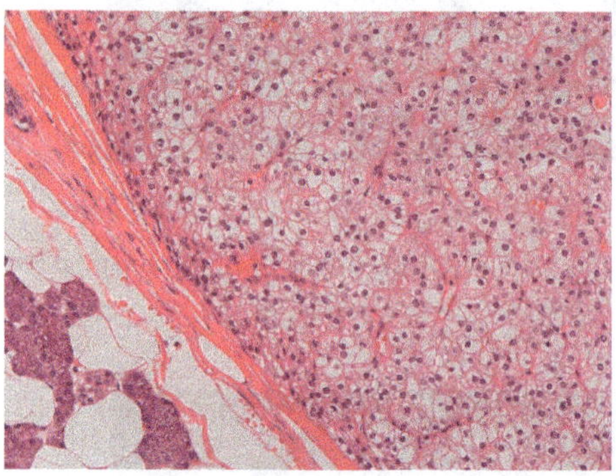

Figure 4: Frozen section of the neoplasm. Clear cells can be seen to form a clear boundary between the normal parotid gland tissues (haematoxylin-eosin, ×100).

surrounded by a fibrous capsule, and the wall of the cyst component was lined by a stratified squamous epithelium, which did not show any atypical changes. Based on the above results, we considered the tumor to be definitely benign. We managed to keep the facial nerve away from the tumor by use of microscissors, and the tumor was removed between the zygomatic and buccal branches.

Histopathological examination showed the tumor contained clear cells, which formed a clear boundary between the normal parotid gland tissues (Figure 4). The Ki-67 labelling index was exceedingly low and the mitotic count was negative. These findings were consistent with oncocytoma of the parotid gland.

Throughout the postoperative period, the nasalis muscle of the affected side was slightly weakened but it was completely recovered at 2 months after surgery. No recurrence was observed during the 18-month follow-up period.

3. Discussion

Oncocytomas are benign neoplasms composed of oncocytes: large cells with abundant granular and eosinophilic cytoplasm [9]. Oncocytomas are rare, comprising only about 0.1 to 1.5% of all salivary gland tumors [8]. The parotid gland is the most common site of oncocytic changes [10], but they have also been noted in the submaxillary gland, sublingual gland, larynx, soft palate, hard palate, and nasal cavities. They often present as solitary slow growing painless masses, which are smooth and with some mobility upon clinical examination. On postcontrast CT, around 50% of oncocytomas demonstrate inhomogeneous enhancement. Some oncocytomas consist of a curved nonenhanced lesion and cystic lesion, corresponding to central scar tissue and cystic degeneration, respectively. As the majority of oncocytomas appear as isointense in comparison to the parotid tissue on MRI with T2 and T1, oncocytomas are often called "vanishing tumors" [9]. However, some oncocytomas show different intensities. In fact, the tumor in our case showed lower intensity on T1-weighted and intermediate signal intensity and partial hyperintensity on T2-weighted images. The usefulness of diffusion-weighted MR imaging for differentiating between oncocytomas and Warthin's tumors has been reported [11]. In this case, we could not obtain accurate diagnosis of the tumor by FNAC. Retrospectively, it is difficult to diagnose oncocytoma based on the findings of FNAC due to only a small number of eosinophilic cells. It has been reported the sensitivity for the detection of oncocytoma by FNAC is 29% [12]. Eventually, surgical management with parotidectomy was essential for diagnosis and treatment. During histopathological examination, it is important to distinguish oncocytomas from oncocytic carcinomas. Oncocytic carcinomas are composed of malignant oncocytes with adenocarcinomatous architectural phenotypes and infiltrative qualities, including local invasion and regional or distant metastases [13]. Furthermore, the frequency of Ki-67-positive cells with nuclear staining was shown to be higher in oncocytic carcinomas than in oncocytomas [13]. These findings were not observed in this case.

Eneroth [14] reported that, in a series of 2,261 patients with parotid tumors, peripheral facial nerve paralysis developed spontaneously in 46 patients. These 46 patients all had malignant parotid tumors, on the basis of which he concluded that facial nerve paralysis must be considered as a criterion of malignancy. However, we encountered a benign parotid gland tumor with facial nerve paralysis. Similar cases have been reported in the literature. Histopathologically, Warthin's tumor is the most commonly reported [1–5], with pleomorphic adenoma [6, 7] and lipoma [15] also reported. Only 2 cases of oncocytoma with facial nerve paralysis have been reported to date [16, 17], with one patient showing painful swelling in the parotid area similarly to that observed in our case [16]. Therefore, our case is considered to be extremely rare. The causes of facial nerve paralysis with benign tumor reported in other studies include the facial nerve being compressed due to a sudden increase in tumor volume. For example, a histological examination of nerve bundles led to the speculation that ischemia of the nerve caused by external compression resulted in facial nerve palsy [3]. A case of spontaneous intratumoral hemorrhage in parotid oncocytoma was also reported [18]. Necrosis, inflammation, and fibrosis surrounding the branches of the facial nerve have also been considered to be a cause of palsy [1]. In our case, the patient suffered serious right parotid pain temporarily. When he visited our hospital, the pain had diminished and CT examination showed that the tumor had become smaller than at the time of the previous scan at our affiliated hospital. As the tumor showed a distinctive dumbbell shape and increased in size somewhat by inflammation (i.e., infection), the facial nerve was pinched by the enlarged tumor. Ischemia and strangulation of the nerve were considered as the reason for the facial nerve paralysis with benign tumor in this case.

4. Conclusion

We reported a parotid gland oncocytoma with facial nerve paralysis. We initially suspected a malignant tumor; however, we later suspected a benign tumor with inflammation based on the reduction in tumor size and pain. We, therefore, planned operative methods to cover either eventuality. As a result, we could resect the tumor while preserving the facial nerve.

Conflicts of Interest

The authors declare that they have no conflicts of interest.

References

[1] R. W. Lesser and J. G. Spector, "Facial nerve palsy associated with Warthin's tumor," *Archives of Otolaryngology*, vol. 111, no. 8, pp. 548-549, 1985.

[2] T. P. O'Dwyer, P. J. Gullane, and I. Dardick, "A pseudomalignant Warthin's tumor presenting with facial nerve paralysis," *Journal of Otolaryngology*, vol. 19, no. 5, pp. 353–357, 1990.

[3] C. Koide, A. Imai, A. Nagaba, and T. Takahashi, "Pathological findings of the facial nerve in a case of facial nerve palsy associated with benign parotid tumor," *Archives of Otolaryngology–Head & Neck Surgery*, vol. 120, no. 4, pp. 410–412, 1994.

[4] G. Marioni, C. de Filippis, E. Gaio, G. A. Iaderosa, and A. Staffieri, "Facial nerve paralysis secondary to Warthin's tumour of the parotid gland," *Journal of Laryngology & Otology*, vol. 117, no. 6, pp. 511–513, 2003.

[5] N. R. Woodhouse, G. Gok, D. C. Howlett, and K. Ramesar, "Warthin's tumour and facial nerve palsy: an unusual association," *British Journal of Oral and Maxillofacial Surgery*, vol. 49, no. 3, pp. 237-238, 2011.

[6] N. H. Blevins, R. K. Jackler, M. J. Kaplan, and R. Boles, "Facial paralysis due to benign parotid tumors," *Archives of Otolaryngology–Head & Neck Surgery*, vol. 118, no. 4, pp. 427–430, 1992.

[7] M. E. Nader, D. Bell, E. M. Sturgis, L. E. Ginsberg, and P. W. Gidley, "Facial nerve paralysis due to a pleomorphic adenoma with the imaging characteristics of a facial nerve schwannoma," *Journal of Neurological Surgery Reports*, vol. 75, no. 1, pp. e84–e88, 2014.

[8] I. Sepulveda, E. Platin, M. L. Spencer et al., "Oncocytoma of the parotid gland: a case report and review of the literature," *Case Reports in Oncology*, vol. 7, no. 1, pp. 109–116, 2014.

[9] N. D. Patel, A. van Zante, D. W. Eisele, H. R. Harnsberger, and C. M. Glastonbury, "Oncocytoma: the vanishing parotid mass," *American Journal of Neuroradiology*, vol. 32, no. 9, pp. 1703–1706, 2011.

[10] M. S. Brandwein and A. G. Huvos, "Oncocytic tumors of major salivary glands. A study of 68 cases with follow-up of 44 patients," *American Journal of Surgical Pathology*, vol. 15, no. 6, pp. 514–528, 1991.

[11] H. Kato, K. Fujimoto, M. Matsuo, K. Mizuta, and M. Aoki, "Usefulness of diffusion-weighted MR imaging for differentiating between Warthin's tumor and oncocytoma of the parotid gland," *Japanese Journal of Radiology*, vol. 35, no. 2, pp. 78–85, 2017.

[12] R. B. Capone, P. K. Ha, W. H. Westra et al., "Oncocytic neoplasms of the parotid gland: a 16-year institutional review," *Otolaryngology–Head and Neck Surgery*, vol. 126, no. 6, pp. 657–662, 2002.

[13] C. X. Zhou, D. Y. Shi, D. Q. Ma, J. G. Zhang, G. Y. Yu, and Y. Gao, "Primary oncocytic carcinoma of the salivary glands: a clinicopathologic and immunohistochemical study of 12 cases," *Oral Oncology*, vol. 46, no. 10, pp. 773–778, 2010.

[14] C. M. Eneroth, "Facial nerve paralysis. A criterion of malignancy in parotid tumors," *Archives of Otolaryngology*, vol. 95, no. 4, pp. 300–304, 1972.

[15] V. Srinivasan, S. Ganesan, and D. J. Premachandra, "Lipoma of the parotid gland presenting with facial palsy," *Journal of Laryngology & Otology*, vol. 110, no. 1, pp. 93–95, 1996.

[16] L. Papangelou, K. Alkalai, and M. Kyrillopoulou, "Facial nerve paralysis in the presence of a benign parotid tumor," *Archives of Otolaryngology*, vol. 108, no. 7, pp. 458-459, 1982.

[17] D. M. Roden and F. E. Levy, "Oncocytoma of the parotid gland presenting with nerve paralysis," *Otolaryngology–Head and Neck Surgery*, vol. 110, no. 6, pp. 587–590, 1994.

[18] E. Iida, R. H. Wiggins 3rd, and Y. Anzai, "Bilateral parotid oncocytoma with spontaneous intratumoral hemorrhage: a rare hypervascular parotid tumor with ASL perfusion," *Clinical Imaging*, vol. 40, no. 3, pp. 357–360, 2016.

Case Report and Literature Review of a Pathologic Mandibular Fracture from Metastatic Esophageal Adenocarcinoma

Daniel C. O'Brien,[1] **Garrett Jones**,[2] **Maggie Yell**,[3] **and Jason McChesney**[1]

[1]*Department of Otolaryngology Head and Neck Surgery, University of West Virginia, Morgantown, WV, USA*
[2]*Department of Medical Education, University of West Virginia, Morgantown, WV, USA*
[3]*Department of Pathology, Anatomy, and Laboratory Medicine, University of West Virginia, Morgantown, WV, USA*

Correspondence should be addressed to Daniel C. O'Brien; daobrien@hsc.wvu.edu

Academic Editor: M. Tayyar Kalcioglu

Distant metastasis to the jaws, including the maxilla or mandible, is very rare. Although the mandible is the preferred sight of these rare metastases, it is extremely rare for oral cavity malignancies to present as pathological mandibular fractures. Here, we present a case of esophageal adenocarcinoma metastasizing to the mandible, and the first reported case presenting with a pathological mandibular fracture secondary to esophageal adenocarcinoma. We also review the 9 other reported cases of metastatic esophageal adenocarcinoma to either the maxilla or mandible.

1. Introduction

Pathological mandibular fractures are rare and account for only 2% of all mandibular fractures. Causes of pathological mandibular fractures have been reported following tooth removal, dental implant placement, secondary to benign and malignant mandibular pathology, osteomyelitis, osteoradionecrosis, bisphosphonate-related osteonecrosis, and Gorham's disease [1]. Even though only 1% of all oral cavity malignancies are metastatic in origin, when these metastases arise, they are the first sign of the primary disease about 25% of the time [2]. Pathological mandibular fractures caused by metastatic disease often present at a late stage. Secondary to advanced stage at presentation, treatment generally consists of chemotherapy or radiation therapy as a means of palliation. If the tumor is resectable, the gold standard of therapy is primary radical surgery [1].

This case report was reviewed by the University of West Virginia Institutional Review Board and found to be exempt and did not require full IRB review.

2. Case Report

A 69-year-old Caucasian male with a past medical history of hypertension, oromandibular dystonia treated with Botox, and recent diagnosis of gastroesophageal reflux disease (GERD) presented to his primary care provider noting an area of his left chin that was numb. The area was small and could be covered with 1 finger. He followed up acutely three weeks later with significant dysphagia for solids, but not liquids. He was urgently referred for an upper endoscopy. Upper endoscopy revealed LA Class D esophagitis with ulceration in the distal esophagus, and biopsies showed inflamed glandular mucosa with at least high-grade dysplasia. These findings were consistent with a diagnosis of Barrett's esophagus secondary to GERD.

Three weeks after his upper endoscopy, he presented to the emergency department with right jaw pain and swelling after hitting his jaw on a work bench. A CT revealed right mandibular angle fracture and coronoid fracture (Figure 1). The facial trauma team was consulted and, secondary to his oromandibular dystonia, he was discharged on a liquid diet with Augmentin, Peridex, and close follow-up. He was seen in the clinic a week later and denied trismus, malocclusion, or difficulty with his liquid diet. On examination, he was found to have an exophytic mass of the right retromolar trigone, which he noted his teeth had been hitting. This mass was present before his fracture and had gotten larger over time. This mass was biopsied in the clinic and came back as likely metastatic adenocarcinoma (Figure 2).

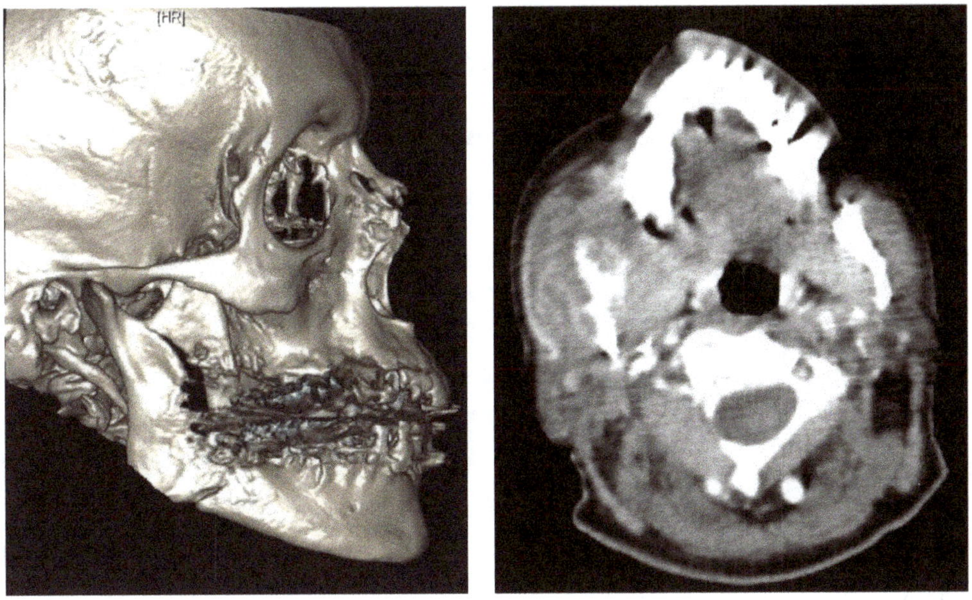

(a) (b)

Figure 1: (a) Three-dimensional reconstruction of patient's pathologic fracture. Note the minimally displaced right mandibular angle fracture and right coronoid fracture. (b) Axial soft tissue of the mandible, displaying the mass of the right retromolar trigone.

The patient underwent a second upper endoscopy. Biopsy taken during this second endoscopy was consistent with a moderately differentiated adenocarcinoma of the distal esophagus. A PET/CT revealed a large, hypermetabolic distal esophageal mass consistent with the given diagnosis of esophageal adenocarcinoma. Hypermetabolic lesions involving the regional lymph nodes, lungs, spine, and right mandible, as shown in Figure 3, were found on PET/CT. These findings were consistent with a Stage IV, TX, NX, M1, and G2, esophageal adenocarcinoma. At that time, he denied smoking, alcohol, illicit drugs, and/or exposure to radiation and carcinogenic chemicals.

The hypermetabolic area of the right mandible, in conjunction with the previous retromolar trigone biopsy, confirmed a likely pathological fracture of the mandible secondary to metastatic esophageal adenocarcinoma. The advanced stage of the cancer made him a poor candidate for surgical intervention for either primary tumor or mandibular metastasis. He was referred for palliative chemoradiotherapy. He passed away one month after diagnosis.

3. Discussion

We are reporting a case of a 69-year-old Caucasian male sustaining a pathological mandibular fracture from metastatic esophageal adenocarcinoma. His pathological mandibular fracture occurred 1 week prior to his diagnosis of esophageal adenocarcinoma. There have been 9 previous cases of metastatic esophageal adenocarcinoma to the jaws reported in the literature and are listed in Table 1. None of these cases were associated with a pathological fracture of the mandible or maxilla [3–11]. The only reported case of metastatic esophageal carcinoma causing a pathologic fracture was secondary to an esophageal squamous cell carcinoma. In this previous case, the primary tumor was diagnosed prior to the pathological mandibular fracture [12].

Only 1% of all oral cavity malignancies arise from metastatic disease, and metastasis to the jaw bones is more common than oral soft tissues [2]. Metastasis to the jaws are thought to be by hematogenous spread, with the posterior portion of the mandible, molar, premolar, and angle of the ramus being the most common sites. Metastasis settles in these areas most commonly secondary to the red bone marrow located in these subsites [2, 13]. Tooth extraction is commonly associated with metastasis to the oral cavity. In some cases, metastatic disease causes loosening of the teeth necessitating extraction, and in other cases, extraction of the teeth provides the inflammatory environment favorable to attract cancer cells. The growth factors provided by the bone marrow stromal cells and gingival inflammation are thought to provide a nurturing environment for cancer cells to thrive [2, 13].

In a review of 453 cases of metastatic disease to the jaw bones, the male-to-female ratio was reported as between 1.2 and 1 with a mean age of 53.4 years old at diagnosis [13]. The most common origin for metastasis to the jaw include lung, kidney, liver, and prostate in men and breast, female genital organs, kidney, and colon in women. Metastatic tumors to the oral cavity most commonly present as exophytic lesions. The survival rate of patients with oral metastasis is reported to be 7 months secondary to the severity and progression associated with metastasis [2]. Secondary to significant disease burden, treatment is generally limited to chemotherapy or radiation therapy as a means of palliation, however, radical resection, if possible, has been described [14]. Classic symptoms of metastatic disease to the jaws include rapid, progressive swelling, pain, and paresthesia.

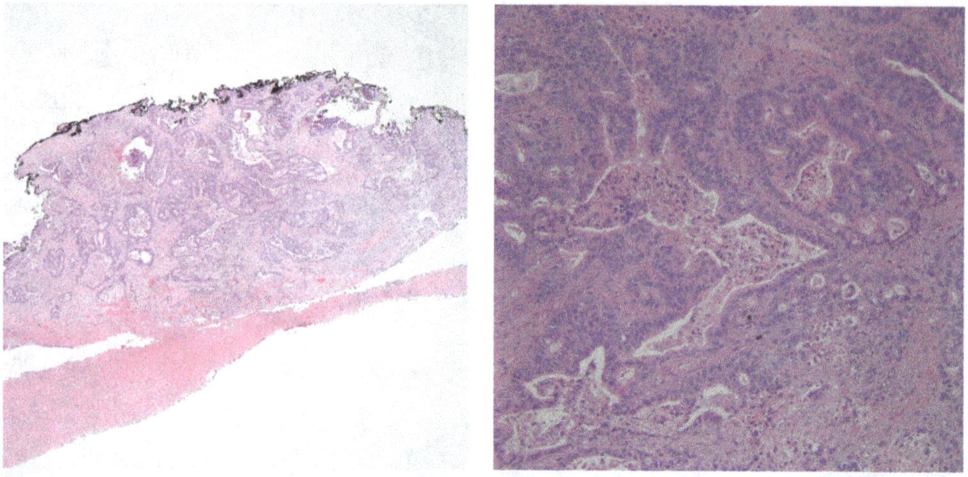

(a) (b)

FIGURE 2: Pathologic specimen of the retromolar trigone biopsy. 2A: 100x magnification of hematoxylin and eosin stain (low power). Back to back gland formation with undermining of squamous mucosa. 2B: 200x magnification hematoxylin and eosin stain (high power). Infiltrating malignant glands containing necrotic debris.

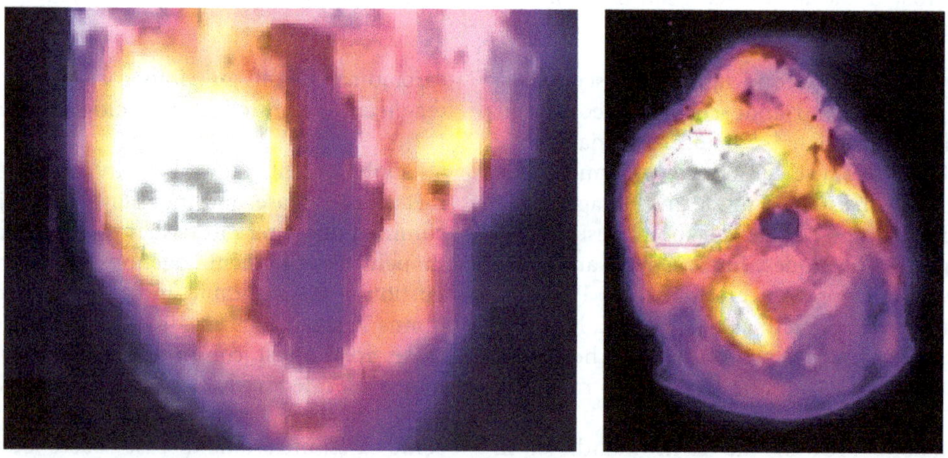

(a) (b)

FIGURE 3: PET/CT of the patient's mandibular mass. This image shows an avidly hypermetabolic mass of the right mandibular angle. (a) Coronal cuts; (b) axial cuts.

TABLE 1: Reported cases of esophageal adenocarcinoma to the maxilla or mandible.

	Authors	Year published	Location of metastasis	Age	Sex	Time between primary diagnosis and metastasis
1	Fontaine et al. [3]	1961	Right mandible	55	Male	Concurrent
2	Tideman et al. [4]	1986	Left posterior maxilla	59	Male	4 weeks
3	Jones [5]	1989	Left mandibular body	54	Male	Concurrent
4	Anderson and Peepler [6]	1990	Left mandibular body and ramus	61	Male	Concurrent
5	Willard et al. [7]	2002	Left posterior maxilla	41	Male	9 months
6	Sanchez-Jimenez et al. [8]	2005	Upper left maxilla	63	Male	4 months
7	Tamiolakis et al. [9]	2007	Mandible	NA	NA	NA
8	Jham and Salama. [10]	2011	Mandible	67	Female	NA
9	Lawes et al. [11]	2013	Left mandible	69	Male	7 years
10	O'Brien et al. (This Case)	2018	Right mandibular angle	69	Male	Metastasis identified prior to primary

Numb chin syndrome or mental nerve neuropathy is characteristic of metastasis to the mandible and includes anesthesia and paresthesia over the chin, lower lip, and submental area. It is worth noting that, in this case, the paresthesia was of the opposite chin from the side of mandibular metastasis. Metastatic disease to the oral cavity should be considered in any patient with symptoms of numb chin syndrome, pain, swelling, or an exophytic lesion [2].

Esophageal adenocarcinoma has become increasingly more common over the last several decades, and it is now more common than esophageal squamous cell carcinoma in the United States. Men have approximately 6-fold higher risk of developing esophageal adenocarcinoma as compared to women [14]. Our patient's only risk factor for developing esophageal adenocarcinoma was being an elderly Caucasian male with GERD. Other risk factors for developing esophageal adenocarcinoma include central adiposity and tobacco consumption, while NSAIDs and H *pylori* are thought to be protective. Alcohol is not considered a risk factor [14]. In recent years, males >65 years old have seen the greatest increase in incidence of esophageal adenocarcinoma [15].

4. Conclusion

We report a case of esophageal adenocarcinoma presenting as a pathological mandibular fracture. Review of the literature shows this is the 10th reported case of esophageal adenocarcinoma metastasizing to either the mandible or maxilla and the first reported case of esophageal adenocarcinoma to present as a pathological mandibular fracture.

Conflicts of Interest

The authors declare that they have no conflicts of interest.

References

[1] P. Boffano, F. Roccia, C. Gallesio, and S. Berrone, "Pathological mandibular fractures: a review of the literature of the last two decades," *Dental Traumatology*, vol. 29, no. 3, pp. 185–196, 2013.

[2] A. Hirshberg, R. Berger, I. Allon, and I. Kaplan, "Metastatic tumors to the jaws and mouth," *Head and Neck Pathology*, vol. 8, no. 4, pp. 463–474, 2014.

[3] R. Fontaine, P. Warter, and G. Lang, "Apropos of a case of the lower thoracic esophagus, until then latent, revealed by an osseous metastasis in a condyle of the inferior maxilla," *Archives des Maladies de l'appareil Digestif et des Maladies de la Nutrition*, vol. 50, pp. 1050–10506, 1961.

[4] H. Tideman, J. F. Arvier, A. G. Bosanquet, and D. F. Wilson, "Esophageal adenocarcinoma metastatic to the maxilla," *Oral Surgery, Oral Medicine, Oral Pathology*, vol. 62, no. 5, pp. 564–568, 1986.

[5] D. C. Jones, "Adenocarcinoma of the esophagus presenting as a mandibular metastasis," *Journal of Oral and Maxillofacial Surgery*, vol. 47, no. 5, pp. 504–507, 1989.

[6] R. S. Anderson and W. J. Peeples, "Mandibular osseous metastasis from esophageal carcinoma: a case report and review of the literature," *Journal of Oral and Maxillofacial Surgery*, vol. 48, no. 2, pp. 188–192, 1990.

[7] C. C. Willard, C. R. Weber, and W. Buche, "Metastatic esophageal adenocarcinoma involving the maxilla," *Journal of Oral and Maxillofacial Surgery*, vol. 60, no. 12, pp. 1496–1499, 2002.

[8] J. Sánchez-Jiménez, F. Acebal-Blanco, R. E. Arévalo-Arévalo, and Molina-MartínezM, "Metastatic tumours in upper maxillary bone of esophageal adenocarcinoma. A case report," *Medicina Oral, Patologia Oral y Cirugia Bucal*, vol. 10, no. 3, pp. 252–257, 2005.

[9] D. Tamiolakis, I. Tsamis, V. Thomaidis et al., "Jaw bone metastases: four cases," *Acta Acta Dermatovenerologica Alpina, Pannonica, et Adriatica*, vol. 16, pp. 21–25, 2007.

[10] B. C. Jham, A. R. Salama, S. A. McClure, and R. A. Ord, "Metastatic tumors to the oral cavity: a clinical study of 18 cases," *Head and Neck Pathology*, vol. 5, no. 4, pp. 355–358, 2011.

[11] K. P. Lawes, M. Danford, and S. Di Palma, "Delayed metastasis to the mandible of esophageal adenocarcinoma," *Head and Neck Pathology*, vol. 7, no. 4, pp. 416–420, 2013.

[12] T. Plath and C. Marks, "Pathologic fracture of the mandible caused by intraosseous metastasis of oesophageal squamous cell carcinoma: a case report," *International Journal of Oral and Maxillofacial Surgery*, vol. 25, no. 4, pp. 282–284, 1996.

[13] S. Irani, "Metastasis to the Jawbones: a review of 453 cases," *Journal of International Society of Preventive and Community Dentistry*, vol. 7, no. 2, pp. 71–81, 2017.

[14] J. H. Rubenstein and N. J. Shaheen, "Epidemiology, diagnosis, and management of esophageal adenocarcinoma," *Gastroenterology*, vol. 149, no. 2, pp. 302–317, 2015.

[15] T. M. Runge, J. A. Abrams, and N. J. Shaheen, "Epidemiology of barrett's esophagus and esophageal adenocarcinoma," *Gastroenterology Clinics of North America*, vol. 44, no. 2, pp. 203–231, 2015.

35

Initial-Stage Primary Intraosseous Squamous Cell Carcinoma Derived from Odontogenic Keratocyst with Unusual Keratoameloblastomatous Change of the Maxilla

Kentaro Kikuchi,[1] Fumio Ide,[1] Shota Takizawa,[2] Seiji Suzuki,[2] Hideaki Sakashita,[2] Tie-Jun Li,[3] and Kaoru Kusama[1]

[1]*Division of Pathology, Department of Diagnostic and Therapeutic Sciences, Meikai University School of Dentistry, 1-1 Keyakidai, Sakado, Saitama 350-0283, Japan*
[2]*Second Division of Oral and Maxillofacial Surgery, Department of Diagnostic and Therapeutic Sciences, Meikai University School of Dentistry, 1-1 Keyakidai, Sakado, Saitama 350-0283, Japan*
[3]*Department of Oral Pathology, Peking University School of Stomatology, 22 South Zhongguancun Avenue, Haidian District, Beijing 100081, China*

Correspondence should be addressed to Kentaro Kikuchi; k-kikuchi@dent.meikai.ac.jp

Academic Editor: Abrão Rapoport

Primary intraosseous squamous cell carcinoma (PIOSCC) is a rare malignant neoplasm derived from odontogenic epithelial remnants in the central jaw bone. Most PIOSCCs originate from odontogenic cysts with a nonkeratinized epithelial lining, especially from radicular/residual and dentigerous cysts. There have been few reports of PIOSCCs derived from the odontogenic keratocyst (OKC), particularly those describing pathological features at the initial stage. The diagnosis of PIOSCC is difficult and based on exclusion of other carcinomas, including metastatic tumors from other primary sites. Here, we report an extremely rare case of initial-stage PIOSCC derived from the OKC with unusual keratoameloblastomatous change of the maxilla.

1. Introduction

Primary intraosseous squamous cell carcinoma (PIOSCC) is a carcinoma arising from the central bone without any initial connection to various epithelia [1]. In 2017, in the World Health Organization (WHO) classification of tumors, the name was changed from PIOSCC to primary intraosseous carcinoma (PIOC), not otherwise specified (NOS) [2]. The diagnosis of PIOSCC requires specific criteria to be met, including the absence of oral ulceration or communication with the overlying mucosa, the absence of a distant primary tumor at the time of diagnosis, and histologic evidence of squamous cell carcinoma [1, 2]. The diagnosis of PIOSCC can be difficult, and it must be differentiated from other malignancies such as ameloblastic carcinoma and metastatic carcinomas; when it causes destruction of the cortical bone and invades adjacent soft tissues, it may be confused with a carcinoma of the oral mucosa. Most PIOSCCs originate from the epithelial lining of odontogenic cysts, especially radicular, residual, and dentigerous cysts [1]. There are about 120 reported cases of PIOSCCs arising from cysts, with 25 of them being derived from odontogenic keratocysts (OKCs) [3, 4]. PIOSCCs arising from OKCs are extremely rare, and fewer than 30 have been reported so far. Few reports have presented clear evidence of histological transition between squamous cell carcinoma and the odontogenic epithelial lining of the cyst wall. Here, we present a very rare case of initial-stage PIOSCC derived from the OKC with unusual keratoameloblastomatous change of the left maxilla.

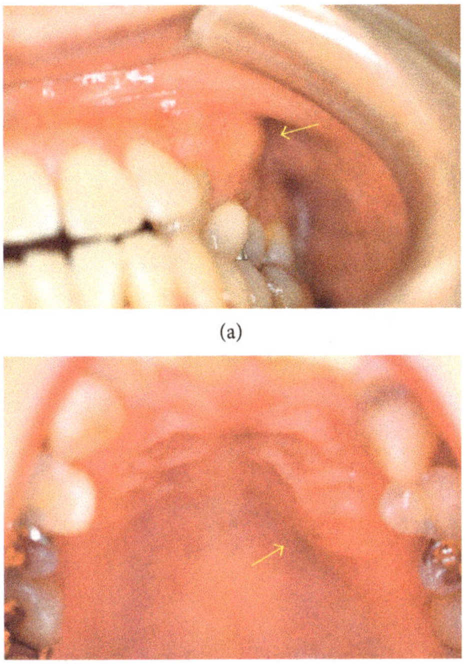

(a)

(b)

Figure 1: Intraoral appearance of the upper jaw. (a, b) Swollen nonulcerative mucosa in the buccal and palatal side gingiva (yellow arrow).

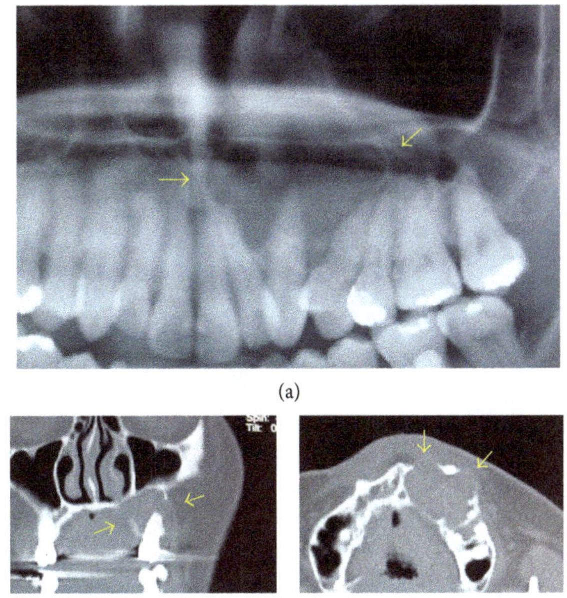

(a)

(b) (c)

Figure 2: Radiologic and computed tomography (CT) findings. (a) Panoramic radiograph showing a well-delineated radiolucent lesion (yellow arrows). (b, c) CT showing expansion and cortical bone osteolysis (yellow arrows).

2. Case Presentation

In January 2016, a 49-year-old Japanese woman visited a local dentist because of gingival swelling in the left upper canine area of the jaw, and a radiolucent lesion was found in the central maxilla. Although she had been aware of dull pain for five years, she had not taken any action because the symptoms improved. In July 2016, she was referred to Meikai University Hospital for detailed examination and treatment because of further gingival swelling and tooth displacement. Intraorally, the lesion involving the area from the upper left canine to the first premolar also showed evident buccal and palatal cortical expansion (Figures 1(a) and 1(b)). The epithelium overlying the mucosa was normal in color and unremarkable. Panoramic radiography showed an extensive, relatively well-delineated radiolucent lesion extending from the left middle incisor to the second premolar with tooth displacement but no root absorption (Figure 2(a)). A computerized tomography (CT) scan also demonstrated expansion and absorptive destruction of both the buccal and palatal cortical plates (Figures 2(b) and 2(c)). Clinically, the findings of a general examination were unremarkable. The clinical diagnosis was a suspected odontogenic tumor, and an incisional biopsy was performed. The histopathological appearance of a biopsy specimen was consistent with the odontogenic keratocyst (OKC) (Figures 3(a) and 3(b)). Surgery for the jaw tumor was performed intraorally under general anesthesia, and the tumor was resected along some peripheral bone tissues. Macroscopically, the surgical specimen was a cystic mass with a fibrous wall measuring 25 × 22 × 15 mm (Figure 4(a)). Microscopically, the lesion was cystic (Figure 4(b)) with a lining of parakeratinized stratified squamous epithelium. Although the pathological findings were almost consistent with the OKC, focally invasive atypical squamous cell epithelia ware noted (Figure 5(a)). Epithelial dysplasia was evident in the areas around the invasive atypical squamous cell nests (Figures 5(b) and 5(c)). Immunohistochemistry showed that the invasive atypical squamous cell nests (Figure 5(d)) were positive for p53 (Figure 5(e)) and that the proliferative activity (MIB 1 index) was about 20% (Figures 5(f)). Unusual ameloblastomatous epithelial elongation with a stellate reticulum was observed in part of the lining epithelium (Figure 6(a)) and also in the epithelium with mitoses (Figure 6(b)). Although postoperative blood tests demonstrated a high level of squamous cell carcinoma antigen (1.6 ng/mL), no tumor lesions were found in other organs by PET-CT and other radiological examinations. The postoperative histopathological diagnosis was most compatible with PIOSCC derived from the OKC.

Additional resection was performed because positivity at the distal surgical margin was suspected. This second surgical specimen measuring 35 × 30 × 25 mm included the left second premolar and maxillary sinus (Figure 7(a)). There was a cystic lesion, 8 × 7 mm in length, located in the palatal side of the second premolar (Figure 7(b)). Microscopically, this lesion appeared to be a typical OKC without malignant components, but there was marked local invasion to the bone marrow (Figure 7(c)). Solid variant OKC-like or keratoameloblastomatous microfollicles with keratin plugs were found in the bone marrow space (Figure 7(d)). The patient underwent additional resection, and the surgical margins were negative. No recurrence and distant metastasis were evident thereafter. The case study protocol was reviewed and approved by the Research Ethics Committee of the Meikai University School of Dentistry (A1321).

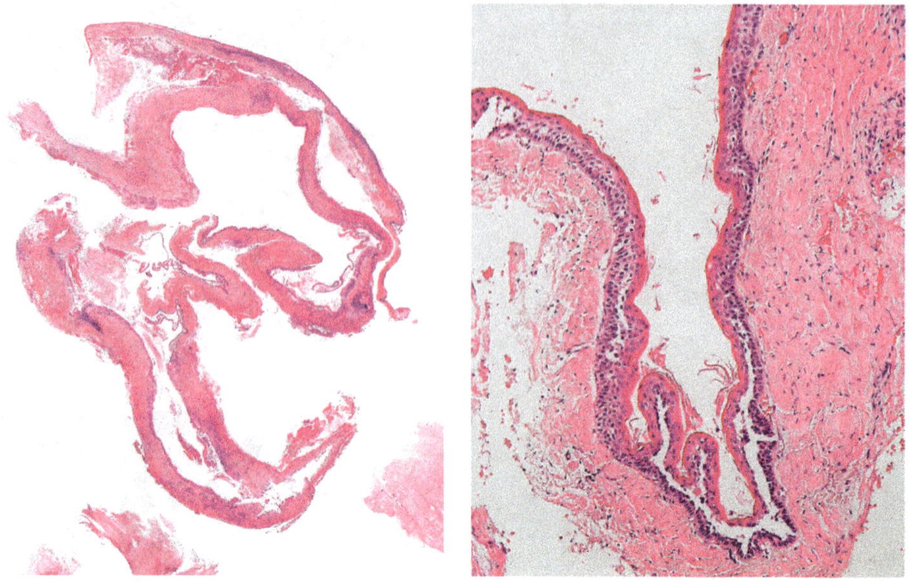

(a) (b)

FIGURE 3: Microscopic features of the biopsy specimen. (a) Survey view of the biopsy specimen. (b) The cyst wall lined by a folded, thin, regular parakeratinized epithelium without rete ridges, and the basal layer lined by palisaded columnar cells with hyperchromatic nuclei (HE; original magnification: ×12.5 (a) and ×100 (b)).

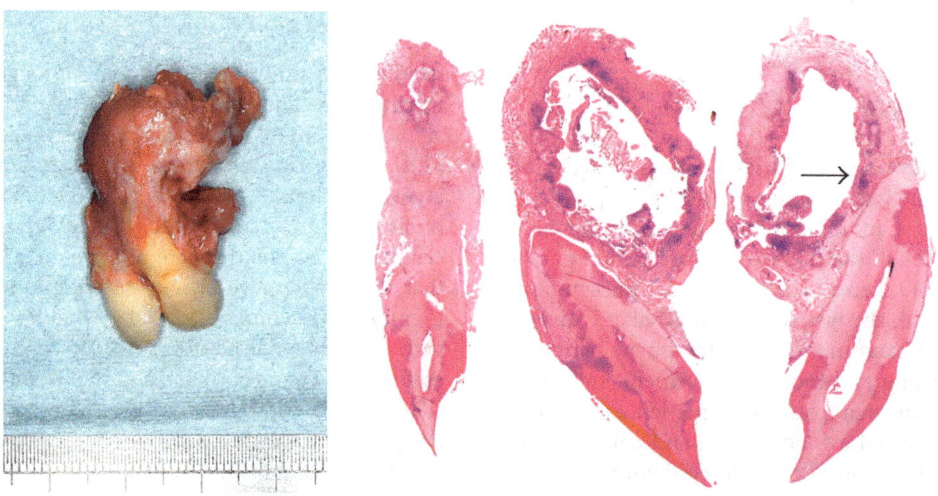

(a) (b)

FIGURE 4: Macroscopic and survey view of the surgically resected specimen. (a) Surgical specimen. (b) Invasive atypical squamous cell nests in the cyst walls (black arrow) (HE; original magnification: ×1 (b)).

3. Discussion

Malignant changes in the epithelial lining of odontogenic cysts have been described previously [1]. Although the exact number of documented cases is difficult to determine, Gardner [5] reviewed all cases documented between 1889 and 1967 and considered 25 of them to be acceptable examples of malignant transformation of the epithelial lining of an odontogenic cyst. Gardner [5] proposed the following definitive criteria for identifying a lesion as PIOSCC derived from the odontogenic cyst: (i) a microscopic area of transition from a benign cystic epithelial lining to SCC, (ii) an intact overlying oral mucosa, (iii) the absence of carcinoma in adjacent structures, and (iv) the absence of metastatic carcinoma from a distant tumor [6]. Our present case fulfills all of these criteria. There are few documented examples of definitive histopathological transition between SCC and the epithelial lining of an odontogenic cyst [7]. In a review of 81 documented cases in the world literature, Woldron and Mustoe [6] considered the incidence of carcinoma arising from the odontogenic cyst to be approximately 1-2 per 1000 [8]. In a recent retrospective study of 116 cases of PIOSCC between 1938 and 2010, Bodner et al. in 2011 [3] found only 16 confirmed cases of PIOSCC arising from the OKC.

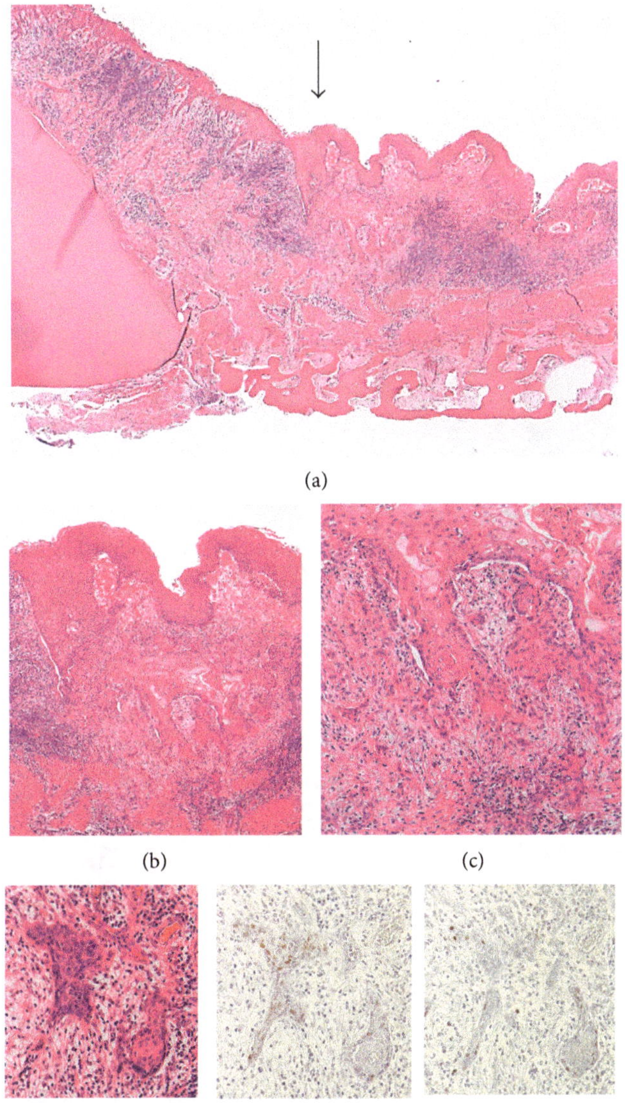

(a) (b) (c) (d) (e) (f)

FIGURE 5: Microscopic features of the surgical specimen. (a) Invasion of atypical epithelium (black arrow). (b) Invasive squamous epithelium irregularly migrating from the epithelial cyst lining similar to SCC. (c) High-power magnification. (d) Invasive nests, (e) p53, and (f) Ki-67 (HE and IHC; original magnification: ×12.5 (a), ×40 (b), ×100 (c), and ×200 (d), (e), and (f)).

PIOSCCs arising from OKCs are extremely rare, accounting for fewer than 30 cases reported so far [3, 4]. Evidence of a cystic component is a prerequisite for the diagnosis of PIOSCC arising from OKCs. The histopathologic criteria employed to document an odontogenic origin are (i) malignant transformation of the cyst lining, with a transition from the normal lining to dysplasia and to carcinoma, (ii) palisaded columnar cells, and (iii) the inductive influence of connective tissue [7]. All of these features were evident in the present case, and the most compatible diagnosis was PIOSCC derived from the OKC.

The pathogenesis of this lesion is still unknown. It has been reported that keratin metaplasia followed by hyperplasia and dysplasia of the cyst epithelium are signature events in the development of SCC in the OKC [9]. Also, the presence of keratinization in the cyst lining suggests a greater risk of malignant change [10]. Furthermore, Gardner [5] and Tamgadge et al. [11] have suggested that long-standing chronic inflammation is a factor related to malignant transformation of benign epithelium. In the present case, chronic inflammatory cell infiltration was seen in the fibrous connective tissue of the cyst wall (Figure 5(a)). The chronic inflammation in the present case was considered due to cyst epithelial damage resulting from degenerated keratins or cortical bone absorption resulting from growth and local invasion. Inflammation would likely occur as a stromal response to such tissue degeneration. In fact, inflammatory cell infiltration was also found in the cystic cavity (Figure 7(d)), and in routine pathological diagnosis, we often observed epidermal cysts with epithelial damage or an inflammatory reaction in response to keratin debris.

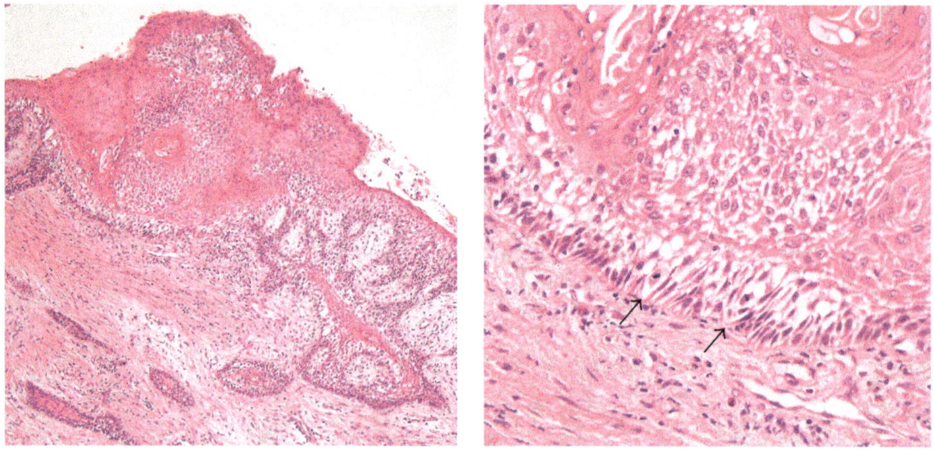

(a) (b)

Figure 6: Unusual ameloblastomatous change of the OKC. (a) Only part of the lining epithelium shows papillary hyperplasia with ameloblastomatous epithelial elongation. (b) The suprabasal layer shows stellate reticulum-like formation, and the basal layer shows palisading tall columnar cell nuclei with focally mitoses (arrowheads) (HE; original magnification: ×40 (a) and ×200 (b)).

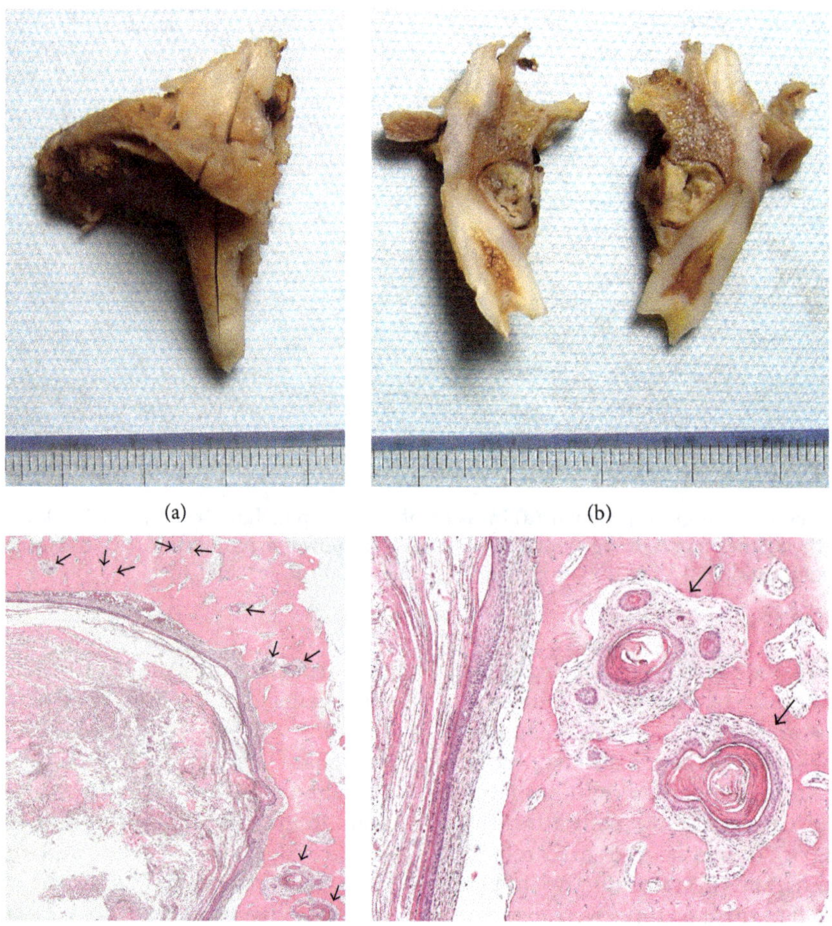

(a) (b) (c) (d)

Figure 7: Macroscopic appearance and microscopic features of the additional surgically resected specimen. (a) Resected specimen. (b) Cystic lesion in the palatal side of the second premolar. (c) Microscopically, locally invasive daughter follicles in many bone marrow spaces (arrows). (d) Invasive solid cystic follicles with a KAB-like growth pattern (arrows) (HE; original magnification ×40 (c) and ×200 (d)).

Unexpectedly, in the specimen obtained at initial surgery, unusual ameloblastomatous epithelial elongation was found in a limited part of the lesion, and in the second resected specimen, very small numerous invasive solid epithelial follicles composed of central lamellar para- or orthokeratin plugs were found in the bone marrow spaces on the outer side of the main cyst (Figures 7(c) and 7(d)). Histologically, these solid epithelial follicles had a keratoameloblastoma (KAB)/solid-OKC- (SOKC-) like growth pattern [12]. Ide et al. suggested that KAB might be derived from a preexisting OKC [13], and Geng et al. presented a supportive case in which the SOKC showed partial transformation to ameloblastomatous change [14]. About 40 years before (1977), Brannon [15] observed mural nodules of ameloblastoma as direct proliferations from the OKC lining, with an incidence of 0.6%. Therefore, we considered that the OKC might have the potential to differentiate into ameloblastoma. In the lining epithelium of odontogenic cysts, pseudoameloblastoma is often seen as a secondary morphological change induced by inflammation. In the additional resected specimen from the present case, no effect of inflammation was evident (Figures 7(c) and 7(d)). It is unknown whether true ameloblastomatous transformation had occurred, but the morphological appearance resembled KAB in part of this additional resected specimen. Therefore, we interpreted this by indicating that the OKC had been partially transformed to benign ameloblastomatous epithelium as associated anaplastic change. Accumulation of further case reports and in vitro studies of odontogenic cysts will be necessary to clarify the mechanism of epithelial differentiation and carcinogenesis caused by various factors including chronic inflammation. Our present case is considered to represent an extremely rare case of initial-stage PIOSCC derived from the OKC showing partial keratoameloblastomatous change in the maxilla.

Consent

Informed consent from a patient has been obtained in this case report.

Conflicts of Interest

The authors declare that there are no conflicts of interest regarding the publication of this article.

References

[1] L. R. Eversole, C. H. Siar, and I. van der Waal, "Primary intraosseous squamous cell carcinoma," in *World Health Organization Classification of Tumours. Pathology and Genetics, Head and Neck Tumours*, L. Barnes, J. W. Everson, P. Reichart, and D. Sidransky, Eds., pp. 290-291, IARC Press, Lyon, France, 2005.

[2] E. W. Odell, C. M. Allen, and M. Richardson, "Primary intraosseous carcinoma, NOS," in *World Health Organization Classification of Head and Neck Tumours*, A. K. El-Naggar, J. K. C. Chan, J. R. Grandis, T. Takata, and P. J. Slootweg, Eds., pp. 207–209, IARC Press, Lyon, France, 2017.

[3] L. Bodner, E. Manor, M. Shear, and I. van der Waal, "Primary intra-osseous squamous cell carcinoma arising in an odontogenic cyst: a clinicopathologic analysis of 116 reported cases," *Journal of Oral Pathology and Medicine*, vol. 40, no. 10, pp. 733–738, 2011.

[4] S. Acharya, A. S. Tayaar, K. Hallkeri, S. Adirajaiah, and K. Gopalkrishnan, "Squamous cell carcinoma emerging in an orthokeratinized odontogenic cyst: a case report and brief review," *Journal of Oral and Maxillofacal Surgery Medicine and Pathology*, vol. 26, no. 4, pp. 563–568, 2014.

[5] A. F. Gardner, "A survey of odontogenic cysts and their relationship to squamous cell carcinoma," *Journal of the Canadian Dental Association*, vol. 41, no. 3, pp. 161–167, 1975.

[6] C. A. Waldron and T. A. Mustoe, "Primary intraosseous carcinoma of the mandible with probable origin in an odontogenic cyst," *Oral Surgery, Oral Medicine, Oral Pathology*, vol. 67, no. 6, pp. 716–724, 1989.

[7] P. R. Elzay, "Primary intraosseous carcinoma of the jaws. Review and update of odontogenic carcinoma," *Oral Surgery, Oral Medicine, Oral Pathology*, vol. 54, no. 3, pp. 299–303, 1982.

[8] P. J. Stoelinga and F. B. Bronkhorst, "The incidence, multiple presentation and recurrence of aggressive cysts of the jaws," *Journal of Cranio-Maxillofacial Surgery*, vol. 16, no. 4, pp. 184–195, 1988.

[9] R. M. Browne and N. G. Gough, "Malignant change in the epithelial lining of odontogenic cyst," *Cancer*, vol. 29, no. 5, pp. 1199–1207, 1972.

[10] K. G. van der Wal, J. G. de Visscher, and H. F. Eggink, "Squamous cell carcinoma arising in a residual cyst. A case report," *International Journal of Oral and Maxillofacial Surgery*, vol. 22, no. 6, pp. 350–352, 1993.

[11] S. Tamgadge, A. Tamgadge, N. Modak, and S. Bhalerao, "Primary intraosseous squamous cell carcinoma arising from an odontogenic keratocyst: a case report and literature review," *Ecancermedicalscience*, vol. 7, p. 316, 2013.

[12] N. A. Said-Al-Naief, H. Lumerman, M. Ramer et al., "Keratoameloblastoma of the maxilla. A case report and review of the literature," *Oral Surgery, Oral Medicine, Oral Pathology, Oral Radiology, and Endodontics*, vol. 84, no. 5, pp. 535–539, 1997.

[13] F. Ide, K. Mishima, and I. Saito, "Solid-cystic tumor variant of odontogenic keratocyst: an aggressive but benign lesion simulating keratoameloblastoma," *Virchows Arch*, vol. 442, no. 5, pp. 501–503, 2003.

[14] N. Geng, D. Lv, Q. M. Chen et al., "Solid variant of keratocystic odontogenic tumor with ameloblastomatous transformation: a case report and review of the literature," *Oral Surgery, Oral Medicine, Oral Pathology, and Oral Radiology*, vol. 114, no. 2, pp. 223–229, 2012.

[15] R. B. Brannon, "The odontogenic keratocyst. A clinicopathologic study of 312 cases. Part II. Histologic features," *Oral Surgery, Oral Medicine, and Oral Pathology*, vol. 43, no. 2, pp. 233–255, 1977.

36

Endovascular Management of a Refractory Pseudoaneurysm of the Sternocleidomastoid Artery Caused by Attempted Internal Jugular Central Line Placement with Long-Term Follow-Up

Yassmeen Abdel-Aty[1] and Michael P. Bellew[2,3]

[1]*Mayo Clinic Arizona, Department of Otolaryngology Head and Neck Surgery, 5777 E Mayo Blvd, Phoenix, AZ 85054, USA*
[2]*Department of Medical Education, Assistant Professor of Neurosurgery, UCF College of Medicine, 6850 Lake Nona Blvd, Orlando, FL 32827, USA*
[3]*Florida Hospital Orlando, 601 East Rollins Street, Orlando, FL 32803, USA*

Correspondence should be addressed to Yassmeen Abdel-Aty; y.abdelaty@gmail.com

Academic Editor: Holger Sudhoff

Introduction. This case report shows successful treatment of a refractory sternocleidomastoid branch of the superior thyroid artery (SBSTA) pseudoaneurysm using endovascular glue embolization in a patient who refused surgery. *Case Presentation.* A 63-year-old female with multiple comorbidities presented with a firm 7 cm tender mass located in the right neck. Ultrasound showed pseudoaneurysm and a $7 \times 3.3 \times 4$ cm multilobular hematoma in the location of the previous central line. CTA showed a corresponding heterogeneous mass. Serial imaging demonstrated enlargement over 2 weeks. Angiogram showed contrast blush off of the SBSTA. *Management and Outcome.* SBSTA was embolized using glue. Repeat angiogram showed embolization and no contrast blush. One month later, the mass was no longer pulsatile but present on physical exam. CTA showed decreased size. 8 months later, her neck was soft without mass. *Discussion.* Pseudoaneurysms of the external carotid artery are rare and usually due to trauma. Pseudoaneurysms after central line placement are documented, but most are complications of femoral central lines. A handful of cases of superior thyroid artery pseudoaneurysms due to several etiologies are reported, but none involving the SBSTA. Therapeutic options include surveillance, compression, thrombin injection, embolization, and surgery. Endovascular management offers an alternative for patients unwilling or unable to undergo open surgery.

1. Introduction

Pseudoaneurysms are a tear though all layers of an artery allowing blood to leak into the surrounding tissue causing a mass that often gradually expands due to its communication with the arterial lumen. Signs and symptoms of pseudoaneurysms in the neck can include a pulsating mass which is the most common presentation, craniocervical pain, dysphagia, hoarseness, and neurologic deficits due to cranial nerve palsy or stroke.

A pseudoaneurysm of the external carotid artery (ECA) is very rare with an incidence of 0.07% and mortality of 30% [1]. It usually occurs if the trunk or branches of this vessel are damaged. This is most likely due to trauma of the neck but can also be due to iatrogenic complications such as surgery in this area and, to a lesser degree, central line placement [2].

Around 7 million central venous catheters are placed yearly in the United States. It is a relatively safe procedure, but complications do occur. The reported incidence of serious complications varies from 0.4% to 9.9%. Accidental arterial puncture occurs in approximately 5% of all central venous catheter placements and is more likely in internal jugular vein catheterization. This can lead to arterial dissection, arteriovenous fistula formation, hematoma,

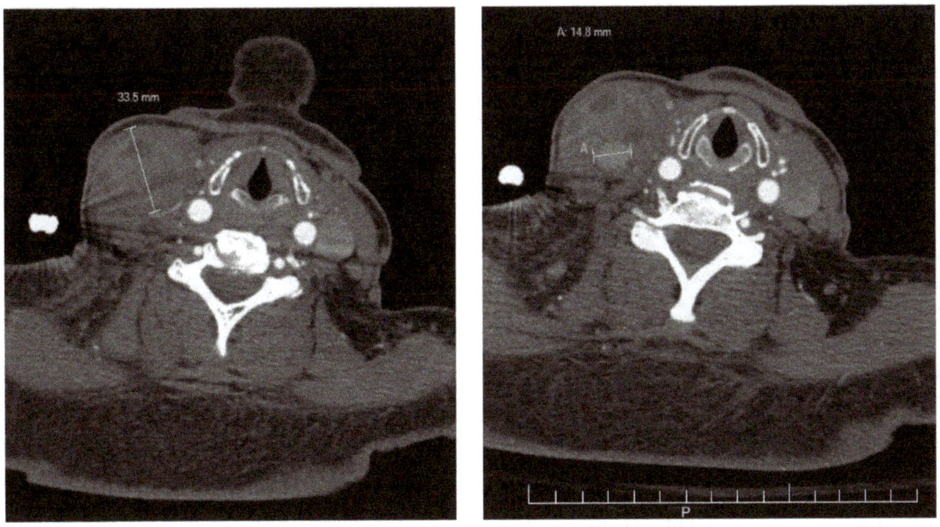

(a) (b)

FIGURE 1: CT angiography of neck: (a) right neck mass measured and (b) right neck pseudoaneurysm measured.

pseudoaneurysms, and stroke [3]. Pseudoaneurysm formation after central line placement has been well documented in the literature but most of these cases are complications of femoral central line attempts [3].

Although cases of ECA pseudoaneurysms have been reported as well as a handful of cases of superior thyroid artery pseudoaneurysm, no cases of a sternocleidomastoid artery pseudoaneurysm have previously been reported to our knowledge. The sternocleidomastoid artery is one of the five branches of the superior thyroid artery which is a branch of the external carotid artery. It can be identified because it is the only branch of the superior thyroid artery that courses laterally [4]. This case study details a management option for aneurysms refractory to standard treatment methods as well as the time course of hematoma resolution during midterm (1 month)/long-term (8 month) follow-up.

2. Case Report

A 63-year-old woman presented with a firm 7 cm multilobular tender mass located in the region of the right sternocleidomastoid directly above the clavicle. She had multiple comorbidities including renal failure, systemic lupus erythematosus, and protein S deficiency, a history of transient ischemic attack, deep vein thrombosis, and pulmonary embolism, and longstanding malnourishment requiring jejunostomy tube placement. The firm mass was identified 1 month after an unsuccessful attempt at placing a right internal jugular vein central line. When the central line was originally placed, she developed pain and swelling of her neck. The swelling was pulsatile at that time and enlarging. She was offered surgery as the standard of care for her condition which she refused because she did not want to undergo an invasive procedure and was aware of the risks involved with holding her anticoagulant medication. She had two thrombin injections in the mass since without success. She complained of right neck pain. She was not having any difficulty breathing and denied shortness of breath.

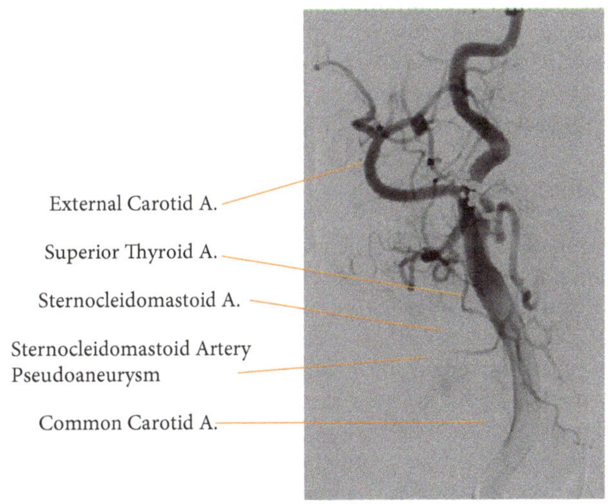

FIGURE 2: Angiogram of right common carotid and its branches. This figure depicts the pseudoaneurysm of right sternocleidomastoid artery prior to embolization as well as shows vascular anatomy rarely identified in the operative setting.

Soft tissue ultrasound after the two thrombin injections showed pseudoaneurysm and a $7 \times 3.3 \times 4$ cm multilobular hematoma at the base of the right neck. CTA of the neck showed a corresponding heterogeneous mass. The pseudoaneurysm was seen measuring 1.5 cm at the internal margin of the hematoma. Serial imaging with CTA demonstrated enlargement over a 2-week interval (Figure 1).

Angiogram showed blush of contrast coming off of the sternocleidomastoid branch of the superior thyroid artery identifying the location of the pseudoaneurysm (Figure 2). This branch was embolized using glue. Repeat angiogram showed successful embolization and no contrast blush.

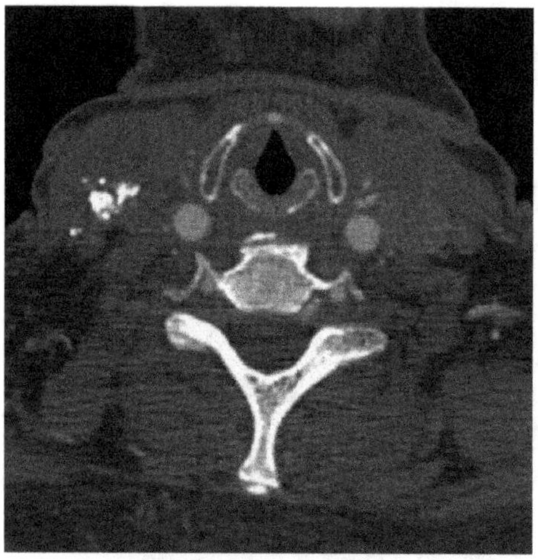

FIGURE 3: CT angiography neck: right neck mass on 1 month follow-up status after right pseudoaneurysm embolized with glue. These can be compared to the preintervention CT in Figure 1 showing that the neck mass has improved.

On follow-up one month later, the mass was no longer pulsatile but still present on physical exam. CTA of the neck showed a decrease in size from the previous CTA (Figure 3).

On follow-up 8 months later, she was found to have a soft neck with no mass on physical exam.

3. Discussion

Diagnostic imaging can be used when history and physical examination point to possible pseudoaneurysm. Doppler ultrasound is a very helpful and benign test that can reveal a pseudoaneurysm as a spindle shape or sac-like dilation. It can show turbulent flow and vessel dilation with a 95% accuracy for pseudoaneurysm. It is less effective for deeper lesions which may be better seen on contrast-enhanced CT or angiography. Using angiography for diagnostic purposes is not first line since it is a more invasive procedure but can be utilized when it is also intended as a therapeutic option after other imaging has been performed [2].

Therapeutic options include surgical resections, conservative surveillance, compression, thrombin injection, and catheter-based embolization. The gold standard treatment of pseudoaneurysm is surgical repair [3]. As with any surgery in the neck, surgical repair does not go without risks. Studies have shown that many iatrogenic pseudoaneurysms will heal spontaneously and as many as 89% of them will resolve spontaneously [2]. This suggests that if the pseudoaneurysm is not causing any major complications it is acceptable to watch it conservatively. However, it must be watched very closely because hemorrhage into the neck or compression of vital structures in the neck could be devastating.

Ultrasound-guided thrombin injection relies on the formation of a clot within the pseudoaneurysm to exclude it from the circulation. Case reports have shown success of ultrasound-guided thrombin injection [1]. This ensures that thrombin is injected directly into the pseudoaneurysm. There is also risk of incomplete occlusion or recannulization which may require additional therapy [5]. Since our patient refused surgery, trying thrombin injections was reasonable but unsuccessful.

A study done at the Ninth People's Hospital, Shanghai Jiao Tong University concluded coil embolization by angiography of pseudoaneurysms coming off the external carotid artery is a useful alternative to standard surgical repair and avoids morbidity associated with performing surgery in the face and neck area [2]. Many case reports have also documented success of endovascular embolization of pseudoaneurysms of the ECA and its branches [6, 7]. In our case, we have shown that glue can also be used to successfully resolve a pseudoaneurysm endovascularly.

4. Conclusion

Pseudoaneurysm should be included in differential for neck mass. A pseudoaneurysm due to central venous catheter placement is a very rare occurrence. Although cases of external carotid artery pseudoaneurysms have been reported, most are due to trauma. A handful of cases of superior thyroid artery pseudoaneurysms have been reported but no cases of sternocleidomastoid artery, a branch of the superior thyroid artery, pseudoaneurysms have previously been reported to our knowledge. This case study shows a successful resolution of a sternocleidomastoid artery pseudoaneurysm using glue endovascularly. Other treatments that were attempted were conservative management and thrombin injections, but these failed to resolve this woman's symptoms. While conservative management and compression may be good therapies to try initially in patients who are not in imminent danger, surgery and endovascular treatment are better therapies in pseudoaneurysms that are resistant to treatment or in unstable patients. Although surgery is the gold standard, endovascular treatment provides a less invasive option when the patient is not a good candidate for surgery or refuses surgical intervention. Thrombin injections may also be attempted but are not as safe without concurrent endovascular cerebral protection.

Conflicts of Interest

The authors declare that they have no conflicts of interest.

References

[1] S. Islam, M. Ali, C. Avery, and J. P. Hayter, "External carotid artery pseudoaneurysm following microvascular free flap reconstruction. The role of endovascular thrombin injection in embolization: a case report and review," *International Journal of Oral and Maxillofacial Surgery*, vol. 43, no. 9, pp. 1069–1072, 2014.

[2] D. Wang, L. Su, Y. Han, and X. Fan, "Embolization treatment of pseudoaneurysms originating from the external carotid artery," *Journal of Vascular Surgery*, vol. 61, no. 4, pp. 920–926, 2014.

[3] J. Momiy and J. Vasquez, "Iatrogenic vertebral artery pseudoaneurysm due to central venous catheterization," *Baylor University Medical Center Proceedings*, vol. 24, no. 2, pp. 96–100, 2011.

[4] P. Gupta, A. S. Bhalla, S. Thulkar et al., "Variations in superior thyroid artery: a selective angiographic study," *Indian Journal of Radiology and Imaging*, vol. 24, no. 1, pp. 66–71, 2014.
[5] C. J. Stapleton, M. R. Fusco, A. J. Thomas, E. I. Levy, and C. S. Ogilvy, "Traumatic pseudoaneurysms of the superficial temporal artery: case series, anatomy, and multidisciplinary treatment considerations," *Journal of Clinical Neuroscience*, vol. 21, no. 9, pp. 1529–1532, 2014.
[6] J. L. Smelt, O. Alhamarneh, J. D. Dyer, and L. Liew, "Endovascular coiling of a mycotic external carotid artery pseudoaneurysm following pharyngolaryngectomy with a free jejunal graft," *Journal of Laryngology & Otology*, vol. 126, no. 2, pp. 214–216, 2012.
[7] J. E. Cohen, J. M. Gomori, S. Moscovici, S. Grigoriadis, F. Ramirez de Noriega, and E. Itshayek, "Endovascular management of postoperative pseudoaneurysms of the external carotid artery," *Journal of Clinical Neuroscience*, vol. 19, no. 5, pp. 649–654, 2012.

37

Acute Mastoiditis Complicated with Concomitant Bezold's Abscess and Lateral Sinus Thrombosis

Aziz Mustafa [1], Burhan Toçi [1], Hajdin Thaçi [1], Bujar Gjikolli [2] and Nehat Baftiu [3]

[1] *ENT Clinic, University Clinical Center of Kosova, Prishtina, Kosovo*
[2] *Radiology Clinic, University Clinical Center of Kosova, Prishtina, Kosovo*
[3] *Anesthesiology/Reanimation Clinic, University Clinical Center of Kosova, Prishtina, Kosovo*

Correspondence should be addressed to Nehat Baftiu; nehatbaftiu777@gmail.com

Academic Editor: Dimitrios G. Balatsouras

Bezold's abscess is a very rare extracranial complication of acute mastoiditis. Lateral sinus thrombosis is another intracranial complication of acute mastoiditis that can occur, but there are only few reports of concomitant ispilateral Bezold's abscess and lateral sinus thrombosis with favorable outcome. We diagnosed and treated successfully a 14-year-old girl suffering from *Streptococcus pneumoniae* acute mastoiditis complicated with Bezold's abscess and lateral sinus thrombosis. Surgical treatment included myringotomy, cortical mastoidectomy, and Bezold's abscess incision and drainage. During the course of treatment, we concluded that lateral sinus thrombosis was not caused from mastoiditis by direct spread but from pressure on internal jugular vein caused from Bezold's abscess.

1. Introduction

Acute otitis media (AOM) is a frequent infection in childhood, mostly with viral etiology, but bacterial AOM and acute mastoiditis (AM) can be complicated with life-threatening either extracranial complication (EEC) or intracranial complication (ICC). Named after German otologist Friedrich von Bezold (1842–1908), who in 1881 was the first author to describe neck abscess along the sternocleidomastoid muscle (SCM) [1], Bezold's abscess (BA) is a severe and very rare ECC of suppurative AOM or cholesteatomatous chronic otitis media (CCOM). In cases of severe bacterial infection of the tip of mastoid, the suppurative content from the mastoid air cells can descent along the upper insertion of sternocleidomastoid muscle and cause collection of the pus between muscle and its fascia. If not treated in time and properly, content from BA can descent to mediastinum, causing acute mediastinitis, another complication with mortality of 70% [2–6]. Comparing with BA, the lateral sinus thrombosis (LST) is an another life-threatening ICC of ear infections, which can be seen more often in combination with other ICCs, but there are only few reports on concomitant ECC/ICC (BA/LST) complications arising from acute mastoiditis [2, 7]. Mainstay in diagnostic of ECC and ICC is clinical imaging, computed tomography (CT), or magnetic resonance imaging (MRI) [8]. Besides the intravenously administered antibiotics, the surgical treatment (mastoidectomy, myringotomy, and abscess drainage) is mandatory for proper management and prevention of sequels. In cases of sinus thrombosis, anticoagulation therapy is not definitively associated with improved outcomes and warrants further research [9–11].

This article describes a favorable outcome case report of concomitant ECC/ICC, BA/LST and discusses management of these complications.

2. Case Presentation

A 14-year-old previously healthy girl was admitted to Infectious Disease Department of University Clinical Center of Kosova in Prishtina, complaining in headache, fever, right earache, and stiffness of the neck and right side torticollis. Diagnosis of meningitis was established according to the symptoms, physical exam, blood analyzes values, and results of lumbar puncture. Blood analyses were as follows: erythrocyte sedimentation rate (ESR) 80 mm/first hour, white blood count (WBC) 22,000 per square mm, and C-reactive protein (CRP) value was 126. Lumbar puncture results showed about 200 cells (leucocytes)/square mm, and manitol 20%, dexamethasone, analgesics-antipyretic, and antibiotics (ceftriaxone and vancomycine) were administered i.v. immediately. Consultation of ENT specialist, 2 days later, revealed right side AOM, with tenderness in mastoid tip palpation. The neck in the right posterior triangle was swollen and tender in palpation. Myringotomy under general anesthesia was performed, and suppurative content is released from middle ear cavity. A swab for bacteriology exam was obtained for culture, and the result, 2 days later, revealed *Streptococcus pneumoniae* as a causative agent. A CT scan, performed two days later, showed right side mastoid cells filled with liquid and thickening of mucosa. Besides this, a collection of possible suppurative content was detected in posterior triangle of right side of the neck, near the mastoid tip (Bezold's abscess). No imaging signs for intracranial spreading of ear infection were detected (Figure 1). The patient was transferred to our department (ENT), and an urgent operation was performed by the first author on the same day: cortical mastoidectomy with neck abscess drainage. The mastoid cells were found to be filled with thick mucosa and suppuration. All mastoid cells were cleaned, and *aditus ad antrum* was widened. A myringotomy procedure was performed, and a ventilation tube was inserted. Bezold's abscess was evacuated from the mastoid side and from neck incision. All mastoid cells from the sinodural angle (Citelli's angle) were cleaned; the bone above sigmoid sinus was thinned and did not show any infiltration of sinus. The bone cover of the lateral sinus was without pathologic changes. A drainage tube was put from the neck incision. The mastoid cavity was tamponed with gauze imbibed in local antibiotic/cortisone and retro auricular incision was not sutured. Metronidazole is added in postoperative medical therapy. Neck drainage from Bezold's abscess was washed out with syringe with saline and antibiotic (gentamicin) twice a day for the next 10 days, and the mastoid tamponade was changed every second day under general anesthesia. The patient showed excellent improvement clinically. Incision was sutured and drainage was removed. Laboratory analyses returned to normal values. Repeated lumbar punctures gave normal result. An MRI of the head was performed two weeks after the operation, and it showed a total thrombosis of lateral (sigmoid) sinus and partial thrombosis of transverse sinus of the right side. An anticoagulant therapy was given for 14 days subcutaneously. After therapy, the control MRI with contrast (magnetic resonance venography, MRV) showed the same picture: total thrombosis of lateral sinus and partial thrombosis of the transverse sinus of the right side with healing of the neck and mastoid cavity (Figure 2). In 30 months of follow-up, the patient has definitive asymptomatic LST and dry normal hearing ear.

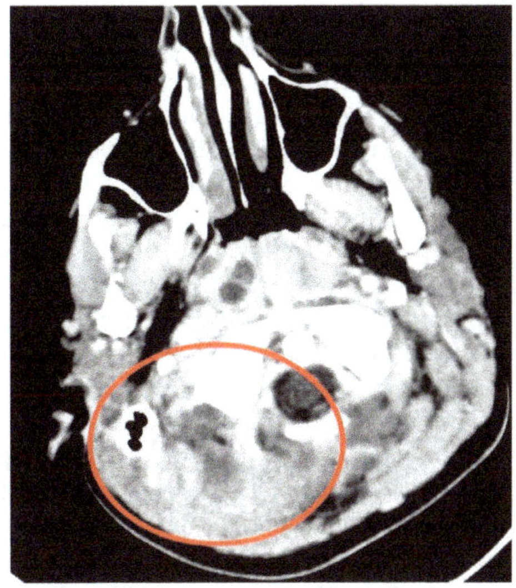

FIGURE 1: Irregular hypodensity below the right mastoid and right half of the occipital bone surrounded with postcontrast (red circle) increase of density represent the abscess formation.

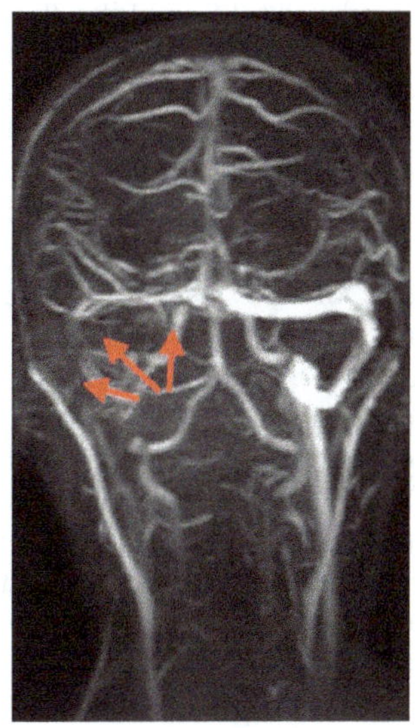

FIGURE 2: Coronal MR venography 3 weeks after operation shows missing right transverse and sigmoid venous sinus.

3. Discussion

The use of antibiotics in treatment of acute otitis media (AOM) reduced the incidence of the acute mastoiditis (AM). During 1950s, 0.4% of episodes of AOM developed into AM, whereas the incidence of AM during 1980s dropped to 0.004% [12]. However, mastoiditis still occurs, and intracranial and extracranial complications can occur if AM is not managed in time. In Britain, only six cases of lateral sinus thrombosis and one case of Bezold's abscess have been reported in the literature in the last decade of the 20th century [13]. In our only tertiary medical center in Kosovo, in a 17-year period (1994–2011), the first author reported 2 cases of BA and 18 cases of LST as complications of cholesteatoma, but none from AM [14, 15]. This presented case is the first reported case of concomitant BA and LST arising from acute mastoiditis.

In all reported cases of BA/LST, the clinical appearance was typical. Earache, tender palpation in the mastoid tip, and neck stiffness and torticollis with high body temperature and clinical appearance of transitory meningitis are first symptoms and signs to raise suspicion on severe complication. If the body temperature changes periodically, the so-called septic temperature, this must warn clinicians of the possible thrombophlebitis, with danger of development of the fatal sepsis [3, 4, 8]. The patient we present in this paper had the all symptoms and signs mentioned above.

The acute mastoiditis is caused by the aerobe or anaerobe bacteria. Au et al. report in a review of 104 cases of pediatric LST from literature that from swabs taken during surgery or during suppuration, in 46% of cases, a single bacterial organism was isolated, with beta hemolytic *Streptococcus*, *Streptococcus pneumoniae*, and *Staphylococcus aureus* being the most common [10]. In our presented case, we took the swab during myringotomy, and the bacteriology result revealed *Streptococcus pneumonia* as the causative agent, and the ordinate antimicrobial therapy was culture based.

In the diagnostic of BA and LST, besides symptoms and signs, laboratory analyses and bacteriology examination, the imaging techniques are mainstay and represent the golden standard. In the cases with BA, on CT imaging, there is usually unilateral opacification of the middle ear and the mastoid cavities, often associated with bone erosion, especially of the mastoid tip. The collection of pus can be detected along the SCM muscle [7]. There are also reports of use of the ultrasound on detection of purulent contents in the neck. MRI and MRV are more sensitive in LST diagnosis and can be used for follow-up of the thrombosis [4, 8–10]. During the management of this particular case, with the help of CT imaging, we diagnosed and treated in time the acute mastoiditis and BA. The diagnosis of LST was made later during postoperative treatment, and the discussion of managing team were in the issue of origin of thrombosis. In the end, we agreed that the cause of thrombosis was the pressure of pus collection on the internal jugular vein (IJV) that subsequently caused the LST. This conclusion was made based on the findings during mastoidectomy, when we found normal bone covering the lateral sinus. Further search on literature must be conducted to conclude or exclude this statement.

Therapy of complications of the acute mastoiditis is medical, and antibiotics are chosen on the basis of the bacteriology exam, empirically and surgically, depending on the complications. All experts who care for the patients with mastoiditis and most of the publications on this topic advocate the administration of i.v. antibiotics and eventually ventilation tube in first 48 hours after the hospitalization and repeat the analyzes. If there is clinical improvement and normalization of analyzes, antibiotics continue for next 5 to 10 days. If there is no improvement, mastoidectomy has to be performed. In case of the complications, especially in the case of multiple complications, surgical treatment must be performed urgently. In our reported case, we first did a ventilation tube insertion and then mastoidectomy and BA evacuation and drainage. The LST was developed in the course of disease, caused from the pressure of pus collection in the neck. This causes the stopping of the blood flow through the venous sinus and causes consecutive thrombosis.

As a conclusion, early detection of developing complication of AM is the cornerstone of effective treatment of these complications. Multiple complications, although rare, still can threaten life of young patients.

Abbreviations

AM: Acute mastoiditis
AOM: Acute otitis media
BA: Bezold's abscess
CCOM: Cholesteatomatous chronic otitis media
CRP: C-reactive protein
CT: Computed tomography
EEC: Extracranial complication
ENT: Ear, nose, throat
ESR: Erythrocyte sedimentation rate
ICC: Intracranial complication
LST: Lateral sinus thrombosis
MRI: Magnetic resonance imaging
MRV: Magnetic resonance venography
WBC: White blood count.

Consent

Informed consent was obtained from the parents of the minor patient included in the study.

Conflicts of Interest

The authors declare that they have no conflict of interest.

References

[1] F. Bezold, "Ein neuer wegfür die ausbreitungeitriger entzündungaus den raumen des mittelohrs auf die nachbarschaft," *Deutsche Medizinische Wochenschrift*, vol. 7, no. 28, pp. 381–384, 1881.

[2] L. H. Govea-Camacho, R. Pérez-Ramírez, A. Cornejo-Suárez, R. Fierro-Rizo, C. J. Jiménez-Sala, and C. S. Rosales-Orozco, "Diagnosis and treatment of the complications of otitis media in adults. Case series and literature review," *Cirugía y Cirujanos*, vol. 84, no. 5, pp. 398–404, 2016.

[3] H. Al-Baharna, H. Al-Mubaireek, and V. Arora, "Bezold's abscess: a case report and review of cases over 14 years," *Indian Journal of Otology*, vol. 22, pp. 148–151, 2016.

[4] I. M. Vlastos, G. Helmis, I. Athanasopoulos, and M. Houlakis, "Acute mastoiditis complicated with Bezold abscess, sigmoid sinus thrombosis and occipital osteomyelitis in a child," *European Review for Medical and Pharmacological Sciences*, vol. 14, pp. 635–638, 2010.

[5] D. Nelson and R. Jeanmonod, "Bezold abscess: a rare complication of mastoiditis," *American Journal of Emergency Medicine*, vol. 31, no. 11, p. 1626, 2013.

[6] G. Marioni, C. de Filippis, A. Tregnaghi, R. Marchese-Ragona, and A. Staffieri, "Bezold's abscess in children: case report and review of the literature," *International Journal of Pediatric Otorhinolaryngology*, vol. 61, no. 2, pp. 173–177, 2001.

[7] M. Lahlou, A. Lazrak, M. Boulaich, A. Oujilal, and M. Kzadri, "Association of Bezold's abscess and sigmoid sinus thrombosis. A case report," *Revue de Laryngologie-Otologie-Rhinologie*, vol. 127, pp. 157–160, 2006.

[8] W. Bou-Assaly, J. Mckellop, and S. K. Mukherji, "Computed

tomography imaging of acute neck inflammatory processes," *World Journal of Radiology*, vol. 2, no. 3, pp. 91–96, 2010.

[9] G. B. Wanna, L. M. Dharamsi, J. R. Moss, M. L. Bennett, R. C. Thompson, and D. S. Haynes, "Contemporary management of intracranial complications of otitis media," *Otology & Neurotology*, vol. 31, no. 1, pp. 111–117, 2010.

[10] J. K. Au, S. I. Adam, and E. M. Michaelides, "Contemporary management of pediatric lateral sinus thrombosis: a twenty year review," *American Journal of Otolaryngology*, vol. 34, no. 2, pp. 145–150, 2013.

[11] E. Novoa, M. Podvinec, R. Angst, and N. Gürtler, "Paediatric otogenic lateral sinus thrombosis: therapeutic management, outcome and thrombophilic evaluation," *International Journal of Pediatric Otorhinolaryngology*, vol. 77, no. 6, pp. 996–1001, 2013.

[12] M. Luntz, A. Brodsky, S. Nusen et al., "Acute mastoiditis–the antibiotic era: a multicenter study," *International Journal of Pediatric Otorhinolaryngology*, vol. 57, no. 1, pp. 1–9, 2001.

[13] J. Jose, A. P. Coatesworth, R. Anthony, and P. G. Reilly, "Life threatening complications after partially treated mastoiditis," *BMJ*, vol. 327, no. 7405, pp. 41-42, 2003.

[14] A. Mustafa, S. Kuçi, and A. Behramaj, "Management of cholesteatoma complications: our experience in 145 cases," *Indian Journal of Otology*, vol. 20, no. 2, pp. 45–47, 2014.

[15] A. Mustafa, C. H. Debry, M. Wiorowski, E. Martin, and A. Gentine, "Treatment of acute mastoiditis: report of 31 cases over a ten year period," *Revue de Laryngologie-Otologie-Rhinologie*, vol. 125, pp. 165–169, 2004.

38

Recurrent Adenomatous Neuroendocrine Tumor of the Middle Ear: A Diagnostic Challenge

J. Vilain, J.-C. Degols, and S. Ledeghen

ENT Department, Clinique Saint-Pierre, 9 Av Reine Fabiola, 1340 Ottignies LLN, Belgium

Correspondence should be addressed to J. Vilain; jacques.vilain@cspo.be

Academic Editor: Harukazu Hiraumi

Middle ear adenomatous neuroendocrine tumor (MEANT) poses a diagnostic challenge. Clinical symptoms are nonspecific. Definite diagnosis is made by histopathological analysis of the tumor after a complete surgical resection based on an extensive computed tomography/magnetic resonance imaging (CT/MRI). Controversial terminology of the neoplasm arises from the differentiation of this tumor composed of both endocrine and exocrine glands. Middle ear (ME) localization is rare and less aggressive than gastrointestinal tract or lung localizations. Nevertheless, clinical and CT/MRI analyses are necessary follow-ups for preventing or detecting recurrence or metastasis. A case of a female patient aged 26 with recurrent middle ear neuroendocrine adenoma is presented herein.

1. Introduction

Known for about 40 years [1, 2], MEANT still challenges pathologists and otorhinolaryngologists. ME localization is rare in comparison with gastrointestinal tract and lungs whose incidence is 2–5/100,000 [3]. Since the first case described in 1976 by Hyams and Michaels, about 150 cases have been reported in the English literature [4].

Clinical symptoms are nonspecific and include hearing loss, aural fullness, tinnitus, otalgia, facial weakness, and the like [5–9].

Anatomical imaging CT and MRI are not specific enough and sufficient for an accurate localization before surgery. Functional imaging (octreoscan™) targets somatostatin receptors, especially SSR2 and SSR5 located on the cell membrane of the tumor, and is much more sensitive [10, 11]. To date, this method is reserved for suspected cases with silent CT/MRI [4].

Definite diagnosis relies on combined histopathology and immunohistochemistry. The authors discuss the controversial terminology of these tumors based on different degrees of glandular or neuroendocrine differentiation [6, 7, 12, 13].

2. Case Report

In February 2008, a 26-year-old female patient consulted us for a second opinion before surgery on a suspected ME cholesteatoma. She had been complaining for several months about right aural fullness and otalgia.

The otoscopy revealed a posterosuperior reddish retrotympanic mass without retraction pockets accompanied by a subnormal audiometry. The well-defined soft tissue mass density observed on the CT scan close to the ossicles but without any bone erosion did not support a diagnosis of cholesteatoma (cf. Figure 1). A surgical exploration was performed, and the tumor easily resected through an ossicle preservation transmastoïd tympanoplasty.

Histological examination revealed an epithelial proliferation with architecture sometimes trabecular, sometimes glandular, embedded in a dense fibrous stroma. The tumor was composed of uniform cuboidal or cylindrical cells with round to oval nuclei and a plasmacytoid morphology. No necrosis or mitotic activity was identified (cf. Figure 2(a)). Periodic acid Schiff (PAS) staining revealed the presence of mucin in some cytoplasms.

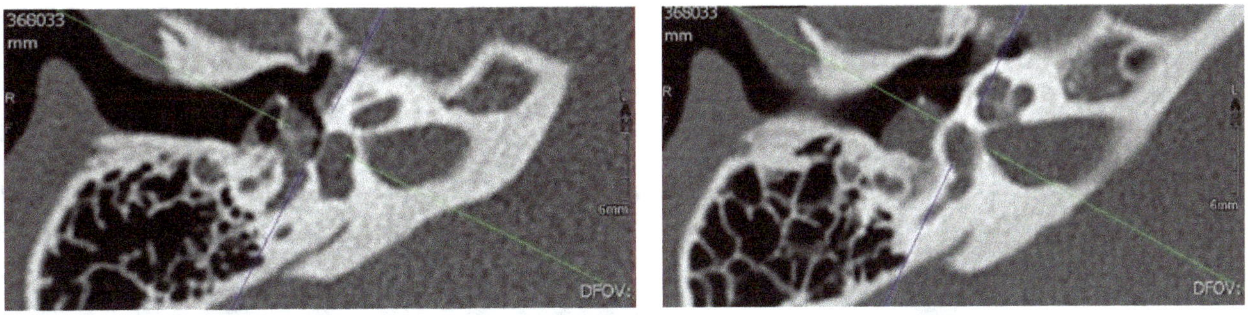

(a) (b)

Figure 1: 2008 high-resolution multidetector computed tomography (MDCT) (axial views) showing nonosteolytic nodular tissue mass in the hypotympanum alongside the promontory.

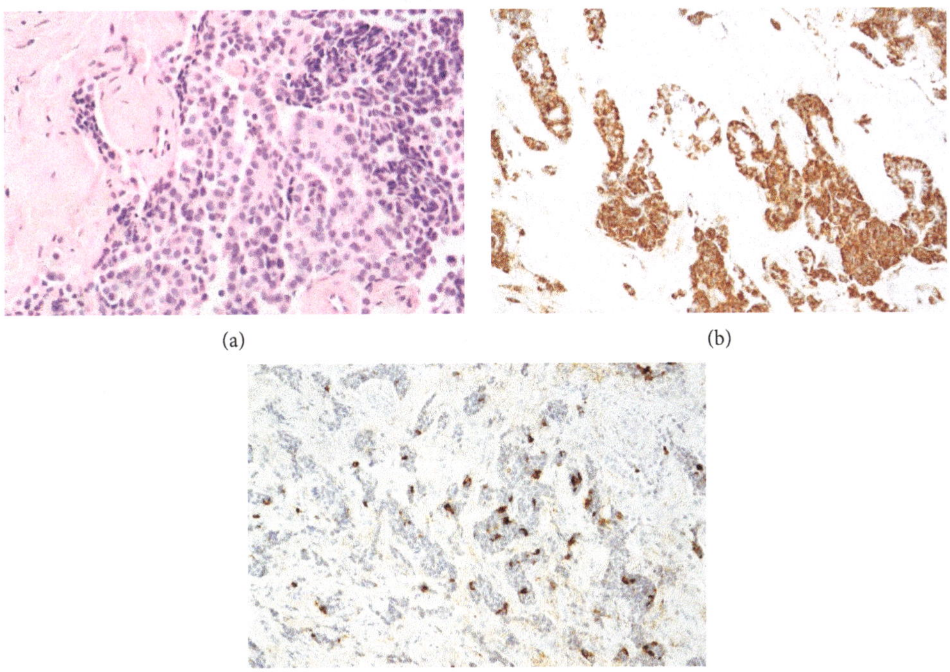

(a) (b) (c)

Figure 2: (a) Hematoxylin-eosin (HE) stain: the pattern of growth is trabecular or glandular. The tumor cells are uniform and cuboidal with a moderately abundant acidophilic cytoplasm. Mitoses are rare and necrosis absent. (b) Immunostaining for synaptophysin. (c) Immunoreactivity: typical immunostaining for chromogranin.

Immunohistochemical staining was strongly positive for synaptophysin (cf. Figure 2(b)), focally positive for chromogranin (cf. Figure 2(c)) and neuron-specific enolase (NSE), reactive for epithelial membrane antigen (EMA) and cytokeratin (AE1/AE3) but was negative for S100 protein. The Ki67 cells proliferation index of 2% was weak. The tumor had the histological and immunohistochemical profile of a "carcinoid tumor."

Two years after the tumor resection, the patient presented an intense right otalgia and a neurosensorial hearing loss. ^{111}Indium-pentetreotide scintigraphy showed an intense activity in the right ME (cf. Figure 3), and the CT scan revealed a soft tissue density mass in the attic of the ME, which confirmed the MEANT recurrence (cf. Figure 4). During a revision surgery, a yellowish tissue was resected by removing the ossicular chain. No adherence or bone erosion was noted. Function was restored by a total ossicular replacement prosthesis (TORP) ossiculoplasty. Histopathology disclosed the neuroendocrine (NE) nature of the tumor.

Scintigraphy and CT scan were free of recurrence two years after the revision surgery. The patient came for her follow-up check 10 years later without any complaint, and follow-up CT scan was negative.

3. Discussion

Histology and immunohistochemistry are the keys for definite diagnosis of the MEANT. These analyses describe

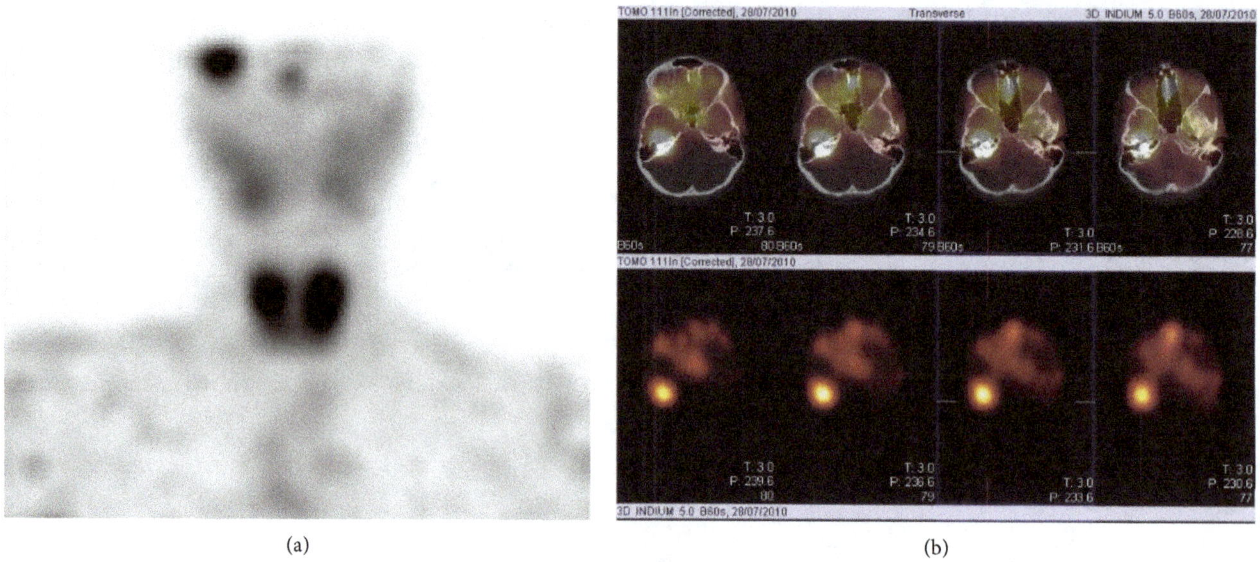

FIGURE 3: (a) ^{111}In-pentetreotide scintigraphy from 2010 (MIP) intense activity in the right ME. (b) ^{111}In-pentetreotide scintigraphy from 2010 (fused transverse SPECT/CT images and transverse SPECT images).

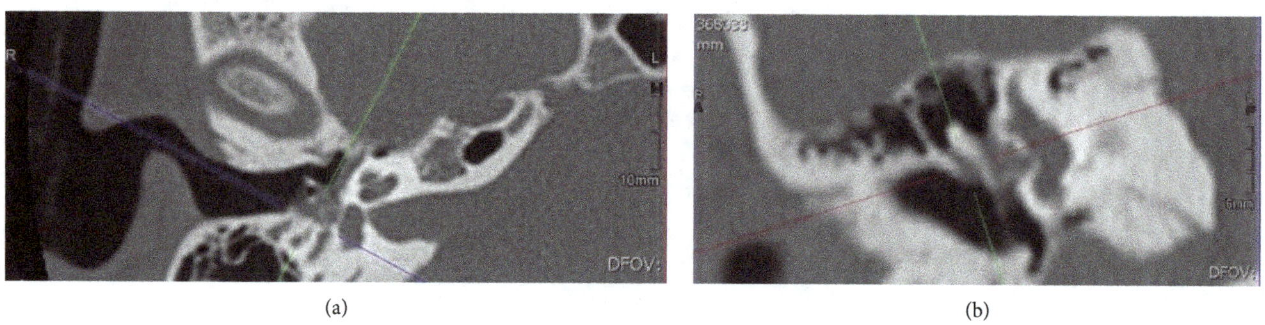

FIGURE 4: High-resolution MDCT from 2010 (coronal and axial views): nodular tissue mass located in the mesotympanum covering the incus and the stapes without osteolysis, suspected of tumor recurrence.

classically both exocrine (mucinous) and/or neuroendocrine differentiation. Immunoreactivity is variously positive for keratin antibodies (cytokeratin, CK7, CK20, and CAM5.2) and neuroendocrine markers (chromogranin, synaptophysin, serotonin, nonspecific enolase, and human pancreatic polypeptide) [6, 12]. Diversity of expression and clinical behavior of these tumors explain the variant terminology used to describe them, including middle ear adenoma, adenomatous tumor, neuroendocrine adenoma, carcinoid tumor, and mixed epithelial and neuroendocrine tumor [13, 14].

Coexistence of cells derived embryologically from both endoderm and mesoderm (neural crest) led some authors to claim either that uncommitted epithelial (endodermal) cells would develop neuroendocrine features, or that uncommitted neural crest cells would acquire exocrine and epithelial characteristics [6].

Most cases of ME localization in literature are described in case reports with local malignancy. Recurrence rate of insufficiently resected tumors occurs between 15 and 22% according to the authors [9, 15]. Even if some authors report cervical nodes and osseous metastases [10, 16], MEANT is less aggressive than gastrointestinal tract or lung localization, as there is absence of necrosis and a low mitotic rate by histologic analysis.

The best treatment is surgery, and the extent of resection depends on the staging, from intact canal wall tympanomastoïdectomy to a subtotal petrosectomy.

Saliba and Evrard [5] reviewed 75 cases and proposed a classification of ME glandular neoplasm based on NE markers immunoreactivity and presence or not of metastases. The average follow-up of the 73 disease-free patients after definitive surgery was 53 months, whereas the average time of recurrence or metastases was 11 years. NE neoplasm behavior remains unpredictable.

More recently, Marinelli et al. [4] proposed through a multi-institutional retrospective study on 32 cases a T/N/M/S staging system for MEANTs. About a third of T2 MEANTs and nearly two-thirds of T3 MEANTs developed local recurrence at a median duration of recurrence of 6 years. According to this staging, our patient is classified as T2a.

MEANTs are listed in the 2017 WHO classification as "middle ear adenoma," arguing that it is always appropriate to designate them as adenomas with neuroendocrine features [17].

Shaverdian et al. [18] studied the clinical relevance of ^{111}In-pentetreotide scintigraphy in the diagnosis and the management of 145 patients with NE tumors (particularly gastrointestinal tract and lung localization). The authors noted that cross-sectional CT/MRI detected 60% of primary or recurrent tumors and suggested that scintigraphy should be reserved for patients with biochemical diagnosis of NE tumor with silent CT/MRI.

4. Conclusions

MEANT is a rare, slow-growing, and low-grade malignancy tumor with nonspecific clinical symptoms. Radical surgery treatment prevents 22% recurrence. Clinical combined with CT/MRI remains actually the best available method for controlling recurrence. Octreotide scintigraphy will be performed in case of doubt. NE neoplasm behavior, however, still remains unpredictable, and a lifelong follow-up is necessary.

Conflicts of Interest

The authors declare that there are no conflicts of interest regarding the publication of this article.

References

[1] E. L. Derlacki and P. L. Barney, "Adenomatous tumors of the middle ear and mastoid," *Laryngoscope*, vol. 86, no. 8, pp. 1123–1135, 1976.

[2] V. J. Hyams and L. Michaels, "Benign adenomatous neoplasm (adenoma) of the middle ear," *Clinical Otolaryngology*, vol. 1, no. 1, pp. 17–26, 1976.

[3] A. Al-Nahhas, "Nuclear medicine imaging of neuroendocrine tumors," *Clinical Medicine*, vol. 12, no. 4, pp. 377–380, 2012.

[4] P. Marinelli John, S. P. Cass, S. E. Mann et al., "Adenomatous neuroendocrine tumors of the middle ear: a multi-institutional investigation of 32 cases and development of a staging system," *Otology and neurotology*, vol. 39, no. 8, pp. e712–e721, 2018.

[5] I. Saliba and A. S. Evrard, "Middle ear glandular neoplasms: adenoma, carcinoma or adenoma with neuroendocrine differentiation: a case series," *Cases Journal*, vol. 2, no. 1, p. 6508, 2009.

[6] K. R. Torske and L. D. Thompson, "Adenoma versus carcinoid tumor of the middle ear: a study of 48 cases and review of the literature," *Modern Pathology*, vol. 15, no. 5, pp. 543–555, 2002.

[7] E. Zan, C. J. Limb, and J. F. Koehler, "Middle ear adenoma: a challenging diagnosis," *American Journal of Neuroradiology*, vol. 30, no. 8, pp. 1602-1603, 2009.

[8] R. Salzman, I. Stárek, V. Tichá, A. Skálová, and J. Kučera, "Metastasizing middle ear carcinoid: an unusual case report, with focus on ultrastructural and immunohistochemical findings," *Otology and Neurotology*, vol. 33, no. 8, pp. 1418–1421, 2012.

[9] M. J. Ramsey, J. B. Nadol Jr., B. Z. Pilch, and M. J. McKenna, "Carcinoid tumor of the middle ear: clinical features, recurrences, and metastases," *Laryngoscope*, vol. 115, no. 9, pp. 1660–1666, 2005.

[10] J. M. Zutenhorst and B. G. Taal, "Metastatic carcinoid tumors: a clinical review," *Oncologist*, vol. 10, no. 2, pp. 123–131, 2005.

[11] R. Martínez-Lázaro, A. Cortes-Blanco, A. Moreno-Selva, and M. B. Morote, "Follow-up of a carcinoid tumor in the middle ear by ^{111}In-pentetreotide scintigraphy," *Clinical Nuclear Medicine*, vol. 32, no. 6, pp. 466-467, 2007.

[12] S. Berns and G. Pearl, "Middle ear adenoma," *Archives of Pathology and Laboratory Medicine*, vol. 130, no. 7, pp. 1067–1069, 2006.

[13] F. A. Cardoso, E. M. R. Monteiro, M. N. D. C. Avila, and B. O. Scarioli, "Adenomatous tumors of the middel ear: a literature review," *International Archives of Otorhinolaryngology*, vol. 21, no. 3, pp. 308–312, 2017 jul.

[14] B. Xu, R. Chetty, and B. Perez-Ordonez, "Neuroendocrine neoplasms of the head and neck: some suggestions for the new WHO classification of head and neck tumors," *Head and Neck Pathology*, vol. 8, no. 1, pp. 24–32, 2014.

[15] D. Bell, A. K. El-Naggar, and P. W. Gidley, "Middle ear adenomatous neuroendocrine tumors: a 25-year experience at MD Anderson Cancer Center," *Virchows Arch*, vol. 471, pp. 667–672, 2017.

[16] C. E. Fundakowski, J. R. Chapman, and G. Thomas, "Middle ear carcinoid with distant osseous metastasis," *Laryngoscope*, vol. 123, no. 3, pp. 779–782, 2013.

[17] A. K. El Naggar, J. K. C. Chan, T. Takata, and P. J. Slootweg, *WHO Classification of the Head and Neck Tumours*, IARC Press, Lyon, France, 2017.

[18] N. Shaverdian, S. N. Pinchot, B. Zarebczan, H. C. Gillis, A. Schiro, and H. Chen, "Utility of ^{111}indium-pentetreotide scintigraphy in patients with neuroendocrine tumors," *Annals of Surgical Oncology*, vol. 20, no. 2, pp. 640–645, 2013.

Diffuse Neurofibroma in a Patient with Unknown History of NF1

Mahmoud A. K. Ebrahim,[1] **Mishal M. AlMutairi**,[2] **Khaled M. Hindi**,[3] **and Jassem M. Bastaki**[4]

[1]*Farwaniya Hospital, Ministry of Health, Kuwait City, Kuwait*
[2]*Zain Hospital, Ministry of Health, Kuwait City, Kuwait*
[3]*Kuwait Institute Medical Specialties, Kuwait City, Kuwait*
[4]*Al-Sabah Hospital, Ministry of Health, Kuwait City, Kuwait*

Correspondence should be addressed to Mahmoud A. K. Ebrahim; ma7moud_ibrahim@hotmail.com

Academic Editor: Abrão Rapoport

Malignant peripheral nerve sheath tumor (MPNST) is a rare disease in the parotid gland with a poor prognosis in most cases. The disease most often develops in the setting of neurofibromatosis type 1 (NF1) but can also occur sporadically. Herein, we report a rare case of MPNST in the parotid gland, in a patient with no previous history of NF1. Initial investigations of the patient, which consisted of laboratory investigations, ultrasound imaging of the swelling, fine-needle aspiration (FNA), computed tomography (CT) scan, and magnetic resonance imaging (MRI) of the neck and swelling, were compatible with a benign pleomorphic adenoma of the parotid gland. However, intraoperatively, the dissection was challenging as the tumor was adherent to the neighboring tissue. A diagnosis of MPNST arising from a diffuse neurofibroma was established based on clinicopathologic features of the disease. The patient, who exhibited clinical features compatible with (NF1), proceeded for radiotherapy following surgery to continue his treatment.

1. Introduction

Malignant peripheral nerve sheet tumors, MPNSTs, are rare spindle cell sarcomas, accounting for 10% of all soft tissue sarcomas [1]. Most MPNSTs occur in the extremities and the trunk, while only 10% develop in the head and neck region [2]. We present a case of low-grade MPNST, arising in a diffuse neurofibroma of the parotid in a patient with no past history of neurofibromatosis type I (NF1). The clinical, histopathologic, and therapeutic aspects of this lesion are detailed in this report.

2. Case Presentation

A 45-year-old male from the Netherlands presented with a painless right parotid swelling that was progressively increasing in size for the past 8 months. Though occasionally he suffered from jaw lock, other symptoms associated with neurologic deficit such as drooling, facial weakness, paresthesia, or auditory defects were absent. Apart from being a social alcohol consumer, there was no history of smoking, prior radiation, or significant family medical history, especially in regard to his present illness.

Physical examination revealed a tender right parotid swelling below the ear lobule, which extended inferiorly to the angle of the mandible (Figure 1). The skin overlying the swelling was slightly erythematous, thickened, and nodular. The swelling was firm, diffused, and fixed to the underlying muscles, and there was no associated lymphadenopathy. Otoscopic examination of both ears was within normal limits.

The patient initially had a neck ultrasound and then a magnetic resonance imaging (MRI) to characterize the nature of the lesion. The neck CT scan revealed a well-defined altered signal enhancing mass measuring $3.5 \times 2.2 \times 2.0$ cm at the posterior aspect of the superficial part of the right parotid gland (Figure 2). The radiologist's impression was an altered signal enhancing mass lesion, likely to be a benign pleomorphic

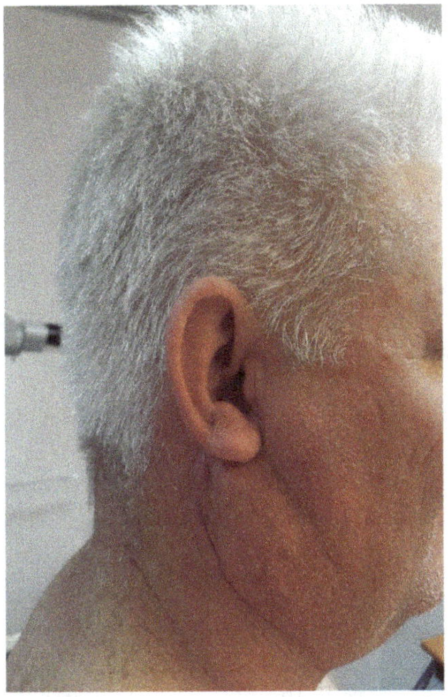

Figure 1: Preoperative clinical photograph showing a right parotid swelling.

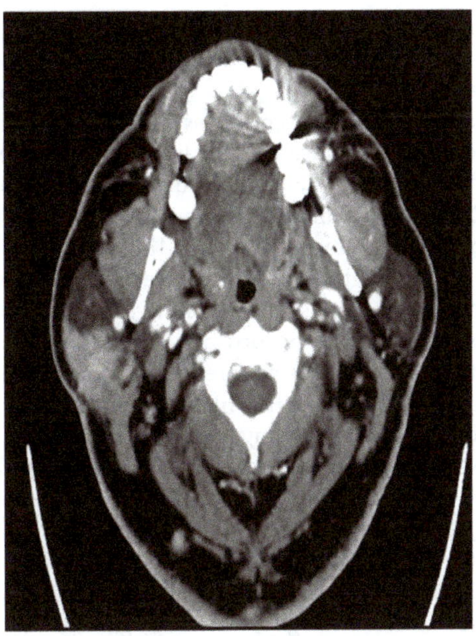

Figure 2: Axial CT with contrast shows a mass in the superficial lobe of the right parotid gland with post-contrast enhancement.

adenoma. The patient then underwent MRI of the parotid glands, which showed a well-defined focal lesion of altered signal intensity at the posterior aspect of the superficial part of the right parotid gland, measuring $3.5 \times 2.2 \times 2.0$ cm along its maximum transverse, craniocaudal, and anteroposterior diameters, respectively. The impression was again benign pleomorphic adenoma of the right parotid gland. However, the radiologist could not exclude other diagnostic possibilities and recommend fine-needle aspiration cytology.

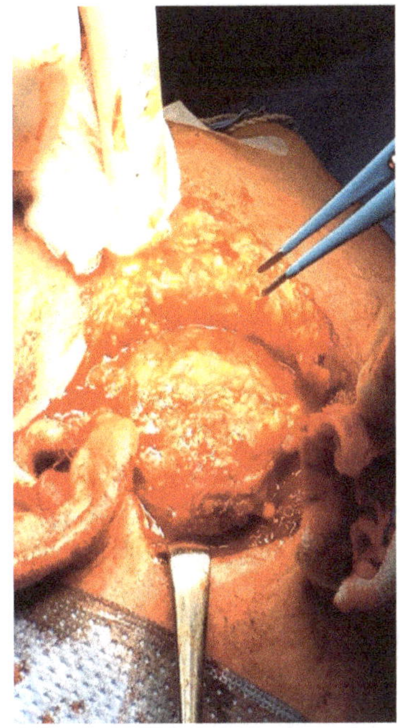

Figure 3: Clinical photograph showing intraoperative view of the parotid swelling.

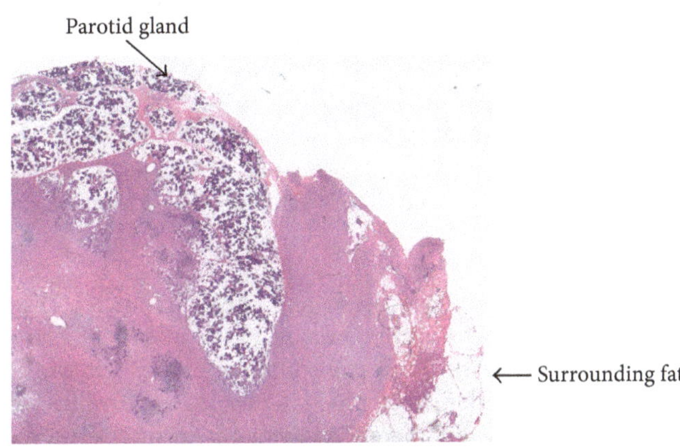

Figure 4: Histologically, diffuse-type neurofibroma arising in the parotid region with diffuse infiltration between salivary gland lobules and surrounding adipose tissue (arrows).

Fine-needle aspiration cytology of the mass was non-conclusive as the smears only showed polymorphous population of lymphoid cells in keeping with intraparotid lymph node. In view of these clinical findings, a superficial parotidectomy with facial nerve monitoring and preservation was planned.

A modified Blair incision was done, with elevation of a skin flap and control of hemostasis during the surgery. The dissection was rather difficult! The superficial parotidectomy was done in piecemeal as the mass was unexpectedly adherent to the skin and underlying fascia (Figure 3). The facial nerve was intact and was examined branch by branch. No frozen section was done during the operation.

Histopathologic examination showed a widely infiltrative tumor involving the parotid parenchyma and extending into

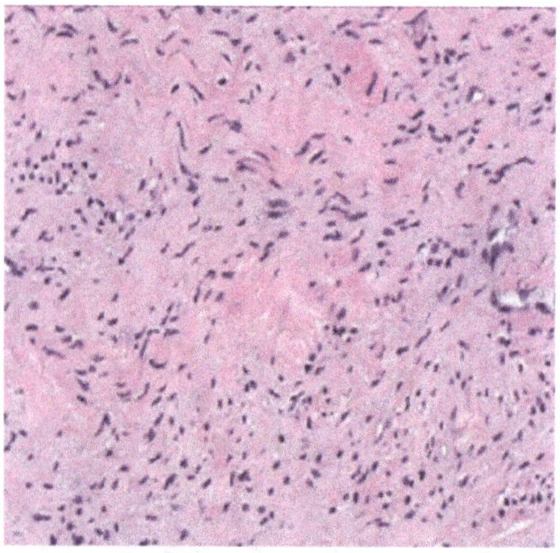

Figure 5: Diffuse-type neurofibroma comprises tumor cells with round to fusiform nuclei in a fine fibrillary collagenous matrix.

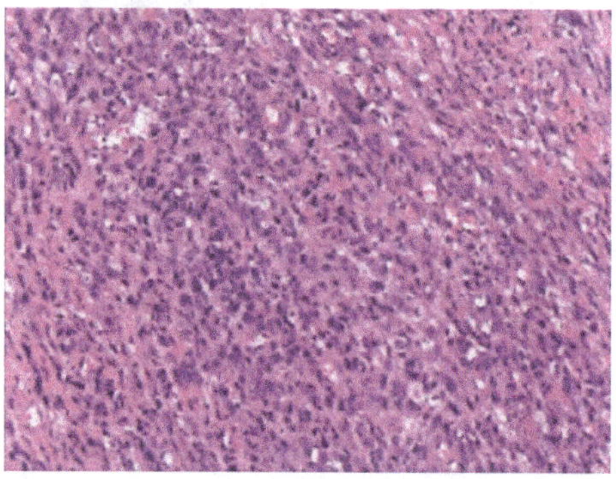

Figure 6: Areas of increased cellularity with epithelioid cells showing nuclear atypia and mitotic activity indicate transition to MPNST.

the surrounding adipose tissue and skeletal muscles (Figure 4). The tumor was predominantly composed of bland spindle cells with wavy nuclear contours, embedded within a fibrillary, pale pink matrix, which resembled a neurofibroma (Figure 5). Of concern, there were evidently distinct scattered more cellular foci of epithelioid tumor cells with nuclear atypia and increased mitotic activity (Figure 6). The tumor was diffusely and intensely positive for the S100 protein and neuron-specific enolase (NSE) immunohistochemical stains, with a low Ki-67 proliferation index. In addition, the CD34 immunohistochemical stain was focally positive in tumor cells. On the other hand, the tumor lacked immunoreactivity for AE1/AE3, p63, EMA, Melan-A, and HMB-45 immunohistochemical stains, thus excluding carcinomas, clear-cell sarcoma, melanoma, and other salivary gland tumors. Based on morphologic and immunophenotypic features of the tumor, the diagnosis rendered was low-grade malignant peripheral nerve sheath tumor (MPNST) arising in a diffuse neurofibroma.

Given the rare presentation and the association of such tumors with NF1, the patient was evaluated clinically for features of the syndrome. Multiple café au lait macules were subsequently discovered on his trunk (Figure 7). The patient was referred to a cancer center for further management and follow-up.

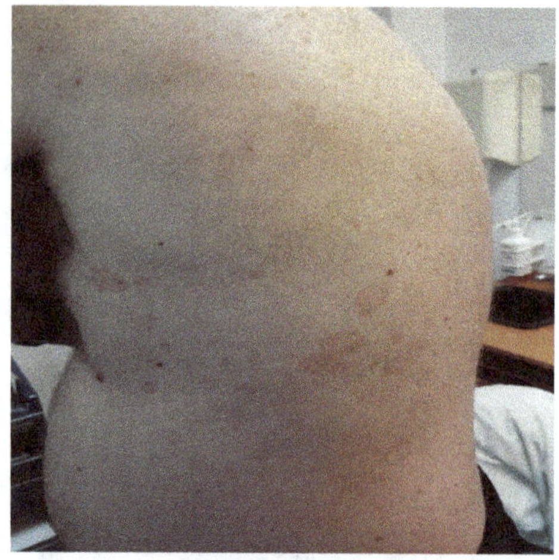

Figure 7: Clinical photograph showing multiple café au lait macules on the patient torso.

Further clinical examination of the patient and MRI revealed no distant metastasis. The patient underwent several courses of radiotherapy and is currently eighteen months' disease free.

3. Discussion

Mesenchymal tumors constitute about 2% to 5% of all salivary gland tumors, most of which (>95%) involve the major salivary glands [3]. Thus, tumors of the peripheral nerve sheath origin presenting as intraparotid masses are even rarer and, when present, are likely to be benign. About one-half of MPNSTs are associated with neurofibromatosis type 1 (NF1) with tendency to arise from preexisting neurofibromas [4]. Sporadic cases of MPNST mostly occur in early middle age, between 30 and 50 years, but a younger age at presentation is usually seen in cases associated with NF1. Most case series show no obvious gender predilection for this disease. Of note, it is apparent that radiation therapy is a risk factor as patients with a history of irradiation are at an increased risk for developing this tumor [5].

MPNST most commonly presents as a mass and is often associated with pain; some patients even experience neurological symptoms, such as weakness or tingling. Sudden enlargement or worsening pain in a preexisting neurofibroma may indicate a malignant transformation to MPNST. These lesions are difficult to diagnose clinically given their rarity and nonspecific clinical presentation. MRI is the preferred choice of imaging modality, which guides diagnosis and assesses tumor extension [6]. Moreover, fine-needle aspiration cytology and histologic tissue examination are necessary for definitive diagnosis [6]; however, even some of these modalities have their limitations and challenges, as was seen in our case.

The histologic features of diffuse neurofibroma involving the parotid region are similar to those seen in diffuse neurofibromas of the skin or other sites. These include an infiltrative growth pattern characterized by extension between salivary gland lobules to the overlying or adjacent skeletal muscle, fascia, and adipose tissue. The tumor consists of bland spindle-shaped cells with ill-defined cell border and fusiform or wavy nuclei [4]. These cells are embedded in a fine fibrillary collagenous matrix, with occasional scattered Meissner corpuscles (eosinophilic lamellar structures) [4]. The histologic diagnosis of low-grade MPNST arising in diffuse neurofibroma is not straightforward. There seems to be a morphologic spectrum between neurofibroma, "atypical" neurofibroma, and low-grade MPNST [4]. No absolute cutoff criteria between these categories have been defined of as yet, making it very difficult to distinguish between them. Most of the low-grade MPNST cases described have 5 or fewer mitotic figures per 50 HPF [4, 7].

The majority of cases of MPNST have spindle cell morphology, with only 5% of cases showing epithelioid morphology [4]. In our case, the majority of the tumor, however, has characteristic histomorphologic features of diffuse-type neurofibroma with rare areas showing transition to frank MPNST, characterized by increased cellularity, nuclear atypia, and epithelioid cytomorphology. Although epithelioid MPNST is regarded as high grade by default, our case was designated as low grade because the epithelioid foci were scant and the bulk of the tumor was low grade in fact.

MPNSTs behave aggressively with frequent distant metastasis and local recurrence [6]. These tumors mostly spread through hematogenous route to the lung, bone, and liver [6]. Therefore, it is crucial that these patients receive prolonged clinical follow-up [6]. Overall, the behavior of MPNSTs depends on a number of factors including tumor location, size, stage, histologic grade, resection quality, necrosis, and association with NF1 [6, 8]. The standard treatment of all sarcomas is a complete surgical excision with clear margins. However, given the complex nature of the head and neck anatomy, complete excision is not always possible [1]. An alternative route would thus be excision combined with high-dose radiotherapy [1], as was done for our patient. It has been described that adjuvant radiotherapy is beneficial in tumors that are high grade, large in size, or with positive surgical margins [6]. There are no randomized studies assessing the role of adjuvant chemotherapy specifically for MPNST [8]. Therefore, the role of adjuvant chemotherapy in the treatment of MPNSTs is debatable and still under assessment [5, 6].

This was a challenging case due to the fact that all preoperative investigations pointed toward a benign entity, namely, pleomorphic adenoma. The rapid increase in size of the tumor, despite the preoperative investigations pointing to a benign disease process, was still worrisome for malignant transformation, especially with the appearance of the overlying skin and the lack of a reason for such a sudden and progressive increase in size (e.g., cystic formation/degeneration due to trauma). The suspicion for malignancy increased tremendously during surgery because of tumor adherence to the surrounding tissue rendering the superficial parotidectomy and tumor dissection very difficult.

4. Conclusion

MPNST is an extremely rare disease in the parotid gland. And when it is low grade, the diagnosis of malignancy can be very difficult and only possible with close examination and correlation of all available data, and histomorphologic, radiologic, and clinical features. In this manuscript, we presented a case of MPNST in the parotid gland, in which all preoperative investigations were suggesting a benign pleomorphic adenoma. But the histologic examination leads to a diagnosis of malignancy and discovering a syndromic association.

The patient underwent postoperative radiotherapy and is currently eighteen months' disease free! Clinicians should be aware of the association of MPNSTs and diffuse neurofibromas with NF1, a diagnosis, if confirmed, with great clinical and genetic implications for the patient and his/her family.

Consent

The consent was taken from the patient before surgery and the same after surgery by the corresponding author.

Conflicts of Interest

The authors declare that there are no conflicts of interest regarding the publication of this article.

References

[1] O. Chis and S. Albu, "Malignant peripheral nerve sheath tumor of the parotid gland," *Journal of Craniofacial Surgery*, vol. 25, no. 5, pp. e424–e426, 2014.

[2] A. Minovi, O. Basten, B. Hunter, W. Draf, and U. Bockmühl, "Malignant peripheral nerve sheath tumors of the head and neck: management of 10 cases and literature review," *Head and Neck*, vol. 29, no. 5, pp. 439–445, 2007.

[3] P. Biswa, "Malignant peripheral nerve sheath tumor in parotid gland-a rare and challenging case," *Journal of Clinical Case Reports*, vol. 3, no. 1, 2012.

[4] I.-M. Schaefer and C. D. Fletcher, "Malignant peripheral nerve sheath tumor (MPNST) arising in diffuse-type neurofibroma," *American Journal of Surgical Pathology*, vol. 39, no. 9, pp. 1234–1241, 2015.

[5] S. Roy, A. K. Gandhi, B. Devnani, L. Singh, and B. K. Mohanti, "Malignant peripheral nerve sheath tumor of the tongue with an unusual pattern of recurrence," *Journal of the Egyptian National Cancer Institute*, vol. 29, no. 2, pp. 115–118, 2017.

[6] H. Touil, S. Briki, F. Karray, and I. Bahri, "Malignant peripheral nerve sheath tumor of the superficial cervical plexus with parotid extension," *European Annals of Otorhinolaryngology, Head and Neck Diseases*, vol. 132, no. 2, pp. 93–95, 2015.

[7] U. Yamaguchi, "Low grade malignant peripheral nerve sheath tumour: varied cytological and histological patterns," *Journal of Clinical Pathology*, vol. 56, no. 11, pp. 826–830, 2003.

[8] M. Farid, E. G. Demicco, R. Garcia et al., "Malignant peripheral nerve sheath tumors," *The Oncologist*, vol. 19, no. 2, pp. 193–201, 2014.

40

Assessment and Retrieval of Aspirated Tracheoesophageal Prosthesis in the Ambulatory Setting

Karuna Dewan, Andrew Erman, Jennifer L. Long, and Dinesh K. Chhetri

Department of Head and Neck Surgery, David Geffen School of Medicine at UCLA, Los Angeles, CA 90095, USA

Correspondence should be addressed to Karuna Dewan; karunadoc@gmail.com

Academic Editor: Marco Berlucchi

Tracheoesophageal prosthesis (TEP) is the most common voice restoration method following total laryngectomy. Prosthesis extrusion and aspiration occurs in 3.9% to 6.7% and causes dyspnea. Emergency centers are unfamiliar with management of the aspirated TEP. Prior studies report removal of aspirated TEP prostheses under general anesthesia. Laryngectomees commonly have poor pulmonary function, posing increased risks for complications of general anesthesia. We present a straightforward approach to three cases of aspirated TEP prosthesis removed in the ambulatory setting. In each case, aspirated TEP was diagnosed with flexible bronchoscopy under local anesthesia at the time of consultation, and all prostheses were retrieved atraumatically using a biopsy grasper forceps inserted via the side channel of the bronchoscope. The aspirated TEP prosthesis can be safely and efficiently removed via bedside bronchoscopy.

1. Introduction

Tracheoesophageal puncture with voice prosthesis placement is the gold standard for voice restoration following total laryngectomy [1]. It provides the most natural voice and is easiest to use compared to other rehabilitation methods [2, 3]. Leakage and malfunction are the most common complications; however, the prosthesis also often becomes dislodged [4]. The dislodged prosthesis may be aspirated, with reported incidence of 3.9% to 6.7% [5, 6]. Aspiration of the voice prosthesis into the trachea may cause significant airway obstruction. Removing aspirated TEPs has traditionally required emergent rigid bronchoscopy under general anesthesia in the operating room. Rao Kadam et al. described the difficult retrieval of an aspirated speaking valve using rigid bronchoscopy under general anesthesia. In a patient with a stoma, difficulties include ventilation issues as well as mechanical issues with the introduction of a rigid bronchoscope into the airway through the neck rather than through the mouth as it was designed to be used [7].

The three cases presented here demonstrate management of an aspirated TEP in the ambulatory setting with flexible bronchoscopy and local anesthetics, avoiding general anesthesia and the associated risk factors and costs. Despite being straightforward, this practice is unfamiliar to community otolaryngologists. Two of the presented patients were previously seen at outside institutions and transferred for a higher care level. The UCLA Institutional Review Board exempted this study.

2. Case 1

A 67-year-old male underwent total laryngectomy and secondary tracheoesophageal prosthesis placement 15 years prior. He was proficient at the use and care of his TEP. He lost his TEP and presented to his speech language pathologist for replacement. He did not recall how or when the TEP was dislodged; thus, it was unclear if he swallowed or aspirated it. After developing mild dyspnea, an emergency room chest X-ray suggested a foreign body. The patient was subsequently transferred to our head and neck surgery office. He reported increased mucus production, coughing, fullness in his chest, and inability to fully catch his breath.

To examine the airway for possible aspirated TEP, topical 4% lidocaine was sprayed into the stoma. With the patient sitting upright in the examination chair, flexible bronchoscopy was performed using a transnasal esophagoscope (KayPentax EE-1580). The prosthesis was found in the left mainstem bronchus (Figure 1).

The TEP's one-way valve orientation allowed air inhalation but not exhalation, trapping air in the lung. The prosthesis was retrieved without difficulty by grasping it with biopsy forceps (Olympus Endobronchial Alligator Jaw Forceps, FB 15C-1) passed through the esophagoscope side channel, then withdrawing the entire bronchoscope out of the trachea-stoma. After removal, the airway was reexamined demonstrating no additional foreign body or injury. The patient tolerated the procedure without discomfort and felt immediate relief of dyspnea. Postremoval chest X-ray failed to show any abnormality.

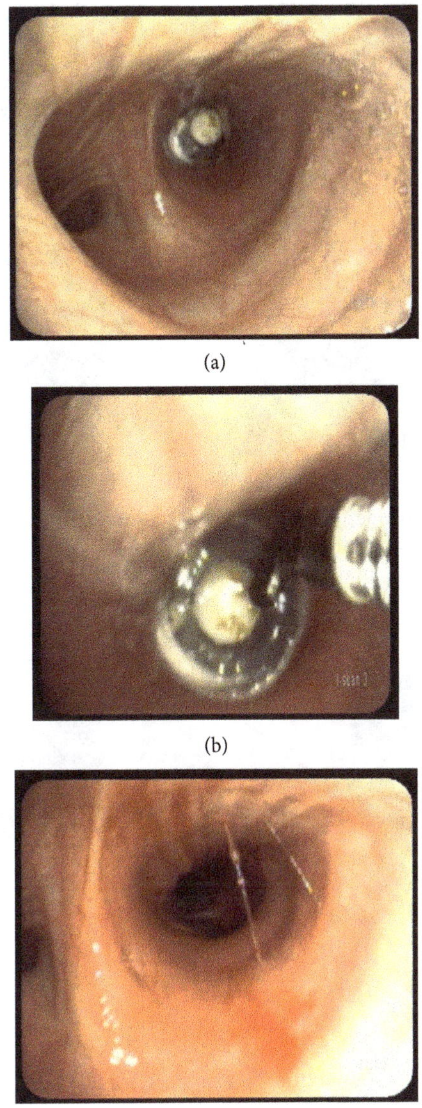

(a)

(b)

(c)

FIGURE 1: (a) Aspirated prosthesis in the left mainstem bronchus. It is situated such that the one-way valve allowed only inspiration. (b) Flexible biopsy forceps grabbing the prosthesis. (c) Left mainstem bronchus after atraumatic prosthesis removal.

3. Case 2

A 72-year-old female 20 years following laryngectomy, free flap reconstruction, and radiation had been using a TEP successfully. While cleaning her prosthesis, it dislodged and was aspirated. She initially presented to an outside hospital acutely short of breath, requiring supplemental oxygen to maintain saturations >90%. CT chest demonstrated a radiopaque foreign body in the right mainstem bronchus (Figure 2).

She was transferred to the emergency department (ED) at our institution as the local consultants recommended "higher level of care." The otolaryngology service evaluated the patient in the ED and performed bedside flexible bronchoscopy (Olympus BF-H190) after topical lidocaine spray. The aspirated prosthesis was found in the right mainstem bronchus (Figure 3).

It was removed atraumatically by grasping with the flexible biopsy forceps then withdrawing the entire bronchoscope. There were no other injuries or remaining foreign bodies. She felt immediate relief. A red rubber catheter was placed through her tracheoesophageal puncture to stent the tract. She was discharged home with next day follow-up with her speech-language pathologist (SLP) for prosthesis replacement.

4. Case 3

A 56-year-old male, 8 years postlaryngectomy with free flap reconstruction, proficient at changing his own prosthesis, presented to our clinic with 2 days of worsening dyspnea. The patient had not noticed aspirating his prosthesis after changing it. He underwent flexible bronchoscopy under topical anesthesia while sitting upright. A TEP lodged in the right mainstem bronchus was removed with biopsy forceps via the endoscope channel (Figure 4). His dyspnea immediately resolved.

5. Discussion

A "lost" tracheoesophageal prosthesis may be swallowed, aspirated, or expelled. Patients with aspirated TEP present with a range of complaints from intermittent cough to more significant airway distress. The prosthesis has a one-way valve, which may compound the airway problem and can potentially lead to pulmonary collapse or overinflation.

All patients who lose their voice prosthesis should undergo a chest X-ray to evaluate for aspirated foreign body. Some prostheses have a radiopaque ring for easy identification. Occasionally, the aspirated TEP may not be reliably demonstrated on imaging, leading to delayed diagnosis. Continued vigilance for airway symptoms must be undertaken by both patient and physician. All TEP patients should be counseled to present in a timely manner to the otolaryngology office in case of lost prosthesis, so that office tracheobronchoscopy can be performed with topical anesthesia and any flexible endoscope. If a prosthesis is found in the airway, it can be removed using flexible biopsy forceps

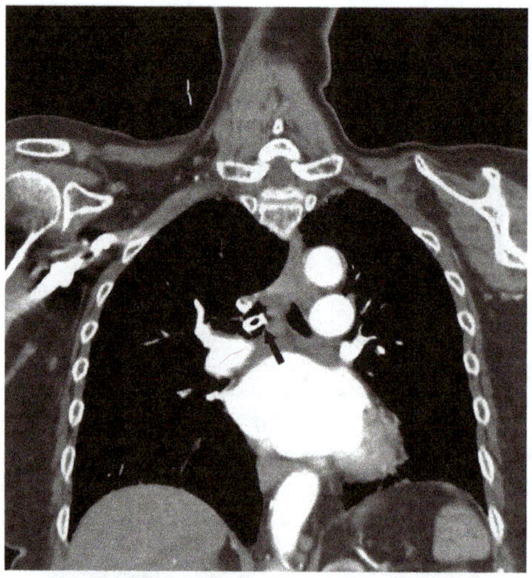

FIGURE 2: Coronal CT scan demonstrating aspirated TEP in the right mainstem bronchus.

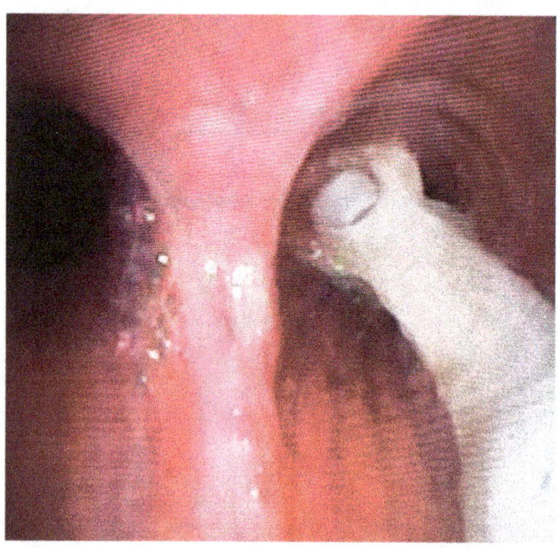

FIGURE 3: Aspirated TEP from the right mainstem bronchus.

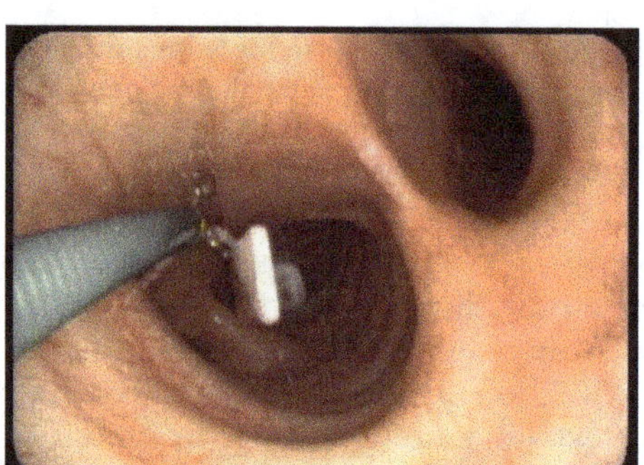

FIGURE 4: Removal of aspirated TEP from the right mainstem bronchus.

that can be placed through the scope channel or just adjacent to the scope. The greatest advantage to this method of TEP recovery is the immediate relief of symptoms. While documented cases of aspirated TEP removal using this method are rare, Chorney et al. report the removal of an aspirated screw in this manner. The patient presented with dysphagia, chest pain, cough, and wheeze. An esophogram demonstrated the presence of a radiopaque foreign body in the right lower lung. The thoracic surgery team was able to remove this with flexible bronchoscopy leading to immediate relief of symptoms [8]. Therefore, the method described in this paper has previously been useful for removal of other airway foreign bodies in the laryngectomy patient.

Failure to present in a timely manner for management of the lost TEP can also lead to closure of the tracheoesophageal puncture tract. This is the most common reason for emergency room presentation after prosthesis loss. Most patients following aspiration of the speech prosthesis are asymptomatic. However, this does not exclude the danger of an aspirated foreign body. Grosu et al. reported the removal of an aspirated speech prothesis, embedded in the carina, using bronchoscopy under general anesthesia. That particular patient was asymptomatic, presenting to the ED after the foreign body was noted on CT scan of the chest [9]. While the patient did not demonstrate any cough, shortness of breath, or hemoptysis, the prolonged presence of the foreign body in the airway places that patient at risk for the development of complications including pneumonia and erosion through the tracheal wall. Therefore, upon loss of a prosthesis, it is important to verify that it is not in the airway, even if a patient is asymptomatic.

6. Conclusions

Tracheoesophageal prosthesis aspiration can lead to significant morbidity. Every case of lost TEP must be assessed minimally with a chest X-ray and ideally also by an otolaryngologist. This report demonstrates the ease and applicability of awake flexible endoscopic removal of aspirated TEP under topical anesthesia. This straightforward procedure can be performed by any otolaryngologist, avoids general anesthesia, and immediately resolves symptoms.

Conflicts of Interest

The authors declare that they have no conflicts of interest.

References

[1] C. G. Tang and C. F. Sinclair, "Voice restoration after total laryngectomy," *Otolaryngologic Clinics of North America*, vol. 48, no. 4, pp. 687–702, 2015.

[2] A. J. Balm, M. W. van den Brekel, I. B. Tan, and F. J. Hilgers, "The indwelling voice prosthesis for speech rehabilitation after total laryngectomy: a safe approach," *Otolaryngologia Polska*, vol. 65, no. 6, pp. 402–409, 2011.

[3] P. V. Pawar, S. I. Sayed, R. Kazi, and M. V. Jagade, "Current status and future prospects in prosthetic voice rehabilitation following laryngectomy," *Journal of Cancer Research and Therapeutics*, vol. 4, no. 4, pp. 186–191, 2008.

[4] D. Ostrovsky, A. Netzer, D. Goldenberg, H. Z. Joachims, and A. Golz, "Delayed diagnosis of tracheoesophageal prosthesis aspiration," *Annals of Otology, Rhinology & Laryngology*, vol. 113, no. 10, pp. 828-829, 2004.

[5] A. I. Kerr, S. Denholm, R. J. Sanderson, and S. J. Anderson, "Blom-singer prostheses-an 11 year experience of primary and

secondary procedures," *Clinical Otolaryngology & Allied Sciences*, vol. 18, no. 3, pp. 184–187, 2007.

[6] J. C. Andrews, R. A. Mickel, D. G. Hanson, G. P. Monahan, and P. H. Ward, "Major complications following tracheoesophageal puncture for voice rehabilitation," *Laryngoscope*, vol. 97, no. 5, pp. 562–567, 1987.

[7] V. Rao Kadam, P. Lambert, H. Pant, and M. O'Reilly, ""Speaking valve" aspiration in a laryngectomy patient," *Anaesthesia and Intensive Care*, vol. 38, no. 1, pp. 197–200, 2010.

[8] M. A. Chorney, R. M. Dubin, and M. S. Levine, "Tracheobronchial foreign body aspiration in laryngectomized patient with tracheoesophageal voice prosthesis," *Clinical Imaging*, vol. 49, pp. 181–183, 2018.

[9] H. B. Grosu, F. J. Esteva, C. A. Jimenez, and R. C. Morice, "Speech prosthesis aspiration," *Emergency Medicine Journal*, vol. 30, no. 1, p. 85, 2013.

41

Grinspan's Syndrome: A Rare Case with Malignant Transformation

Numan Kökten,[1] Lokman Uzun,[1] Ayşe Serap Karadağ,[2] Tülay Zenginkinet,[3] and M. Tayyar Kalcıoğlu[1]

[1]*Department of Otolaryngology, Istanbul Medeniyet University Medical Faculty, Goztepe Training and Research Hospital, Istanbul, Turkey*
[2]*Department of Dermatology, Istanbul Medeniyet University Medical Faculty, Goztepe Training and Research Hospital, Istanbul, Turkey*
[3]*Department of Pathology, Istanbul Medeniyet University Medical Faculty, Goztepe Training and Research Hospital, Istanbul, Turkey*

Correspondence should be addressed to M. Tayyar Kalcıoğlu; mtkalcioglu@hotmail.com

Academic Editor: Abrão Rapoport

Aim. Oral lichen planus (OLP) is one of the common chronic inflammatory, noninfectious, and precancerous oral mucosal diseases that affect the stratified squamous epithelium in adults. Grinspan et al. reported an association of OLP with diabetes mellitus and vascular hypertension and called that Grinspan's syndrome in 1966. We aim to present a case of Grinspan's syndrome with malignant transformation. *Case Presentation.* A 60-year-old man who presented with a ten-year history of OLP diagnosed clinically and histologically was referred to our otolaryngology department with a painless swallowing in the left buccal mucosa for 3 months. Clinical examination revealed several plaques, striated white lesions in the buccal mucosa bilaterally, and an exophytic tumor in the left buccal mucosa. Histopathological examination showed lichen planus bilaterally and oral squamous cell carcinoma in the left buccal mucosa. The tumor had been developed on the preexisting areas of lichen planus which had been histologically proven before. The tumor was removed completely, and the tissue defect on the buccal mucosa was repaired with a split-thickness skin graft. *Conclusion.* Patients with OLP should be followed up periodically in a long term at close intervals for early diagnosis of malignant transformation.

1. Introduction

Oral lichen planus (OLP) is one of the common chronic inflammatory, noninfectious, and precancerous oral mucosal diseases that affect the stratified squamous epithelium in adults [1, 2]. In general population, OLP prevalence is about 0.5–2% worldwide and more common in females [2]. OLP can present as painless white streaks, raised, lacy-like lesions, or painful and persistent ulcers or plaques or papules and can resemble leukoplakia [2, 3]. In OLP patients, buccal mucosa, gingiva, tongue, labial mucosa, and vermilion of the lower lip are the most common affected sites [1–4]. The buccal mucosa is affected most commonly, and the tongue and gingiva follow buccal mucosa [4]. The lesions are mostly bilateral [5].

Although the etiopathogenesis is still unknown, immunological mechanisms are blamed [1, 6]. Autocytotoxic T lymphocytes were arraigned to trigger apoptosis of epithelial cells resulting in chronic inflammation. Civatte bodies, acanthosis, and parakeratosis are the results of lymphocytic infiltration of subepithelial tissue, basal membrane impairment, and degenerations of keratinocytes [1]. Malignancy potential of OLP is reported between 0.3 and 10% [7, 8]. The release of inflammatory cytokines caused by oxidative stress is supposed to activate transcription factors that affect premalignant cells to turn into malignant cells [1, 3, 4].

OLP diagnosis can be made with clinical features like classic oral white lesions, but to confirm diagnosis and exclude the dysplasia or malignancy, the histopathological examination is recommended [5, 6].

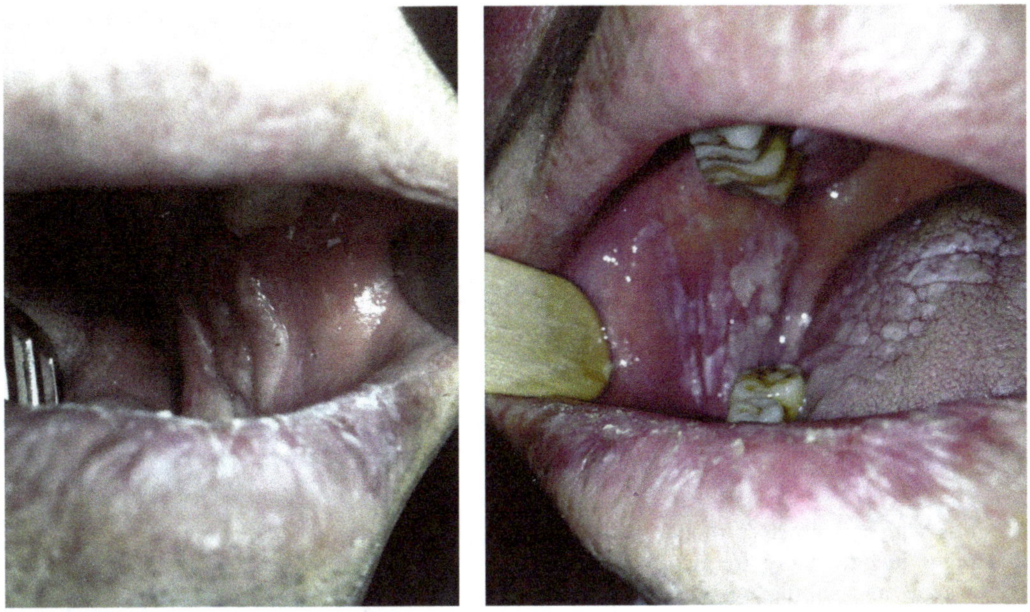

(a) (b)

Figure 1: (a) Exophytic tumor with a smooth whitish surface on the left buccal mucosa. (b) Lichen planus in the right buccal mucosa and on the tongue; actinic cheilitis is also seen on the lips.

OLP has been associated with different systemic diseases such as primary biliary cirrhosis, thymoma, ulcerative colitis, chronic active hepatitis, and myasthenia gravis and with several viruses such as hepatitis C virus (HCV), human papillomavirus (HPV), human herpes virus 6 (HHV-6), and Epstein-Barr virus (EBV) [6]. The lesions related with an identifiable aetiology which resemble OLP clinically and histopathologically are called lichenoid reaction [9]. Some dental materials, chronic graft versus host disease, and drugs such as angiotensin-converting enzyme inhibitors, antimalarial drugs, and nonsteroidal anti-inflammatory drugs are some examples that cause lichenoid reactions [6, 9].

Anti-inflammatory agents such as the topical corticosteroids are mainly preferred for OLP treatment; if lesions are widespread, systemic agents may be required [1, 5, 6].

Patients with OLP should be followed up periodically in a long term at close intervals for early diagnosis of malignant transformation. Malignant transformation after 40 years from the initial diagnosis of OLP has been reported [6, 10].

Grinspan et al. reported an association of OLP with diabetes mellitus (DM) and vascular hypertension (VHT) and called that Grinspan's syndrome [11]. We present a case of Grinspan's syndrome with malignant transformation.

2. Case Presentation

A 60-year-old man who presented with a 10-year history of OLP diagnosed clinically and histopathologically was referred to our otolaryngology department from dermatology department. The complaints of the patient were burning sensation after hot or spicy foods in the left buccal mucosa and painless swallowing in the left buccal mucosa for 3 months (Figure 1(a)). There was no history of using tobacco, drinking alcohol, or any other harmful habits. Medical history of the patient represents diabetes mellitus of 5 years and newly diagnosed hypertension accompanying OLP.

Clinical examination revealed several plaques and striated white lesions on the tongue and in the left and right buccal mucosae (Figure 1(b)) and an exophytic tumor with a smooth whitish surface on the left buccal mucosa. There was also actinic cheilitis on his lips. A complete otolaryngologic examination was done, and a blood sample was sent to laboratory for hematological examination. Incisional biopsies were taken from each buccal mucosa. Histopathological examination of the lesions showed lichen planus in the right and left buccal mucosae (Figure 2(a)) and oral squamous cell carcinoma (OSCC) in the left buccal mucosa (Figure 2(b)).

The tumor had been developed on the preexisting areas of lichen planus which had been histologically proven before. The tumor was removed completely, and the tissue defect on the buccal mucosa was repaired with a split-thickness skin graft. Figure 3 represents the situation of the left buccal mucosa one year after the operation.

3. Discussion

OLP may clinically demonstrate various forms such as reticular, erosive and ulcerated, atrophic, hypertrophic, bullous, and pigmentous forms [5, 6]. Reticular form is the most frequent form with small white papules or white lines network which is known as Wickham's striae [6]. Erosive and atrophic forms are less common but often associated with malignancy development [2, 4, 6].

The incidence of oral mucosa malignancies is reported about 0.004% per year with an 80% rate of OSCC in Europe [2]. OSCC may present like nonhealing, indurated ulcers or hyperkeratotic, exophytic masses or as submucosal, slightly

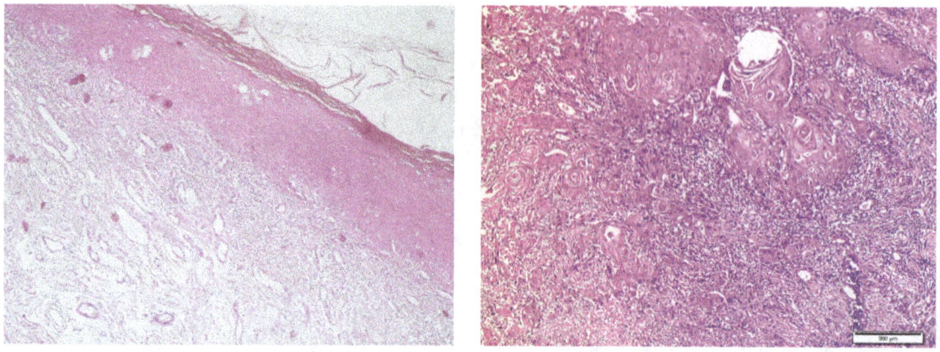

(a) (b)

Figure 2: (a) H&E ×100: lichen planus with hyperkeratosis, parakeratosis, epidermal hyperplasia, eosinophilic colloid bodies (Civatte), and lymphocytic infiltration at superficial dermis. (b) H&E ×10: areas infiltrated with OSCC.

indurated, red lesions with an intact epithelium less frequently [12]. Red areas include more frequent dysplastic features than white areas and should be biopsied preferentially [13]. Known external risk factors are poor nutrition, alcohol abuse, tobacco exposure, erythroplakia, and leukoplakia [12].

Nowadays, the malignant transformation of OLP is still a controversial subject [2, 5, 8]. The atrophic and erosive forms have more risks for malignant transformation [2, 4, 6]. In these forms of OLP, carcinogenic agents are supposed to react more easily because of the atrophy or absence of the epithelium [6]. Degeneration-healing cycles of cells in the OLP region are also assumed to facilitate neoplasm development.

Both OLP and lichenoid reactions can cause OSCC. In a recent meta-analysis of 57 studies with the data on 19,676 OLP and 419 oral lichenoid reaction cases, Aghbari et al. [14] reported that the rate of malignant transformation for OLP was 1.1% and 2.5% for the oral lichenoid reactions. They also reported that smokers, alcoholics, and HCV-infected patients have a higher incidence of malignant transformation.

Krutchkoff et al. had established the criteria of malignant transformation of OLP as follows: there must be a 2-year follow-up period after the initial clinical and histological diagnosis of OLP and the absence of carcinogenic factors such as exposure to tobacco and alcohol history [15]. Our patient had been followed up for OLP for 10 years and had not any external carcinogenic factor.

Diabetes mellitus (DM) is a clinical entity with hyperglycemia due to insulin defect. Disregulation of insulin, glucose, and lipids can lead to skin lesions in some DM patients [16]. Grinspan et al. reported an association of OLP with DM and VHT and called that Grinspan's syndrome [11]. However, with the presentation of three cases, drug therapy for VHT and DM was blamed to produce lichenoid reactions for Grinspan's syndrome [17]. In our case, OLP is associated with DM, VHT, and OSCC. Our patient had been followed up for OLP for 10 years and for DM for 5 years being treated with saxagliptinum 5 mg/day for 3 years and insulin 25 units/day at nights for 5 years. VHT is diagnosed just before the surgery and treated with perindoprilat-indapamide (5–12.5 mg/day). So, he did not use any DM or VHT drugs before the OLP

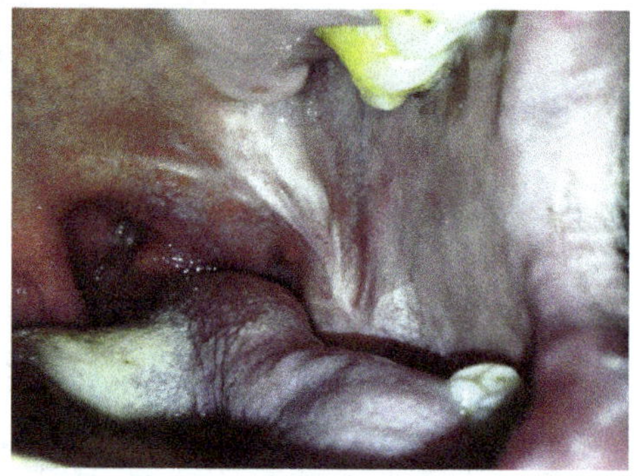

Figure 3: Left buccal mucosa one year after the operation. A scar tissue is present, and there is no sign for relapse.

appeared. Blood glucose levels of our patient are under control about 94–142 mg/dL at near-normal preprandial levels, and hemoglobin A1C levels are under 7% with the treatment. Systolic and diastolic blood pressures of our patient are under control with the treatment with a range of 122–166 mm·Hg and 78–115 mm·Hg, respectively. He continues the same treatment.

In our case, the patient was followed up for lichen planus earlier by dermatologists; after recognition of mass in the left buccal mucosa, he was referred to us. Hematological and histopathological investigations showed that the patient has Grinspan's syndrome with malignant transformation. The patient underwent surgical treatment and followed up monthly for the first year after the operation. Now, no relapse or any sign of metastasis was observed in the patient 33 months after the operation.

4. Conclusion

Malignant transformation is the most important complication of long-standing and nonhealing lichen planus. Close follow-up and repeat biopsies are mandatory for prevention and early recognition of malignant transformation. It is still controversial about Grinspan's syndrome that DM and VHT are accompanying OLP or medication of DM and VHT leads to oral lichenoid lesions. We presented a case with Grinspan's syndrome which appeared before DM and VHT medication and with malignant transformation.

Conflicts of Interest

The authors declare that there are no conflicts of interest regarding the publication of this article.

References

[1] E. M. Otero-Rey, F. Suarez-Alen, M. Peñamaria-Mallon, J. Lopez-Lopez, and A. Blanco-Carrion, "Malignant transformation of oral lichen planus by a chronic inflammatory process: use of topical corticosteroids to prevent this progression?," *Acta Odontologica Scandinavica*, vol. 72, no. 8, pp. 570–577, 2014.

[2] R. Laeijendecker, T. van Joost, M. C. Kuizinga, B. Tank, and H. A. Neumann, "Premalignant nature of oral lichen planus," *Acta Dermato-Venereologica*, vol. 85, no. 6, pp. 516–520, 2005.

[3] A. Marini, M. Wagenmann, E. Ting, and U. R. Hengge, "Squamous cell cancer and human papillomavirus infection in oral lichen planus: case report and literature review," *Dermatologic Surgery*, vol. 33, no. 6, pp. 756–760, 2007.

[4] S. G. Fitzpatrick, S. A. Hirsch, and S. C. Gordon, "The malignant transformation of oral lichen planus and oral lichenoid lesions: a systematic review," *Journal of the American Dental Association*, vol. 145, no. 1, pp. 45–56, 2014.

[5] J. B. Epstein, L. S. Wan, M. Gorsky, and L. Zhang, "Oral lichen planus: progress in understanding its malignant potential and the implications for clinical management," *Oral Surgery, Oral Medicine, Oral Pathology, Oral Radiology, and Endodontology*, vol. 96, no. 1, pp. 32–37, 2003.

[6] G. Abbate, A. M. Foscolo, M. Gallotti, A. Lancella, and F. Mingo, "Neoplastic transformation of oral lichen: case report and review of the literature," *Acta Otorhinolaryngologica Italica*, vol. 26, no. 1, pp. 47–52, 2006.

[7] R. W. Katz, J. S. Brahim, and W. D. Travis, "Oral squamous cell carcinoma arising in a patient with long-standing lichen planus: a case report," *Oral Surgery, Oral Medicine, Oral Pathology*, vol. 70, no. 3, pp. 282–285, 1990.

[8] P. F. Petti, J. V. Bagán, C. Scully, and N. Chaparro, "Malignant turn of oral planus in three new cases," *Acta Otorrinolaringológica Española*, vol. 55, no. 1, pp. 41–44, 2004.

[9] A. K. Ramachamparambathu, L. Chatra, and P. S. K, "Malignant transformation of a potentially low risk lichenoid reaction," *Journal of the College of Physicians and Surgeons-Pakistan*, vol. 22, no. 3, pp. 184-185, 2012.

[10] M. De Vincentiis, A. Gallo, A. Minni, R. Turchetta, and G. Acquaviva, "Le precancerosi del cavo orale," in *Proceedings of de Campora E. I Tumori del Cavo Orale, V Convegno Internazionale*, pp. 20-21, Isola Tiberina, Roma, Italy, November 1992.

[11] G. Colella, A. Itro, and G. Corvo, "A case of a carcinoma arising in lichen planus in a subject with diabetes mellitus and arterial hypertension (Grinspan's syndrome)," *Minerva Stomatologica*, vol. 41, pp. 417–420, 1992.

[12] I. van der Waal, "Tumours of the oral mucosa," *Ned Tijdschr Derm Venereol*, vol. 12, pp. 368–370, 2002.

[13] C. Scully, "The oral cavity," in *Textbook of Dermatology*, R. H. Champion, J. L. Burton, D. A. Burns, and S. M. Breathnach, Eds., vol. 4, pp. 3074–3076, Blackwell Science, Oxford, UK, 6th edition, 1998.

[14] S. M. H. Aghbari, A. I. Abushouk, A. Attia et al., "Malignant transformation of oral lichen planus and oral lichenoid lesions: a meta-analysis of 20095 patient data," *Oral Oncology*, vol. 68, pp. 92–102, 2017.

[15] D. J. Krutchkoff, L. Cutler, and S. Laskowski, "Oral lichen planus: the evidence regarding potential malignant transformation," *Journal of Oral Pathology and Medicine*, vol. 7, no. 1, pp. 1–7, 1978.

[16] T. Naheed, N. Akbar, M. Shehzad, S. Jamil, and T. Ali, "Skin manifestations amongst diabetic patients admitted in general medical ward for various other medical problems," *Pakistan Journal of Medical Sciences*, vol. 18, no. 4, pp. 291–296, 2002.

[17] P. J. Lamey, J. Gibson, S. C. Barclay, and S. Miller, "Grinspan's syndrome: a drug-induced phenomenon?," *Oral Surgery, Oral Medicine, Oral Pathology*, vol. 70, no. 2, pp. 184-185, 1990.

42

A Rare Case of Large Schwannoma of the Parapharyngeal Space

Nora Siupsinskiene,[1,2] Irina Arechvo,[3] Rimante Lapinskaite,[4] Evaldas Padervinskis,[1] Silvija Ryskiene,[5] and Saulius Vaitkus[1]

[1]*Department of Otorhinolaryngology, Academy of Medicine, Lithuanian University of Health Sciences, Eiveniu 2, LT-50161 Kaunas, Lithuania*
[2]*University of Klaipeda, Herkaus Manto 84, LT-92294 Klaipeda, Lithuania*
[3]*Department of Ear, Nose and Throat Diseases, Republican Vilnius University Hospital, Siltnamiu 29, LT-04130 Vilnius, Lithuania*
[4]*Raseiniu Hospital, Ligonines 4, LT-60127 Raseiniai, Lithuania*
[5]*Department of Radiology, Academy of Medicine, Lithuanian University of Health Sciences, Eiveniu 2, LT-50161 Kaunas, Lithuania*

Correspondence should be addressed to Irina Arechvo; arechvo@gmail.com

Academic Editor: Seckin Ulualp

Schwannoma originating from the peripheral nerves is a rare lesion of the parapharyngeal space. The special traits of the presented case included the following: the patient presented with slowly progressing dysphagia, speech difficulties, jaw numbness, and taste dysfunction. A dislocated lateral pharyngeal wall with mild inflammatory changes of the oropharyngeal mucosa was observed during pharyngoscopy. The radiological and histological characteristics of the neoplasm are consequently presented. Special emphasis is placed on the surgical treatment of the tumor.

1. Introduction

The parapharyngeal space is an inverted pyramid-shaped area of the deep tissues of the neck. The pyramid is based in the skull base, and its top extends to the greater horn of the hyoid bone. Clinically, the styloid process divides the parapharyngeal space into two segments. The prestyloid and poststyloid compartments are separated by the fascia of the tensor veli palatini muscle. The anterolateral prestyloid compartment contains the retromandibular portion of the deep lobe of the parotid, adipose tissue, small or ectopic salivary glands, a small branch of the trigeminal nerve supplying the tensor veli palatini muscle, the ascending pharyngeal artery, the pharyngeal venous plexus, and lymph nodes. The largest part of the posteromedial poststyloid compartment consists of fat. This space also contains the internal carotid artery and jugular vein, as well as cranial nerves IX–XII, the cervical sympathetic trunk, and lymph nodes.

Schwannoma is a relatively rare, slow-growing benign tumor that develops from a myelinated coating of the peripheral nerve [1]. Schwannoma may appear in any part of the body. The literature reveals that in 25 to 45 percent of cases, the tumor develops in the head and neck area, while it is rarely found in the parapharyngeal space [2]. Most tumors of the parapharyngeal space are benign and form from the salivary gland tissue [2, 3]. The tumors of neural origin are characterized by an insidious course and are consequently often delayed in diagnosis. The treatment depends on the size and location of the tumor [4].

The aim of this paper was to present an exceptionally rare and difficult case of large schwannoma of the parapharyngeal space possibly of the small branch of the mandibular nerve (V3) and to review the scientific literature.

2. Case Report

A 32-year-old man was referred to the Lithuanian University of Health Sciences Kaunas Clinics Hospital with the symptoms of throat discomfort on the left side and dysphagia. The symptoms persisted for approximately 2 months. At arrival,

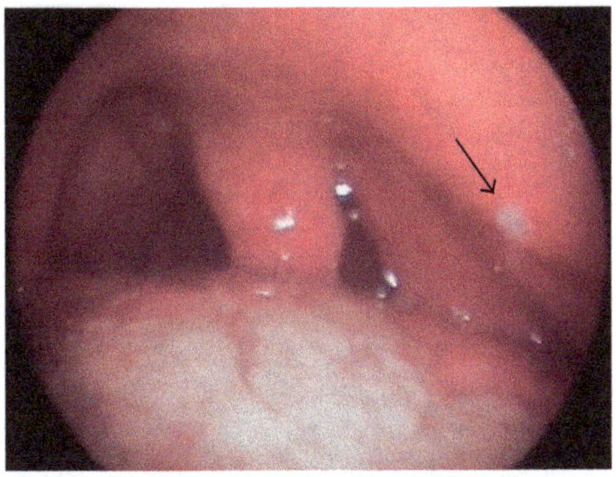

FIGURE 1: The oropharyngeal lumen is narrowed by a mass in the left parapharyngeal space. A small area of fibrin is visible at a previous puncture point (arrow).

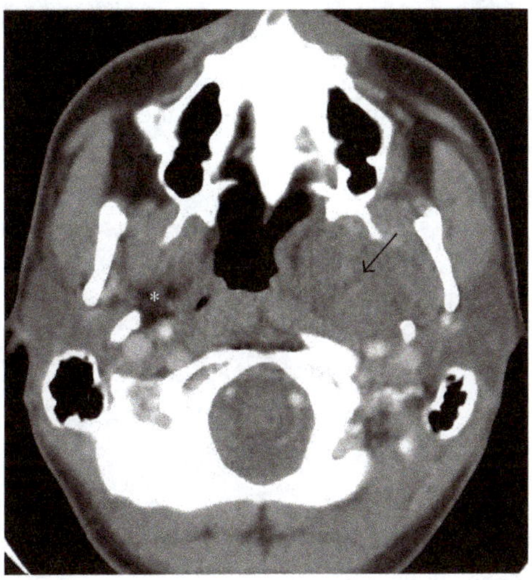

FIGURE 2: The contrast-enhanced axial CT scan shows the nonhomogeneous tumor within the left parapharyngeal space with a narrowing pharyngeal lumen (arrow). Note the normal fat contour in the right prestyloid compartment (asterisk).

the patient had no fever and there were no other signs of acute infection. Anamnestically, the patient was treated with antibiotics due to a suspected peritonsillar abscess on the left side for a period of 1 month. His left peritonsillar area was repeatedly punctured. However, only blood was obtained with a puncture. The prescribed antimicrobial therapy was not effective—dysphagia progressed, the patient started to report more speech difficulties, his lower jaw became numb, and taste dysfunction appeared. During pharyngoscopy, a dislocated lateral pharyngeal wall with mild inflammatory changes of the oropharyngeal mucosa was observed. The palate tonsil was displaced towards the uvula (Figure 1)

The fibronasolaryngoscopic investigation revealed that the left side of the nasopharynx was narrowed by a large mass covered with an intact smooth mucous membrane. No pathology was observed in the larynx—the color of mucosa was normal, and the vocal cords were mobile and smooth. No additional structures were seen. Neck lymph nodes could not be palpated.

Due to the suspected pharyngeal tumor, the patient underwent a contrast-enhanced computed tomography (CT) study, which showed a clearly limited, oval-shaped lesion in the left parapharyngeal space (Figure 2).

The size of the tumor was $4.2 \times 3.3 \times 6.7$ cm. It was characterized by a nonhomogeneous structure with multifocal intratumoral hemorrhages of varying ages. The tumor encased the carotid arteries and the styloid process, while it stretched the pterygoid muscles on the left side and remodeled the pterygoid processes of the sphenoid bone. The medial part of the tumor pushed the palatal tonsil and uvula towards the centerline, as well as the root of the tongue to the front and the middle. Moreover, it significantly deformed the oropharyngeal and nasopharyngeal cavities. The upper part of the tumor ascended and tapered to the bone surface of the base of the skull and extracranial oval foramen. The lower pole of the tumor reached the submandibular salivary gland level and dislocated it slightly laterally.

To clarify the diagnosis, the patient underwent a magnetic resonance imaging (MRI) study. The study showed that due to its localization and tumor-specific features, the most likely diagnosis was schwannoma of the small branch of the mandibular nerve (V3) since a limited formation of specific localization with a component of cystic degeneration was found. Deformed from the medial part, the lateral pterygoid muscle with the V3 is shown in Figure 3.

To determine a final diagnosis and plan a further treatment, a biopsy with histological verification of the tumor was performed. Under local anesthesia, a punch biopsy was carried out. A histological examination confirmed the diagnosis of schwannoma. Transoral removal of the tumor was planned. During an angiographic study prior to the surgery, the tumor-feeding blood vessels, of which the main vessel was the left ascending pharyngeal artery, were identified and embolized (Figure 4).

After the preparation of the patient, the schwannoma extirpation through a 5 cm incision at the left wall of the pharynx from the hard palate to the root of the tongue was performed under general anesthesia, while the widening of the oropharynx was done with a throat gag. The tissues were bluntly separated and the tumor capsule was reached, while the bloodstream of the surrounding area was externally disconnected. The tumor was removed in parts, thus reducing its volume. Later, it was totally removed with a capsule. No postoperative complications were observed. The wound healed by primary intention. The patient was discharged for further outpatient treatment on the sixth postoperative day. Antibiotic therapy with penicillin and painkillers was prescribed postoperatively.

Histological examination of the operating material revealed a tumor that formed by monomorphic, mitotically inactive spindle-shaped cells with oval nuclei and an eosinophilic cytoplasm, which were positive for S100 calcium-binding protein P (Figure 5).

Cells were either fascicular or palisade in structure. Larger individual cells with large and irregularly shaped nuclei were found. Furthermore, thick-walled blood vessels, xanthoma accumulations of macrophages, and abundant groups of hemosiderophages with several foci of necrosis were also visible. The diagnosis of schwannoma was confirmed.

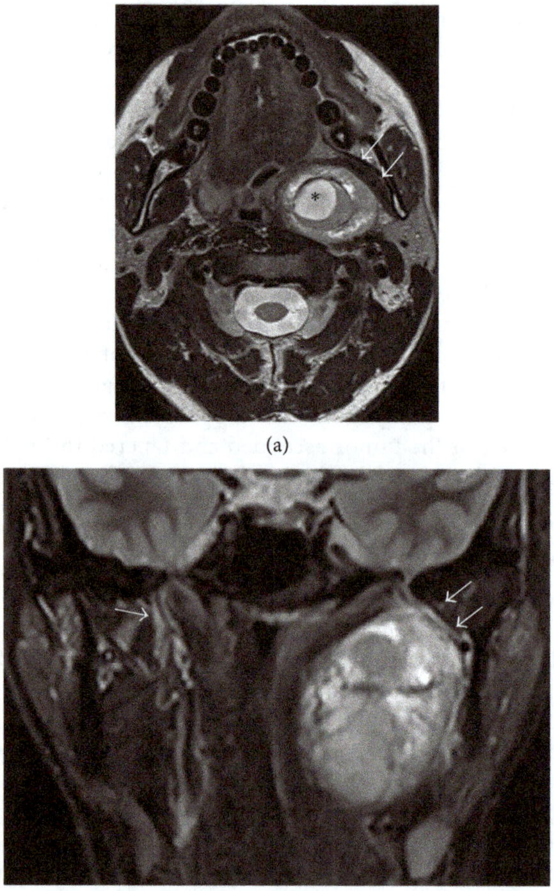

Figure 3: (a) Magnetic resonance imaging, axial projection. A large mass with cystic degeneration (asterisk) dislocating the root of the tongue is seen in the left parapharyngeal space. Stretched pterygoid muscles are shown with arrows. (b) Coronal projection shows the limits of the tumor (upper: the skull base; lower: the level of the submandibular salivary gland). Double arrow shows the laterally dislocated third branch of the trigeminal nerve on the left side. Note the normal proximal segment of the V3 on the right side (thin arrow).

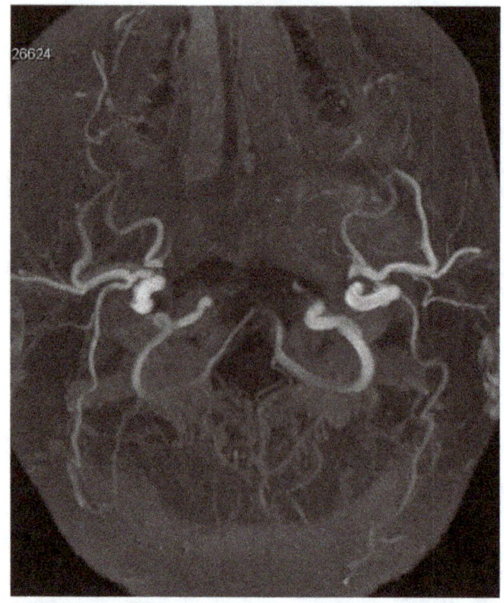

Figure 4: An angiographic study showed the tumor contour and contrasted tumor-feeding blood vessels—the ascending pharyngeal artery was the main vessel.

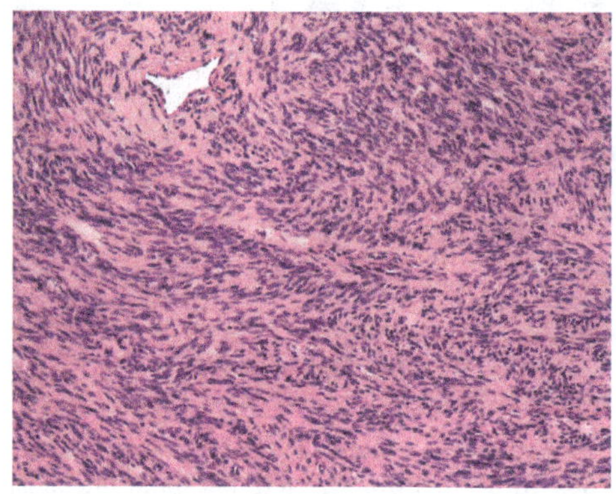

Figure 5: Histopathology showing monomorphic spindle cells with oval nuclei and eosinophilic cytoplasm positive for S100 calcium-binding protein P. The tumor cells formed palisade structures.

Six months postoperatively, no tumor relapse was observed during either physical examination or the repeated CT study (Figure 6).

Currently, the patient has been observed for a period of two years. There are no signs of schwannoma relapse.

3. Discussion

According to the literature, tumors of the parapharyngeal space are rare. It was reported previously that only 0.5 percent of all head and neck tumors are located in the parapharyngeal space [2]. Neurogenic tumors more often occur in the poststyloid compartment of the parapharyngeal space than in the prestyloid compartment [4]. In the majority of cases, cervical schwannomas are found in young and middle-aged people [2], while very rare in children [5].

Usually, schwannomas grow slowly and for a long time without causing any symptoms. However, a fully formed tumor causes pressure on the surrounding tissues. Clinical symptoms depend on the anatomy of the area of a growing tumor. Moreover, during visual inspection, a volumetric formation without mucositis in the lateral pharyngeal wall is observed. In the presented case, the redness of the pharyngeal mucosa was likely related to the previous multiple punctures. The diagnosis is confirmed by biopsy and histologic tumor examination. Histologically, schwannoma is a limited and well-encapsulated tumor occasionally presenting with a cystic degeneration component [6]. Such a cystic component was clearly delineated on the magnetic resonance image (Figure 3). Histologically, the tumor is differentiated from possible malignant tumors—fibrosarcomas, leiomyosarcomas, and fibrotic histiocytomas.

Radiological studies are very important for the diagnosis of the disease and surgical planning. Different authors [2, 7] recommend an initial evaluation of the tumor with contrast-enhanced CT examination, which was first performed in our case (Figure 2). MRI remains the "gold standard" for the diagnosis of these tumors. Radiological diagnostic methods

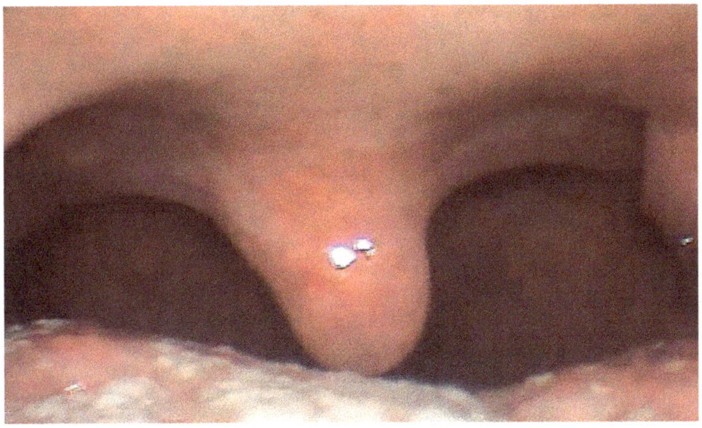

(a)

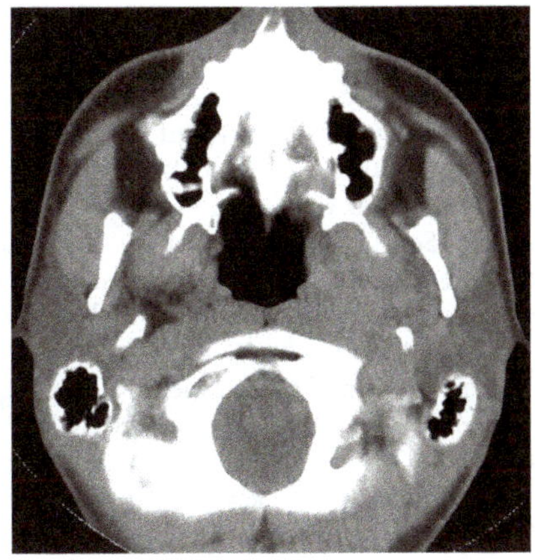

(b)

FIGURE 6: (a) Normal contour of the oropharynx six months postoperatively. (b) Computed tomography axial image: no tumor relapse is seen.

can be used to identify the source-nerve of a growing tumor and to reduce the risk of postoperative nerve damage. Typical radiological diagnostic characteristics of schwannomas are the following: well-limited formation that deploys the surrounding structures without invading the surrounding tissue. Cystic and fatty degeneration, as well as signs of hemorrhage and calcification, can also be observed.

The preferred treatment of schwannomas is surgical in nature. Schwannomas are largely resistant to radiotherapy. Therefore, this method of treatment is of limited applicability. There are different removal techniques of the parapharyngeal space lesions: transoral, transcervical, transparotid, transcervical-transmandibular, and lateral skull base approaches. The transoral approach can only be used for benign prestyloid space tumors. However, this approach is considered to be unsafe since it is related with many postoperative complications such as hemorrhage, fistulas, and nerve damage [8]. A transcervical-transparotid approach identifies and preserves not only the facial nerve but also the external and internal carotid arteries, the internal jugular vein, the cranial nerves IX, X, XI, and XII, and the sympathetic nervous system chain. Most deep-lobe parotid gland tumors can be removed with this approach, and it is particularly effective for small tumors. The transcervical-transmandibular approach provides good control of tumor extension towards the skull base, the pterygomaxillary fossa, and large neck vessels [9]. We chose the transoral approach, since the larger part of the tumor was located in the prestyloid compartment of the parapharyngeal space. We also preferred this method since the patient has anatomically large oral cavity. Preoperatively, we discussed with the patient the possibility of the intraoperative switch to a transmandibular approach in case of insufficient space to remove the tumor totally. However, according to the literature data, transoral removal of the tumor might increase the risk of complications (nonradical tumor removal, massive bleeding, infection, and IX–XII cranial nerve damage), although no neurological complications or complications of other types were observed after the operation in the discussed case. In all cases, a radical removal of the tumor is recommended. After the removal of the tumor capsule, the risk of relapse is significantly reduced. When an external tumor removal technique is used, the tumor is accessed through the neck, parotid gland, cheekbones, lower jaw, the mastoid part of the temporal bone, and the infratemporal space, or a combination of these access methods is used [7]. After the removal of the tumor, the most common postoperative complication is vocal cord paralysis, which occurs in up to 85 percent of all the cases and results in hoarseness [7].

The literature data indicate that the prognosis of encapsulated schwannomas is good because radical removal of the tumor results in the full recovery of a patient. Relapses and malignant transformation of the tumor are very rare. If the tumor is removed nonradically, a re-excision is appropriate.

4. Conclusions

Schwannomas of the parapharyngeal space are very rare. The majority of patients experience painless pressure phenomena without neurological deficit. Computed tomography and magnetic resonance imaging studies are the main diagnostic methods to determine the exact diagnosis, and thus should be performed before planned management treatment of the tumor, which is usually radical removal of the tumor with its capsule.

References

[1] M. Campanacci, F. Bertoni, and P. Bacchini, "Benign tumors of peripheral nerves," in *Enzinger and Weiss's Soft Tumors*, pp. 1111–1207, Mosby, St. Louis, MO, USA, 2001.

[2] J. G. Batsakis and N. Sneige, "Parapharyngeal and retropharyngeal space diseases," *Annals of Otology, Rhinology, and Laryngology*, vol. 98, no. 4, pp. 320-321, 1989.

[3] G. Giraddi, S. Shrinivas, S. Vanaki, and R. S. Puranik, "Schwannoma of parapharyngeal space," *Journal of Maxillofacial and Oral Surgery*, vol. 9, no. 2, pp. 182–185, 2010.

[4] D. O. Mangukiya, A. Reza, M. Topno, R. Gautam, P. Mullerpattan, and R. Jadhav, "A case report on parapharyngeal nerve cell tumor (schwannoma)," *Indian Journal of Surgery*, vol. 73, no. 1, pp. 58–60, 2011.

[5] H. S. Gilmer-Hill and D. G. Kline, "Neurogenic tumors of the cervical vagus nerve: report of four cases and review of the literature," *Neurosurgery*, vol. 46, no. 6, pp. 1498–1503, 2000.
[6] J. G. Batsakis, *Tumors of Head and Neck: Clinical and Pathological Consideration*, Lippincott Williams and Wilkin, Philadelphia, PA, USA, 1979.
[7] A. Khafif, Y. Segev, D. M. Kaplan, Z. Gil, and D. M. Fliss, "Surgical management of parapharyngeal space tumors: a 10-year review," *Otolaryngology and Head and Neck Surgery*, vol. 132, no. 3, pp. 401–406, 2005.
[8] K. D. Olsen, "Tumors and surgery of the parapharyngeal space," *Laryngoscope*, vol. 104, pp. 1–28, 1994.
[9] F. Bossa, M. G. Vigili, P. Ruscito, A. Marzetti, and F. Marzetti, "Surgical management of parapharyngeal space tumours: results of 10-year follow-up," *Acta Otorhinolaryngologica Italica*, vol. 29, no. 1, pp. 10–15, 2009.

43

Diagnosis and Treatment of Paracoccidioidomycosis in the Maxillofacial Region

Antonio Dionízio De Albuquerque Neto, André Vitor Alves Araújo, Daniel Assunção Cerqueira, Lorenzzo De Angeli Cesconetto, Nilton Provenzano, and Eder Magno Ferreira de Oliveira

Oral and Maxillofacial Surgery, Dr. Mário Gatti Municipal Hospital, Campinas, SP, Brazil

Correspondence should be addressed to Antonio Dionízio De Albuquerque Neto; antonioalbuquerque.bmf@gmail.com

Academic Editor: Abrão Rapoport

Paracoccidioidomycosis is a fungal infection initially described in Brazil in 1908 by Adolfo Lutz. Manifestation of this disease depends on numerous factors, such as microorganism virulence, hormonal profile, genetic predisposition, nutrition, and immune system. It is characterized classically by cutaneous lesions, lymphadenopathy, and pulmonary involvement. It presents male predilection, which can be explained by the protective effect of female hormones. Classic presentation within oral cavity is a superficial ulcer characterized by hemorrhagic dots of moriform aspect. Treatment should be established individually and closely monitored. This manuscript aims at reporting five cases of this pathology.

1. Introduction

Paracoccidioidomycosis (PMC) is a fungal infection caused by *Paracoccidioides brasiliensis*, and it affects mainly patients living in the South and Central America. It has male predilection (M : F ratio was 15 : 1), preferably middle-aged rural workers (30 to 50 years) [1, 2].

Primarily, PMC occurs in the lung due to the mechanism of aspiration of spores, which can be spread through lymphatic or hematogenous routes to other organs of the body. Oral lesions manifest as ulcers with hemorrhagic dots of moriform aspect. Clinically, due to healing difficulty, differential diagnoses of PMC are squamous cell carcinoma, traumatic ulcer, lymphoma, oral tuberculosis, sarcoidosis, Wegener's granulomatosis, leishmaniasis, actinomycosis, and primary syphilis [1, 3–7].

Treatment is based on three groups of drugs: amphotericin B (from the group of polyenic antibiotics); sulfadiazine and other sulfanilamide compounds; and the group of azolic drugs. Duration of treatment varies from 6 to 24 months, and if not treated properly it can be fatal [5, 8, 9].

This study aims at reporting five cases of paracoccidioidomycosis in the facial region, diagnosed and treated in a hospital in the countryside of São Paulo, Brazil. The first case will be exposed in details, and other cases will be summarized on Table 1.

2. Case 1

A 47-year-old male patient who was a rural worker reported "wounds in the mouth" and persistent cough for about 6 months. He reported chronic smoking and denied comorbidities.

A granulomatous ulcer with hemorrhagic dots and moriform aspect was observed in the posterior mandibular alveolar ridge and in the right jugal mucosa (Figure 1). Some dental elements presented severe mobility, which began after lesion emergence. He had an ulcerated lesion in the right cervical region with serous exudate (Figure 2). Cervical contrast CT scan revealed images compatible with cervical lymphadenopathy in the right side and exteriorization of the infectious process through cutaneous fistula (Figure 3).

Table 1: Details of the clinical cases reported in the study.

Case	Gender	Age	Habitation	Habits and addictions	Treatment	Comorbities	Anatomic region	Follow-up
1	Male	47	Rural	Drug addiction, alcoholism,and smoking	Sulfamethoxazole + trimethoprim	Malnutrition	Oral mucosa + pulmonary + lymph node	18 months
2	Male	68	Rural	Smoking	Itraconazole	Negative	Oral floor	12 months
3	Male	57	Rural	Smoking	Sulfamethoxazole + trimethoprim	Arterial hypertension	Lips + oral mucosa	24 months
4	Male	48	Rural	Smoking	Sulfamethoxazole + trimethoprim	Negative	Oral mucosa	20 months
5	Male	38	Rural	Smoking	Sulfamethoxazole + trimethoprim	Negative	Alveolar ridge	8 months

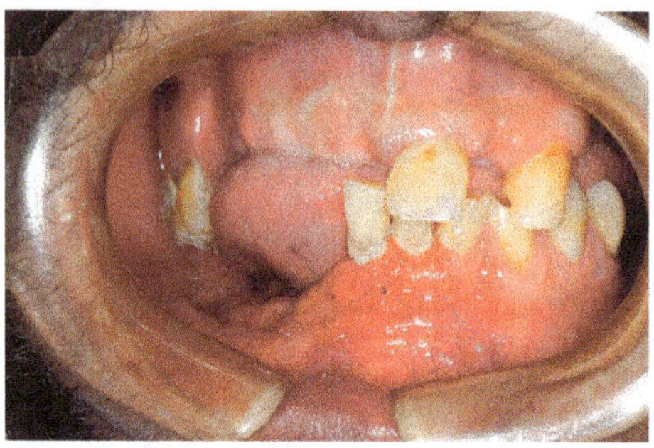

Figure 1: Initial intraoral clinical appearance showing the moriform aspect in the right buccal floor and alveolar ridge.

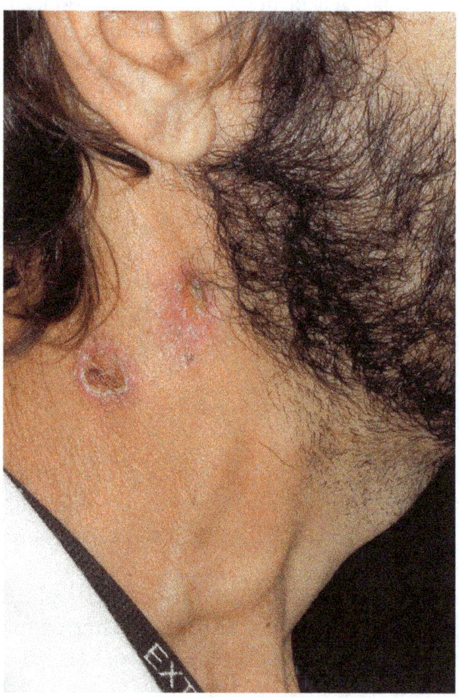

Figure 2: Ulcerated lesion in the right cervical/submandibular region.

Chest X-ray showed infiltrative lesions with reticulonodular aspect in butterfly-wing shape.

A direct mycological examination was performed from cervical lymph node puncture, sputum, and intraoral mucosal

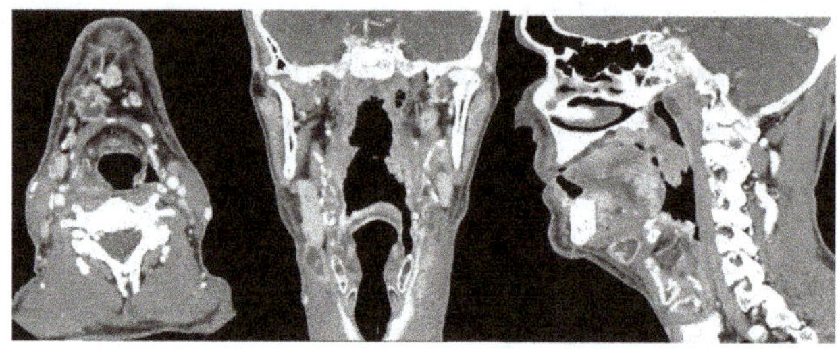

Figure 3: Computed tomography cuts showing lymph node enlargement as a hypodense and heterogeneous image in the right submandibular region.

scraping. The result was positive for the presence of yeasts with multiple buds surrounding mother cells, suggestive of *P. brasiliensis*. Thus, culture with fungal isolation was carried out, and the final result was *Paracoccidioides* spp. DNA-PCR examination for *Mycobacterium tuberculosis* was negative, and the result was nonreagent for the rapid HIV test, revealing leukocytosis (13,500/mm^3), without left deviation.

Incisional biopsy of the intraoral lesion was performed under local anesthesia. Histological sections revealed a mucosal fragment coated with parakeratinized stratified squamous epithelial tissue, exhibiting pseudoepitheliomatous hyperplasia constituted by dense connective tissue. An intense granulomatous inflammatory infiltrate with predominance of eosinophils and formation of granulomas and microabscesses were observed, as well as numerous multinucleated giant cells. Spherical fungi of different diameters and birefringent membrane located both within multinucleated giant cells or dispersed through the tissue were also present. In depth, there were fragments of mineralized tissue and hemorrhagic areas (Figure 4).

The patient was referred to an infectologist who followed up the case. An association of sulfamethoxazole 2400 mg + trimethoprim 480 mg was prescribed three times a day during 12 months. After 1-year follow-up, the patient was asymptomatic and presented remission of the oral and cervical lesions (Figures 5 and 6).

3. Case 2

A 68-year-old male patient who had melanoderma and was a chronic smoker and resident of the rural region was

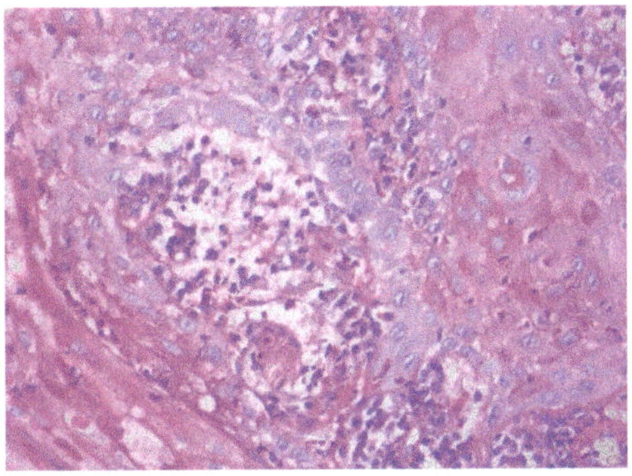

FIGURE 4: Anatomopathological examination image.

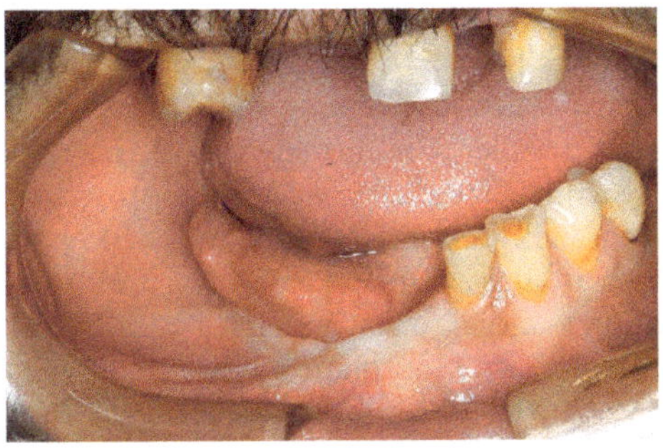

FIGURE 5: Intraoral oral appearance after antifungal therapy demonstrating lesion regression.

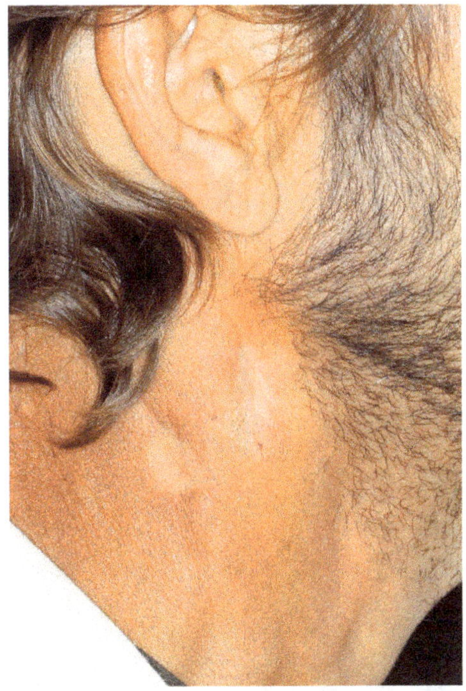

FIGURE 6: Clinical aspect of the submandibular/cervical region showing the remission of the ulcerated lesion and associated fistula.

referred to the surgery outpatient clinic with "mouth sore" complaint. Clinical examination verified an ulcerated lesion with hemorrhagic dots, a classic aspect of PCM (Figure 7). Biopsy was performed under local anesthesia, and the hypothesis was confirmed. Itraconazole therapy was initiated by the infectious team.

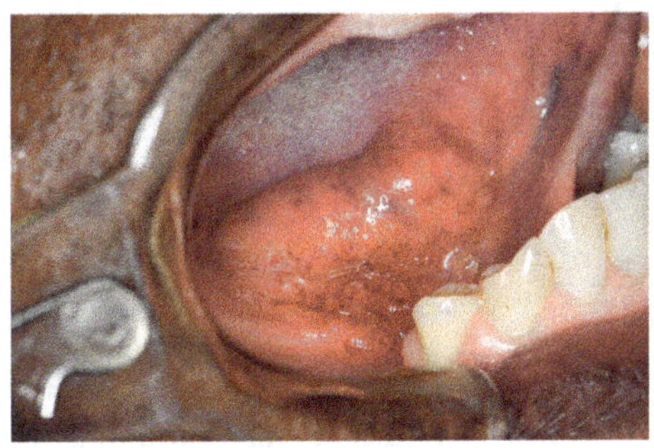

FIGURE 7: Classical presentation of PMC as exuberant hemorrhagic dots.

4. Case 3

A 57-year-old male patient who was a rural worker and smoker with systemic arterial hypertension attended the outpatient clinic complaining about "sore and pain in the lips and mouth." Clinical examination revealed the presence of erythematous ulcers in the lips and oral mucosa; the patient had a slight limitation of mouth opening due to the inflammatory process installed in the lips (Figures 8 and 9). Diagnostic suspicion of malignant neoplasia or paracoccidioidomycosis was raised. After anatomopathological examination of multiple fragments collected under local anesthesia, PMC was confirmed. Antifungal therapy with Bactrim (trimethoprim + sulfamethoxazole) was conducted.

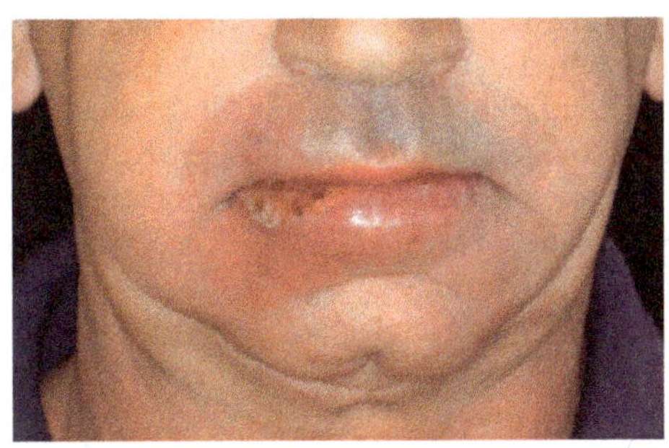

FIGURE 8: Frontal view of the patient presenting ulcers on the lips and associated cutaneous erythema.

PMC was confirmed after anatomopathological examination. Therapy started promptly with trimethoprim + sulfamethoxazole.

5. Case 4

A 48-year-old male patient who was a rural worker presented to the clinic, and he denied habits, addictions, or comorbidities. His main complaint was a "bleeding wound in the mouth." Clinical examination revealed an ulcer lesion of approximately 4 cm associated with hemorrhagic dots (Figure 10).

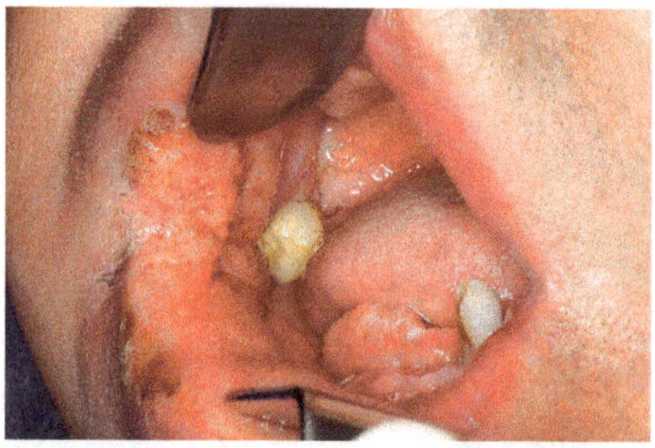

Figure 9: Ulcerated lesion in the jugal mucosa, lips, and buccal commissure.

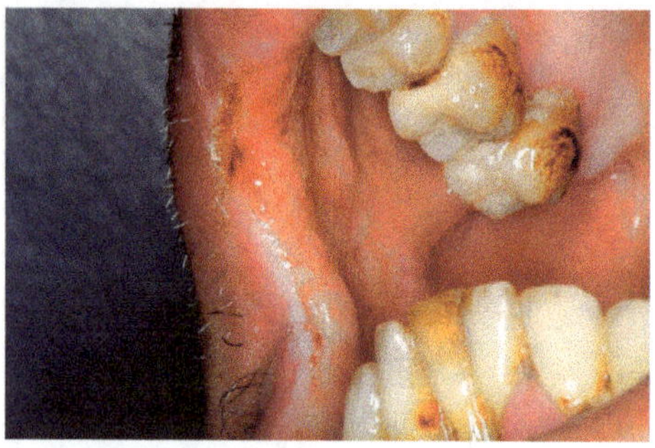

Figure 10: Ulcerated lesion of approximately 4 cm in the right jugal mucosa and buccal commissure.

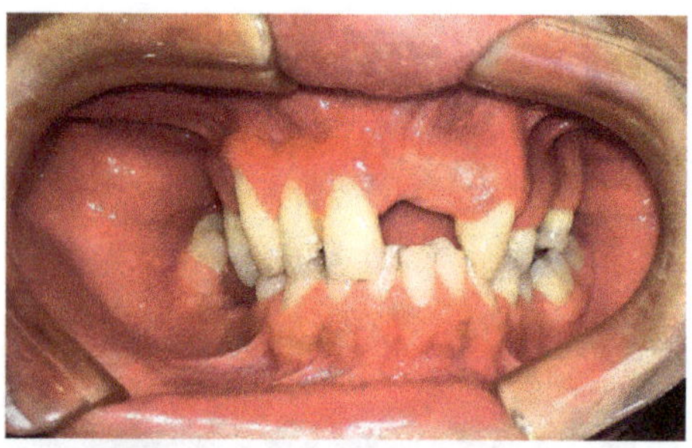

Figure 11: Erythematous lesion in the gums of the right maxilla and associated dental mobility.

6. Case 5

A 38-year-old male patient who was a rural worker and smoker presented to the clinic, and he denied comorbidities and complained about gingival bleeding when he brushed his teeth (Figure 11). Biopsy was performed since the lesion did not disappear after basic periodontal treatment. Pathologic examination revealed PMC; thus, antifungal therapy with Bactrim was initiated.

7. Discussion

Paracoccidioidomycosis was first described in Brazil in 1908 by Adolfo Lutz. Years later, in 1911, Alfonse Splendore reported other clinical cases and studied in detail its microbiology. PMC is also known as Brazilian blastomycosis, South American blastomycosis, Lutz's disease, Lutz–Splendore–Almeida disease, and Lutz's mycosis. Despite being a disease that does not require compulsory notification in Brazil (absence of precise data of its incidence), most cases were reported in the southern, southeastern, and center-western regions, closely related to rural dwellers. All patients listed in Table 1 reside in the countryside [7, 8].

Infective propagules (microconidia) reach the lower airways, where they constitute a primary complex, and possible dissemination of the fungus via lymphatic vessels and hematogenous spread to other organs are likely to happen. Manifestation of the disease depends on numerous factors, such as microorganism virulence and hormonal, genetic, nutritional, and immune system issues. Approximately 10 million people are infected worldwide by this fungus, but only 2% develop the active disease. Although transmission between humans is possible, it is very rare because the fungi switch to yeast form which cannot pass through the cell wall, differently from the unmodified mycelial form found in the nature [4, 5, 10, 11].

PMC has predilection for male gender in a ratio of 15 : 1; this difference can be explained by the protective effect of female hormones. Beta-estradiol seems to have a protective effect which inhibits transformation of the mycelium into yeast. Among individuals under 14-year-old or during menopause, the microorganism does not present predilection to gender due to decreased hormonal influence. Bicalho et al. [12] observed in a sample of 62 Brazilian patients the ratio of 30 : 1 between men and women. All five cases reported in this article were from male patients [1, 8, 13, 14].

The classic presentation of PMC in the oral cavity is a superficial ulcer characterized by hemorrhagic dots that usually affect the gums, palate, and mucous membranes. When ocular and genital mucosae are affected, they present the same characteristics of the classic oral lesion. Gingiva may be erythematous with consequent periodontal bone loss, mobility, and tooth loss. Bone destruction can be perceived through panoramic radiography, usually characterized by osteolytic areas in the alveolar region. This bone involvement can reach the maxillary sinus causing its opacification and destruction of the anterior wall. Palate perforation with oral-nasal communication rarely occurs. Cutaneous lesions can be caused by continuity, hematogenous contamination or, less often, by direct inoculation; in addition, contamination might happen through fistulas related to infected lymph nodes or osteomyelitis. Lesions in the nasal region are described in the literature; usually, they are continuity of lesions in the upper lip, mainly as a consequence of macrocheilia or related to direct contamination by sinus drainage [1–6, 15].

Lymph nodes are more frequently involved in young patients (less than 30 years old); they are initially firm, painful, and hypertrophic, and later, they develop phlogistic signs and suppuration [1, 2]. In case 1, the patient evolved with cutaneous lesion associated with cervical fistula in the right side and lymph node involvement, and the infection by ganglionic paracoccidioidomycosis was confirmed by aspiration. Cervical chain involvement was evident in the CT with contrast.

Bones and joints can be affected in about 6–20% of the reported cases, which is usually asymptomatic. Bone/joint lesions are predominant in the thorax, scapular region, and upper limbs. Paracoccidioidomycosis can affect any organ/region, including the central nervous system, for example, as cerebral granuloma and meningoencephalitis. Thus, possible lesions should be investigated through imaging and clinical findings [2, 5, 16]. In our article, three cases (60%) evolved with alveolar osteolysis, substantial dental mobility, and multiple dental losses.

Reports of paracoccidioidomycosis in HIV patients are less frequent than expected; this is still not well understood, but epidemiological differences between HIV and *P. brasiliensis* infections among rural and urban populations may be related. Morejón et al. [17] observed a discreet association between HIV and *P. brasiliensis* in only 1.4% of the analyzed cases. In general, the patients were farmers and the majority had less than 200 CD4+/μL. Thus, PMC can be considered an opportunistic infection among HIV positive population of endemic regions. Eight cases were reported among immunosuppressed patients after renal transplantation, in which latent foci were reactivated due to immunologic depression. There was no association with immunosuppression in the cases reported in our article [2, 13].

Radiographic findings in the posteroanterior thoracic incidence consist of reticulonodular pulmonary infiltrate, mainly in the upper two-thirds; it was bilateral and asymmetric. Computed tomography of the thorax shows nodules, ground-glass opacities, acinar lesions, parenchymal bands, peribroncovascular interstitial thickening, paracicatricial emphysema, and traction bronchiectasis [8, 16]. Similar findings were found in two patients in our study of cases (40%).

Facing the infection by paracoccidioidomycosis, an immune response is generated as granulomatous epithelial growth, which is a way to contain the progression of the fungal infection. This structure is formed by macrophages that surround the pathogen. Anatomopathological examination revealed an ulcer with pseudoepitheliomatous hyperplasia, as well as a granulomatous structure composed by giant multinucleated cells and macrophages. Fungi can be found inside giant cells or free. This fungus classical appearance is similar to "Mickey Mouse ears" or "boat steering wheel," which represents multiple yeasts with associated buds [1, 4, 5].

Diagnosis can be achieved through some complementary exams, such as direct microscopy and mycological examinations, which aim to identify microorganism in the sputum, purulent exudate, or material collected from lesions. Fungal culture may be useful but impaired due to slow fungal growth or sample contamination and its low sensitivity. Visualization of fungal particles can be obtained from pathological examination with Gomori–Grocott dye or PAS (periodic acid-Schiff). Exfoliative cytology is a diagnostic option, and it is also interesting to follow-up infection evolution during treatment. More recent options aim to identify antigenic/antibodies material and to evaluate quantity/type of antibodies present, such as direct/indirect immunofluorescence, immunoelectrophoresis of serum proteins, immunodiffusion technique, ELISA, and immunoblotting/western blot. In general, PCR to identify *P. brasiliensis* DNA has high sensitivity and specificity [1, 4, 5, 7].

Treatment should be instituted on an individualized basis and rigorous follow-up; special attention should be given to comorbidities, nutritional status, and drug use by patients starting treatment, besides, adherence of the patient to the pharmacotherapy. Medications of choice depend on the severity of the condition. Itraconazole is considered the gold standard in mild and moderate conditions, with a dosage of 200 mg/day for 6 to 18 months. Combination of sulfamethoxazole 2400 mg + trimethoprim 480 mg (Bactrim), daily, from 12 to 24 months is a viable option with excellent results. In severe cases, amphotericin B is the drug of choice, at doses of 0.75 mg/kg/day; it presents high toxicity, side effects, possible hospitalization, and renal function monitoring. *In vitro* studies demonstrate strains of *P. brasiliensis* resistant to various types of drugs; thus, new treatment protocols are necessary [2, 4–7, 9, 12, 15]. In our case reports, 80% of patients were treated successfully with the combination of sulfamethoxazole + trimethoprim.

Disease cure is difficult due to the risk of relapse; treatment success must be analyzed through clinical, radiographic, and immunological examination. Recurrence should be considered, although it is more common among immunosuppressed patients. Estimated mortality rate is 30% among patients with HIV, which can be decreased with early treatment with amphotericin B followed by life-long prophylaxis with some antifungals from the group of azoles or sulfonamide. Vaccine based on *P. brasiliensis* GP43 antigen requires more studies and greater applicability [4, 5, 13, 14].

8. Final Considerations

Paracoccidioidomycosis represents an important public health problem due to its high morbidity and mortality potential. Long and costly treatments in addition to recurrent episodes demand PMC treatment innovations. It should be considered as differential diagnosis in cases of opportunistic infection in immunosuppressed patients. Our study reported a range of presentations of the same infection, from complicated cases to cases that did not present classically as PMC.

Conflicts of Interest

The authors declare that they have no conflicts of interest.

References

[1] B. W. Neville, D. D. Damm, and C. M. Allen Jeb, *Oral and Maxillofacial Pathology*, Elsevier, Amsterdam, Netherlands, 4th edition, 2016.

[2] S. A. Marques, R. C. Leite, and S. Paulo, "Paracoccidioidomycosis," *Clinics in Dermatology*, vol. 30, no. 6, pp. 610–615, 2012.

[3] J. Regezi and J. Sciubba, *Patologia Oral Correlações Clinicopatológicas*, Elsevier Editora Ltda, Rio de Janeiro, RJ, Brazil, 6th edition, 2012.

[4] M. Ameen, C. Talhari, and S. Talhari, "Advances in paracoccidioidomycosis," *Clinical and Experimental Dermatology*, vol. 35, no. 6, pp. 576–580, 2009.
[5] M. A. D. Abreu, F. G. Salum, M. A. Figueiredo, and K. Cherubini, "Important aspects of oral paracoccidioidomycosis–a literature review," *Mycoses*, vol. 56, no. 6, pp. 189–199, 2013.
[6] F. M. Girardi and M. L. Scrofernecker, "Clinical image oral paracoccidiodomycosis mimicking lip carcinoma," *Brazilian Journal of Infectious Diseases*, vol. 20, no. 1, pp. 103-104, 2015.
[7] M. Palmeiro, K. Cherubini, and L. S. Yurgel, *Paracoccidioidomicose-Revisão da Literatura*, Sci Medica, PUCRS, Porto Alegre, RS, Brazil, Vol. 15, 2005.
[8] B. Wanke and M. A. Aidê, "Paracoccidioidomycosis," *Jornal Brasileiro de Pneumologia*, vol. 35, no. 12, pp. 1245–1249, 2009.
[9] M. A. Shikanai-Yasuda, "Paracoccidioidomycosis treatment," *Revista do Instituto de Medicina Tropical de São Paulo*, vol. 57, no. S19, pp. 31–37, 2015.
[10] C. Talhari, J. V. B. D. Souza, V. J. Parreira, D. Reinel, and S. Talhari, "Oral exfoliative cytology as a rapid diagnostic tool for paracoccidioidomycosis," *Mycoses*, vol. 51, no. 2, pp. 177-178, 2007.
[11] M. R. Azenha, R. Caliento, L. G. Brentegani, and S. A. D. Lacerda, "A retrospective study of oral manifestations in patients with paracoccidioidomycosis," *Brazilian Dental Journal*, vol. 23, no. 6, pp. 753–757, 2012.
[12] R. N. Bicalho, M. F. Santo, M. C. F. Aguiar, and V. R. Santos, "Oral paracoccidioidomycosis: a retrospective study of 62 patients," *Oral Diseases*, vol. 7, no. 1, pp. 56–60, 2001.
[13] M. V. Radisic, L. Linares, J. Afeltra et al., "Acute pulmonary involvement by paracoccidiodomycosis disease immediately after kidney transplantation: case report and literature review," *Transplant Infectious Disease*, vol. 19, no. 2, 2017.
[14] A. C. S. De Azevedo Izidoro, P. C. D. Silva, M. D. O. Ribas et al., "Case of recurrent paracoccidioidomycosis in female 10 years after initial treatment," *Bulletin of Tokyo Dental College*, vol. 48, no. 2, pp. 67–72, 2007.
[15] S. S. Neto, L. F. B. de Paulo, and R. R. Rosa, "Oral paracoccidioidomycosis as a differential diagnosis of oral cancer," *Images in Infectious Diseases*, vol. 45, no. 6, 2012.
[16] F. V. A. Lima Júnior, L. G. Savarese, L. M. Monsignore, R. Martinez, and M. H. Nogueira-barbosa, "Computed tomography findings of paracoccidioidomycosis in musculoskeletal system," *Radiologia Brasileira*, vol. 48, no. 1, pp. 1–6, 2015.
[17] K. M. L. Morejón, A. A. Machado, and R. Martinez, "Paracoccidioidomycosis in patients infected with and not infected with human immunodeficiency virus: a case-control study," *American Society of Tropical Medicine and Hygiene*, vol. 80, no. 3, pp. 359–366, 2009.

44

Concomitant Extramedullary Plasmacytoma in the Oropharynx and Hypopharyngeal Squamous Cell Carcinoma

Hiroki Sato, Shoko Yoshimasu, Isaku Okamoto, Akira Shimizu, Yasuaki Katsube, Hideki Tanaka, and Kiyoaki Tsukahara

Department of Otorhinolaryngology, Head and Neck Surgery, Tokyo Medical University, Tokyo, Japan

Correspondence should be addressed to Hiroki Sato; satohiro@tokyo-med.ac.jp

Academic Editor: Abrão Rapoport

We report a rare case of hypopharyngeal squamous cell carcinoma occurring synchronously with extramedullary plasmacytoma (EPM) of the oropharynx in which radiotherapy was used as the curative treatment. A 73-year-old man presented with a sore throat that had persisted for 6 months. Examination revealed a superficial, smooth tumorous lesion at the base of his tongue with a red hue in the oropharynx. In addition, a protruding tumor was observed on the mucosal surface in the right piriform recess of the hypopharynx, and computed tomography revealed thickening of the pharyngeal wall at the right tongue base and in the right piriform recess of the hypopharynx. Because no definitive diagnosis could be reached for the lesion at the base of the tongue, the entire tongue-base tumor was resected by transoral surgery under endoscopy. Proliferation of plasma cells in the tumor was detected, and a bone marrow puncture test ruled out multiple myeloma leading to a definitive diagnosis of Stage I (cT1N0M0) squamous cell carcinoma in the right piriform recess of the hypopharynx and primary extramedullary plasmacytoma in the oropharynx. Radiotherapy was selected for curative treatment with a complete response for both cancers. No recurrences have been observed as of 12 months postoperatively.

1. Introduction

Extramedullary plasmacytoma (EPM) is a tumor that originates from plasma cells. EPM develops in soft tissues other than bone marrow, frequently in the head and neck area. A large number of the malignant tumors developing in the head and neck area are squamous cell carcinomas, and such carcinomas often occur together with other malignant tumors, either synchronously or metachronously [1, 2]. However, head and neck squamous cell carcinoma occurring synchronously with EPM is extremely rare. A search in PubMed revealed only 3 cases of EPM coexisting with head and neck squamous cell carcinoma: a case of maxillary sinus EPM together with lingual squamous cell carcinoma; a case of laryngeal EPM together with laryngeal cancer; and a case of nasopharyngeal EPM together with nasopharyngeal cancer [3–5]. The present case of EPM coexisting with hypopharyngeal carcinoma is the first such case to be reported. Generally, surgery or radiotherapy is considered curative treatment for both EPM and head and neck squamous cell carcinomas. When EPM and head and neck squamous cell carcinomas are present together, adequate consideration of the treatment modality is necessary. We report a case of hypopharyngeal squamous cell carcinoma occurring synchronously with EPM of the oropharynx in which radiotherapy was used as the curative treatment.

2. Case Presentation

The patient was a 73-year-old man. He was examined at our hospital for a sore throat that had persisted for 6 months. He had a drinking habit of one 500 ml bottle of beer daily and no history of smoking. Diabetes, hypertension, and hyperlipidemia were noted in his previous medical history.

Pharyngolaryngoscopy revealed a superficial, smooth tumorous lesion with a red hue in the oropharynx at the base of the tongue. In addition, a protruding tumor with atypical blood vessel formation was observed on the mucosal surface

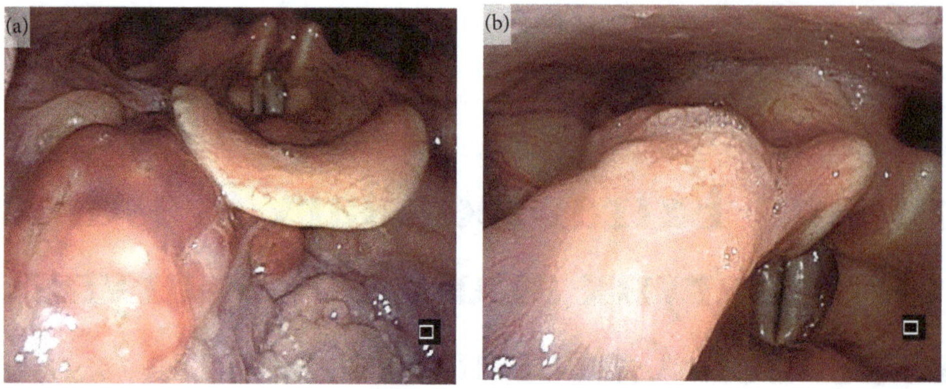

Figure 1: Pharyngolaryngoscopy. A superficial, smooth tumorous lesion with red color is observed (a). A protruding lesion with atypical blood vessel formation in the mucosa surface is also observed (b).

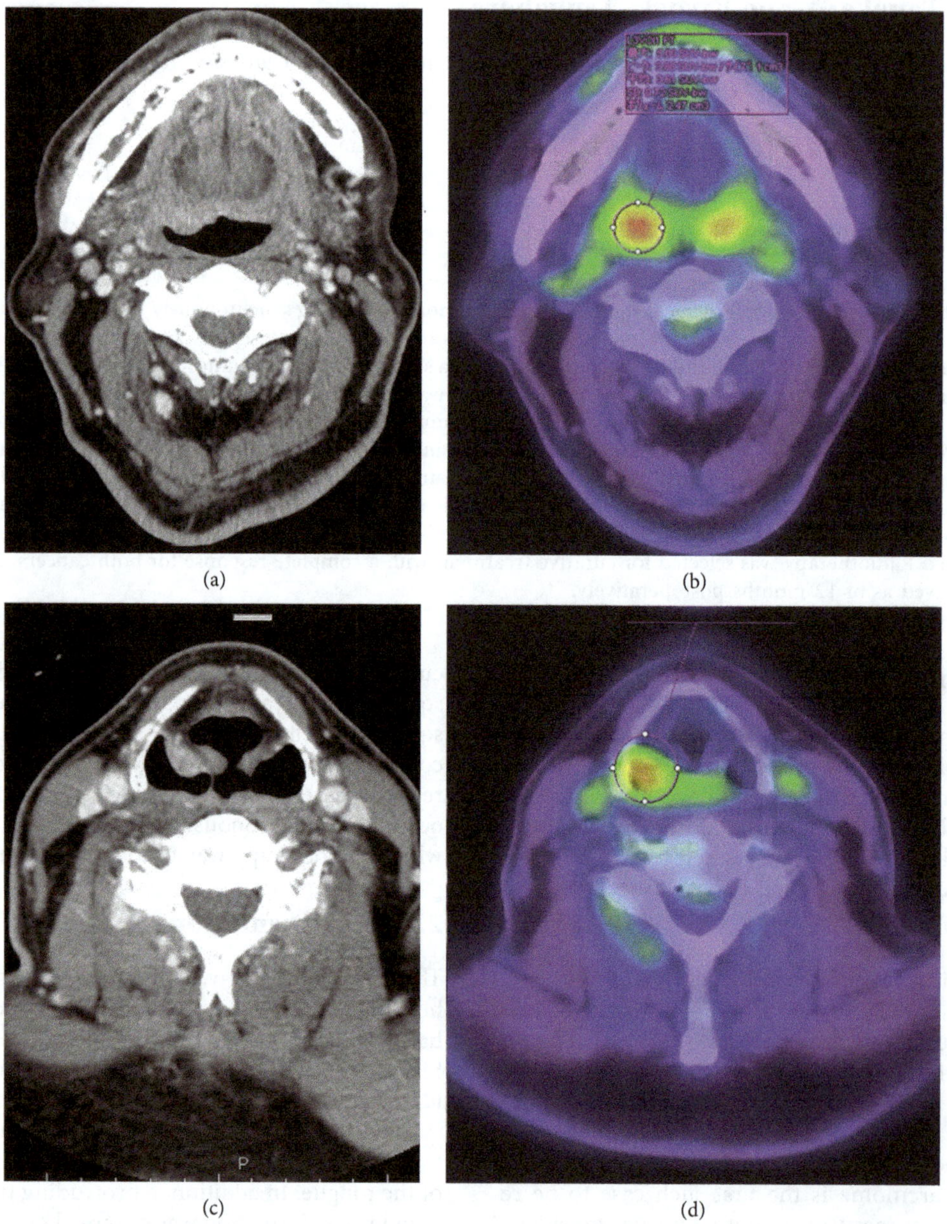

Figure 2: Contrast-enhanced CT and FDG PET/CT. Thickening of the pharyngeal wall with irregular contrast enhancement is observed on the right side of the tongue base and in the right piriform recess. SUVmax is 2.0 on the right side of the tongue base and 4.2 in the right piriform recess.

in the right piriform recess of the hypopharynx (Figure 1). On contrast-enhanced CT, thickening of the pharyngeal wall showing irregular contrast enhancement was observed at the right tongue base and in the right piriform recess of the hypopharynx (Figure 2). No swelling of neck lymph nodes was observed. On fluorodeoxyglucose positron emission tomography/computed tomography (FDG PET/CT), accumulation was observed for maximum standardized uptake values (SUVmax) of 2.0 and 4.2 in the lesions of the oropharynx and hypopharynx, respectively (Figure 2). No accumulation was observed in neck lymph nodes or other parts.

Based on tissue biopsies, the histopathological diagnosis for the lesion in the right piriform recess of the hypopharynx was squamous cell carcinoma (Figure 3). While the lesion at the base of the tongue was suspected to represent malignant lymphoma on histopathological examination, no definitive diagnosis could be reached. To achieve a definitive diagnosis, the entire tongue-base tumor was resected by transoral surgery under endoscopy. Subsequent histopathological examination revealed proliferation of plasma cells in the tumor, and immunostaining findings were as follows: $\kappa(-)$, $\lambda(+)$, CD3(−), CD20(−), CD138(−), CD79a(+), and MUM-1(+) (Figure 4). A bone marrow puncture test ruled out multiple myeloma. Based on the above, a definitive diagnosis of Stage I (cT1N0M0) squamous cell carcinoma in the right piriform recess of the hypopharynx and primary extramedullary plasmacytoma in the oropharynx was made. In the treatment plan, radiotherapy was selected for curative treatment. After irradiating the whole neck with 40 Gy in 20 fractions, the irradiation field was reduced to target the tumor in the hypopharynx only, and additional radiotherapy comprising 30 Gy in 15 fractions was conducted (Figure 5). Treatment outcome was complete response for both cancers, and no recurrences have been observed as of 12 months postoperatively.

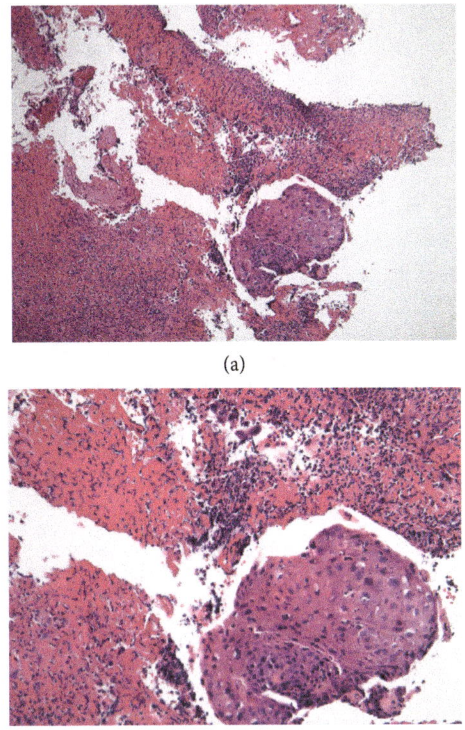

(a)

(b)

FIGURE 3: Histopathological findings for hypopharyngeal tumor biopsy. Features observed include increased nuclear chromatin, disparity between large and small nuclei, and signs of mitosis. These findings are indicative of squamous cell carcinoma.

3. Discussion

Locations where other cancers frequently occur together with head and neck squamous cell carcinomas are the esophagus, head and neck, stomach, and lungs. In 20% of esophageal cancer patients, other malignancies arise in the upper aerodigestive tract, and in 10%, they occur in the head and neck area [6, 7]. Synchronously occurring squamous cell carcinomas are thus generally suspected when multiple cancers are identified in the head and neck region. However, while accounting for just 3% of plasmacytomas as an extremely rare type of cancer, around 80% of EPMs develop in the head and neck region [8]. They mostly occur in the oral cavity, nasal cavity, pharynx, and larynx, so the frequency is higher in the upper respiratory tract [8]. Occurrence rates are 40% for the nasal cavity, 20% for the nasopharynx, and 18% for the oropharynx [9].

As stated in Introduction, among head and neck cancers, reported cases of concomitant squamous cell carcinoma and EPM are extremely rare, and this represents the first report of synchronous EPM and hypopharyngeal carcinoma. The mechanisms underlying joint occurrence of EPM and squamous cell carcinomas in the head and neck region have been unknown in all cases reported to date [3–5]. This is because the risk factors for both pathologies differ. When dual malignancies are observed in the head and neck area, EPM should be considered as a candidate for differential diagnosis, despite its rarity.

The National Comprehensive Cancer Network (NCCN) guidelines recommend radiotherapy or surgery for Stage I hypopharyngeal cancer [10]. Transoral resection is also increasingly being selected for patients with Stage I or II hypopharyngeal cancer. However, radiotherapy alone is frequently used for EPM because of its favorable radiosensitivity. Skóra et al. reported high response rates for radiotherapy alone in 17 cases of primary EPM in the head and neck, with 75% achieving complete response and 25% achieving partial response [11]. In the present case, we resected the EPM for biopsy purposes, and as a safety margin was not obtained at resection, we considered radiotherapy as warranted. Also, as the hypopharyngeal cancer was able to be treated under the same irradiation field, the hypopharyngeal carcinoma was also treated by radiotherapy.

EPM is an extremely rare disease that occurs mostly in the head and neck area, making this an important differential diagnosis for head and neck malignancies. Although no definitive diagnosis could be determined for the primary tumor in the oropharynx in the present case through

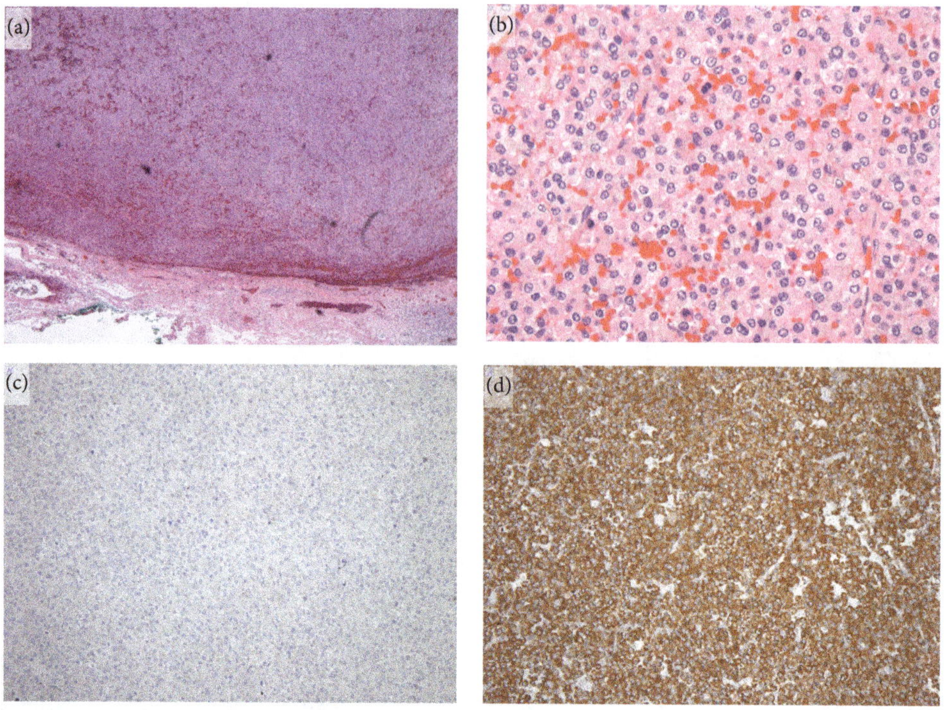

FIGURE 4: Histopathological findings for transorally resected nasopharyngeal tumor. HE staining: low magnification (a) and high magnification (b). Proliferation of plasma cells and unevenly distributed nuclei are observed. Immunostaining shows negative results for κ (c) and positive results for λ (d).

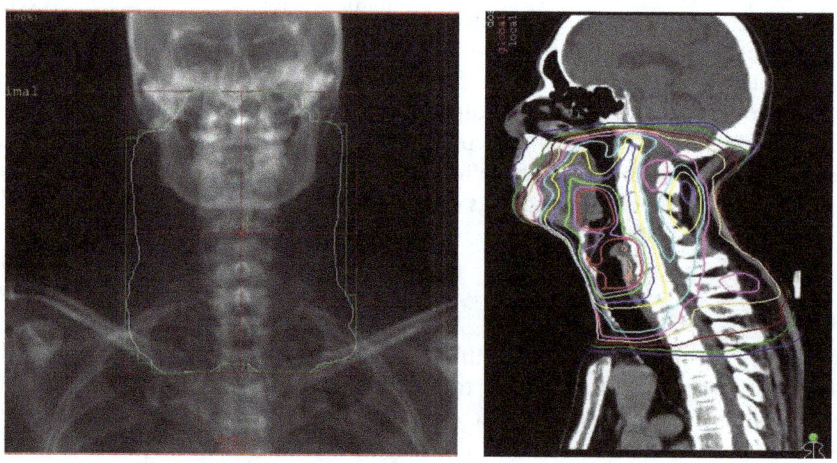

(a) (b)

FIGURE 5: Distribution map of radiotherapy.

the initial biopsy, complete resection for biopsy purposes enabled definitive diagnosis. As EPM may be locally recurrent or develop into multiple myeloma after treatment, pretreatment diagnosis is crucial. The follow-up protocol is that local recurrence, metachronous head and neck carcinoma, locoregional lymph node metastasis, and distant metastasis are assessed every 2–3 months by performing fiberscopy, CT, or cervical ultrasonography. In addition, metachronous esophageal and gastric carcinoma is assessed once a year by performing esophagogastroduodenoscopy. The screening for recurrence of the EPM is done using serum-free light chains every 6 months. After treatment, not only recurrence of the EPM but also of squamous cell carcinomas has to be kept in mind, as the latter frequently recur metachronously, necessitating rigorous follow-up.

Conflicts of Interest

The authors declare that they have no conflicts of interest.

References

[1] W. F. McGuirt, "Panendoscopy as a screening examination for simultaneous primary tumors in head and neck cancer: a prospective sequential study and review of the literature," *Laryngoscope*, vol. 92, no. 5, pp. 569–576, 1982.

[2] M. Morita, H. Kuwano, S. Ohno et al., "Multiple occurrence of carcinoma in the upper aerodigestive tract associated with esophageal cancer: reference to smoking, drinking and family history," *International Journal of Cancer Banner*, vol. 58, no. 2, pp. 207–210, 1994.

[3] L. Junquera, L. Gallego, A. Torre, J. Hernando, and M. F. Fresno, "Synchronous oral squamous cell carcinoma and extramedullary plasmacytoma of the tonsil," *Oral Surgery, Oral Medicine, Oral Pathology, Oral Radiology, and Endodontology*, vol. 108, no. 3, pp. 413–416, 2009.

[4] X. L. Zhang, D. Q. Li, J. J. Li, S. S. Li, and X. M. Yang, "Synchronous occurrence of extramedullary plasmacytoma and squamous cell carcinoma in situ in the larynx: a case report," *Chinese Journal of Cancer*, vol. 29, no. 12, pp. 1029–1034, 2010.

[5] R. C. Du, H. N. Li, W. Huang, X. Y. Tian, and Z. Li, "Unusual coexistence of extramedullary plasmacytoma and nasopharyngeal carcinoma in nasopharynx," *Diagnostic Pathology*, vol. 10, no. 1, p. 170, 2015.

[6] The Japanese Society for Esophageal Diseases, *Comprehensive Registry of Esophageal Cancer in Japan (1998-1999)*, 3rd edition, Secretariant of the Japan Esophageal Society, Tokyo, Japan, 2002.

[7] A. Watanabe, M. Hosokawa, M. Taniguchi, H. Tsujie, and S. Sasaki, "Head and neck cancer associated with esophageal cancer," *Auris, Nasus, Larynx*, vol. 34, no. 2, pp. 207–211, 2007.

[8] R. C. Gromer and A. J. Duvall III, "Plasmacytoma of the head and neck," *Journal of Laryngology and Otology*, vol. 87, no. 9, pp. 861–872, 1973.

[9] R. H. Liebross, C. S. Ha, J. D. Cox, D. Weber, K. Delasalle, and R. Alexanian, "Clinical course of solitary extramedullary plasmacytoma," *Radiotherapy and Oncology*, vol. 52, no. 3, pp. 245–249, 1999.

[10] NCCN Clinical Practice Guidelines in Oncology (NCCN Guidelines®), *Head and Neck Cancers Version 2.2018*, NCCN, Fort Washington, PA, USA, 2018.

[11] T. Skóra, K. Pudełek, J. Nowak-Sadzikowska, M. Pietrasz, B. Szyszka-Charewicz, and J. Jakubowicz, "Effect of definitive radiotherapy on the long-term outcome in patients with solitary extramedullary plasmacytoma," *Hematological Oncology*, vol. 35, no. 3, pp. 317–322, 2017.

45

Paraganglioma Presenting as a Nasal Septal Mass

James H. Kim,[1] **Nathan Tu**,[2] **and Bozena Barbara Wrobel**[3]

[1]*Keck School of Medicine of the University of Southern California, Los Angeles, CA, USA*
[2]*University of Southern California LAC+USC Medical Center Department of Otolaryngology, Los Angeles, CA, USA*
[3]*Associate Professor of Clinical Otolaryngology Head and Neck Surgery, Keck School of Medicine, Los Angeles, CA, USA*

Correspondence should be addressed to James H. Kim; kim883@usc.edu

Academic Editor: Richard T. Miyamoto

Objectives. To describe a rare case of a paraganglioma arising from the nasal septum and review the diagnosis and management of paragangliomas in the nasal cavity and paranasal sinuses. *Methods.* We present a case of a 70-year-old female presenting with persistent nasal congestion and obstruction. Nasal endoscopy revealed a posterior septal mass approaching the sphenoid sinuses and partially obstructing the nasopharynx. A biopsy of the mass was taken, and histologic analysis confirmed a diagnosis of paraganglioma. *Results.* The patient underwent an endoscopic resection of the tumor. There has been no evidence of disease recurrence after 3 months of follow-up. *Conclusions.* Paragangliomas arising from the nasal septum are exceedingly rare, but should be considered in the differential diagnosis in patients presenting with nasal septal masses. These tumors are typically benign, although few cases of malignant sinonasal paragangliomas have been reported. Treatment requires surgical excision with close follow-up as several cases of tumor recurrence have been reported.

1. Introduction

Paragangliomas are rare, slow-growing neuroendocrine tumors arising from cells of neural crest origin. They typically originate from the adrenal gland, but occur extra-adrenally in 5–10% of cases [1]. In the head and neck region, paragangliomas make up only 0.6% of all tumors, most commonly in the carotid body and jugular-tympanic regions [1–3]. Though rare, there are few reported cases of paragangliomas arising in the nasal cavity and paranasal sinuses [4–8]. To our knowledge, there has only been one previously reported case of a paraganglioma originating from the nasal septum [8].

2. Case Report

A 70-year-old female complaining of persistent nasal congestion and obstruction presented to our clinic for evaluation. She denied any headache or epistaxis. Nasal endoscopy was performed which showed a posterior septal mass approaching the sphenoid sinuses bilaterally and partially obstructing the view of the nasopharynx. The overlying mucosa was intact except for a small area superiorly which showed a soft granulomatous mass protruding into the left nasal cavity.

The patient was taken to the operating room for septoplasty with biopsy of the mass at an outside institution. Microscopic examination of the biopsy specimen demonstrated clusters of epithelioid-appearing cells separated by bands of fibrillary stroma. The epithelioid cells were noted to have abundant amphophilic cytoplasm, uniform, rounded nuclei with "salt and pepper" chromatin, and small nucleoli. No mitotic activity, invasion, necrosis, or calcification was seen. Immunohistochemical staining demonstrated positivity for neuron-specific enolase (NSE), chromogranin A, synaptophysin, and CD56 cell markers within the epithelioid cells. Fibrillary cells were positive for NSE, chromogranin A, S-100, glial fibrillary acid protein (GFAP), and CD56 cell markers. Based on the histological appearance and immunohistochemical staining, a diagnosis of paraganglioma was made.

The patient was referred to our institution for further management. Preoperative CT imaging showed a smoothly marginated, soft tissue density mass centered at the posterior nasal septum with extension into the nasopharynx and bulging into the right sphenoid sinus (Figure 1). Severe thinning and smooth remodeling of the anterior wall of the sphenoid sinus and anterior clivus were seen. MRI imaging demonstrated hyperintense signaling of the mass on T1-weighted images with a peripheral rim of hypointense signaling on T2-weighted imaging suggestive of a capsule.

An endoscopic resection of the mass was performed. Intraoperatively, a large mass was seen in the posterior aspect of the septum, bulging into the bilateral nasal cavities and extending into the sphenoid sinuses (Figure 2). Erosion of the bone of the rostrum and anterior face of the sphenoid were also seen. Complete resection of the mass was achieved through a posterior septectomy and bilateral sphenoidotomy with tissue removal. Postoperative histologic analysis of the specimen was consistent with a paraganglioma (Figure 3).

The patient has been symptom free without local recurrence 3 months following tumor resection.

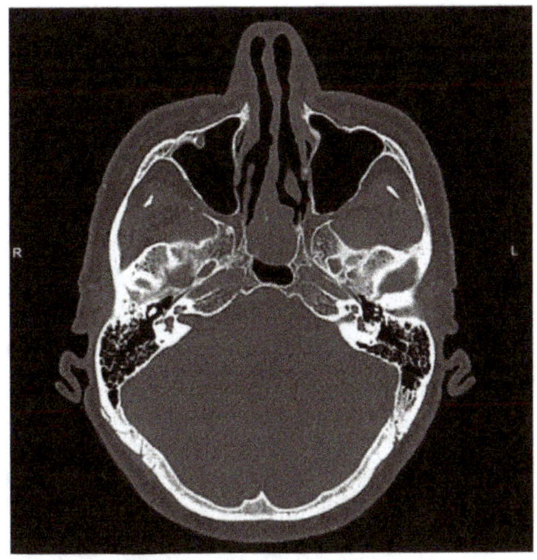

Figure 1: Axial CT image showing a soft tissue mass centered at the posterior nasal septum with extension into the nasopharynx.

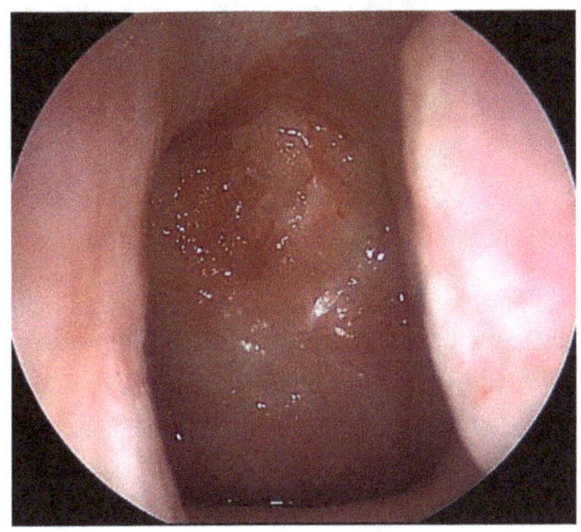

Figure 2: Intraoperative image of the mass protruding from the posterior septum within the left nasal cavity.

3. Discussion

Paragangliomas arising from the nasal cavity and nasal sinuses are extremely rare. Only 48 total cases of paragangliomas occurring in the nasal cavity or paranasal sinuses have been reported to date, occurring in patients with ages ranging between 8 and 89 years old, with an average age of 49 years old. These tumors are slightly more prevalent amongst females (60.4%). Twelve were reported to be malignant in nature, demonstrating either intracranial extension or metastasis to the cervical lymph nodes, brain, and bone. These masses were most frequently reported to originate from the ethmoid sinuses, middle turbinate, and maxillary sinuses. Other less common locations of origin reported include the superior and inferior turbinates, and the sphenoid and frontal sinuses. To the best of our knowledge, there has only been one other reported case of a paraganglioma originating from the nasal septum (Table 1) [8].

The most commonly reported symptoms included nasal obstruction, headache, and recurrent epistaxis. The vast majority of reported cases were functionally inactive, with no evidence of catecholamine or adrenocorticotropic hormone (ACTH) secretion. However, there have been a few reported cases of metabolically active tumors secreting ACTH and catecholamines, causing hypertension and other cushingoid features in the affected patient [12, 13, 30]. As such, testing for catecholamine and metanephrines is recommended in symptomatic patients [29, 33].

The origin of paragangliomas in the nasal cavity and paranasal sinuses remains unclear. Although paraganglionic tissue has never been demonstrated in the nasal cavity, a wider distribution of paraganglionic tissue is thought to exist in fetuses and neonates, degenerating after birth [42, 43]. Some authors have suggested that the migration of these embryonic paraganglionic cells accounts for the occurrence of paragangliomas in areas with no known paraganglionic tissue like the nasal cavity [13, 29, 42, 44]. Additionally, it has been shown that paraganglionic tissue exists around the terminal portion of the maxillary artery in infants and could possibly represent a point of origin for paragangliomas in the nasal cavity due to its anatomic proximity [19, 45]. Others have suggested that the paraganglionic tissue may exist in the pterygopalatine fossa due to the close relationship of paraganglionic tissue with arteries and cranial nerves [18, 19, 22].

In contrast, chondrocytes of the cartilaginous septum develop from neural crest cells between the nasal cavities by the ninth week of embryonic development [46, 47]. This is evident by the expression of various neural crest stem cell markers in nasal septum progenitor cells [48]. Several studies have demonstrated that these neural crest-derived chondrocytes in an adult septum retain pluripotent properties, with the capacity for osteogenic, chondrogenic, and neurogenic differentiation [48, 49]. It is possible that the neural crest origin of septal chondrocytes plays an important factor in the development of nasal septal paragangliomas.

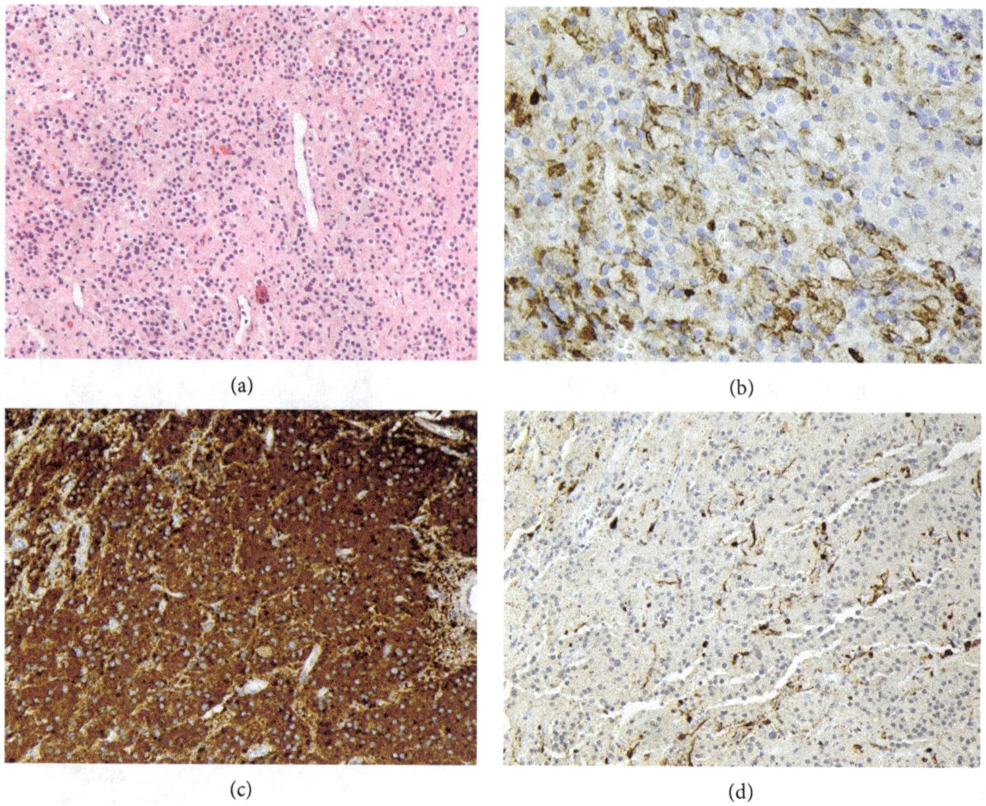

FIGURE 3: (a) H&E of the septal mass showing a "zellballen" pattern of clusters of epithelioid cells between bands of fibrillary stroma (20x). IHC staining showing positivity for (b) chromogranin A within epithelioid cells (40x), (c) synaptophysin within epithelioid cells (20x), and (d) S-100 within fibrillary cells (20x).

TABLE 1: Review of reported cases of sinonasal paragangliomas.

Case	Author	Year	Sex	Age	Location	Biological behavior	Therapy	Follow-up
1	Harkins [9]	1957	F	52	Ethmoid sinus	Benign	Exc, RT, lig ECA	NED at 1 year
2	Moran [10]	1962	F	89	Nasal cavity	Benign	Exc, ligation of external carotid artery	NED at 2 years
3	Lack [3]	1976	F	50	High nasal vault	Benign (local recurrence x3)	Exc, ligation of external carotid artery	NED at 11 years following final exc
4			F	50	Middle turbinate	Benign	Exc	No f/u
5			M	8	Middle turbinate	Benign	Exc	NED at 7 years
6	Gosavi [11]	1978	M	65	Middle turbinate	Benign	Exc, RT (incomplete cycle)	NED at 2 years
7	Apple [12]	1982	F	50	Ethmoid, sphenoid, and maxillary sinuses	Benign; ectopic ACTH production	Exc, RT, hormonal pharmacotherapy	NED at 6 years
8	Koegel [13]	1982	F	71	Maxillary and sphenoid sinuses	Malignant (extension into temporal lobe); catecholamine secretion	RT	No follow-up available
9	Himelfarb [14]	1985	M	41	Middle turbinate	Benign	Exc	NED at 1 year
10	Straehler [15]	1985	M	42	Maxillary sinus	Benign	Exc	No follow-up available
11	Ueda [16]	1985	F	31	Maxillary and ethmoid sinuses	Benign	Exc	NED at 2.5 years
12	Watson [17]	1988	M	56	Inferior turbinate	Benign	Exc, RT	NED at 3 years
13	Branham [18]	1989	F	25	Maxillary and ethmoid sinuses	Malignant (brain metastasis)	Exc, RT, CT	DOD at 3 years
14	Kuhn [19]	1989	M	62	Superior nasal cavity, ethmoid sinus	Benign	Exc	NED at 1 year

Table 1: Continued.

Case	Author	Year	Sex	Age	Location	Biological behavior	Therapy	Follow-up
15	Shimoda [20]	1989	M	58	Ethmoid sinus and bilateral frontal fossa	Malignant (cervical lymph nodes metastasis)	Exc, RT	NED at 2 years
16	Talbot [21]	1990	F	17	Maxillary sinus	Benign	Embolization of internal maxillary artery, exc	NED at 3 months
17	Nguyen [22]	1995	F	32	Ethmoid sinus	Malignant (bone metastasis)	Exc, RT	DOD at 15 years
18	Biswas [23]	1999	F	45	Middle turbinate	Benign	Exc	NED at 1 month
19	Sharma [24]	1999	M	33	Frontal sinus (primary); orbit, optic nerve, cavernous sinus, maxillary and ethmoid sinuses (recurrent)	Malignant (recurrence, intracranial invasion)	CT, RT, exc; vessel embolization, exc 8 months later for recurrence	DOD at 19 months
20	Welkoborsky [25]	2000	F	54	Nasal cavity	Benign	Exc	NED at 3 years
21			F	56	Ethmoid sinus	Malignant (brain metastasis)	Exc, RT	DOD at 28 months
22			M	57	Ethmoid sinus	Benign	Exc, RT	NED at 2 years
23	Scott [26]	2001	M	24	Nasal cavity, ethmoid sinus	Benign	Exc	NED at 15 months
24	Lecuna [27]	2002	F	72	Ethmoid sinus (primary); maxillary sinus (recurrent)	Malignant (recurrence, submandibular lymph nodes metastasis)	Exc	No follow-up available
25	Ketabchi [28]	2003	F	72	Nasal cavity	Benign	Exc	NED at 8 months
26	Mouadeb [29]	2003	M	72	Ethmoid sinus	Benign	Exc	NED at 4 years
27	Lieberum [30]	2003	M	64	Frontal and ethmoid sinuses	Benign; ectopic ACTH production	Exc	NED at 2 years
28	Askar [31]	2003	M	47	Middle turbinate	Benign	Exc	NED at 2 years
29	Rocha [32]	2005	M	45	Nasal cavity	Benign	Exc	NED at 5 months
30	Liess [33]	2007	F	64	Sphenoid sinus, sella, cavernous sinus	Benign	Partial exc, RT	Residual tumor stable at 2 years
31	Morales [7]	2007	F	41	Sphenoid and ethmoid sinuses	Benign	No information available	No follow-up available
32	Jin [34]	2008	F	23	Superior turbinate	Malignant (questionable transformation simulating Ewing's sarcoma/primitive neuroectodermal tumor)	Exc	NED at 3 years
33	Fasunla [35]	2008	F	39	Lateral nasal wall	Benign	Exc	NED at 1 year
34	Kisser [6]	2012	F	36	Maxillary sinus	Benign	Exc	NED at 1 year
35	Zainine [36]	2012	F	43	Middle turbinate	Benign	Exc	NED at 2 years
36	Papaspyrou [4]	2013	F	33	Nasal cavity	Benign	Exc	NED at 15 years
37			M	64	Ethmoid sinuses, anterior skull base, frontal lobe dura (primary); ethmoid, sphenoid, cavernous sinus, orbit (recurrent)	Malignant (recurrent, intradural metastases)	2 exc, RT, CT	DOD at 60 months
38			F	56	Ethmoid sinus	Malignant (brain metastasis)	Exc, RT	DOD at 28 months
39			F	80	Nasal cavity, maxilloethmoidal angle, maxillary, ethmoid, and sphenoid sinuses (primary); nasal cavity, anterior skull base, frontal lobe (recurrent)	Malignant (recurrent, intracranial invasion)	Exc	DNOD 17 months after 2nd surgery
40			M	57	Ethmoid sinus	Benign	Exc	NED at 2 years
41			F	54	Nasal cavity	Benign	Exc	NED at 3 years
42	Granato [5]	2013	F	61	Nasal cavity	Benign	Exc	NED at 2 years

Table 1: Continued.

Case	Author	Year	Sex	Age	Location	Biological behavior	Therapy	Follow-up
43	Michel [37]	2013	M	47	Maxillary sinus	Malignant (cervical lymph node metastasis)	Exc, RT	NED at 1 year
44	Amiraraghi [38]	2013	M	29	Cribriform plate and fovea ethmoidalis presenting as nasal polyps	Benign	Exc	NED at 3 years
45	Arora [39]	2014	F	40	Lateral nasal wall	Benign	Exc	NED at 2 years
46	Yamaguchi [40]	2015	F	66	Ethmoid sinus	Benign	Exc	NED at 1 year
47	Aydin [41]	2015	F	32	Nasal cavity, ethmoid sinus	Benign (local recurrence x2)	Exc	NED 5 years after final exc
48	Srivastava [8]	2016	M	60	Anterior nasal septum	Benign	Exc	NED at 18 months

RT, radiation therapy; CT, chemotherapy; Exc, surgical excision; NED, no evidence of disease; DOD, died of disease.

Despite the neural crest origins of nasal chondrocytes, paragangliomas arising from the nasal septum are extremely rare.

Masses arising from the nasal septum represent a broad spectrum of diagnoses including polyps, chondromas, hematomas, and hemangiomas. Less common septal lesions include sarcomas, melanomas, and other neoplasms [46, 50]. Patients with septal masses typically present with nonspecific symptoms of nasal obstruction or epistaxis, making it difficult to diagnose these masses based on clinical evaluation alone. CT imaging and MR imaging are useful tools in determining exact locations and boundaries of lesions, as well as identifying any erosion or extension into surrounding structures, though imaging features of most masses are nondiagnostic. Diagnosis of such masses requires a combination of clinical history and histopathologic findings. Although paragangliomas of the nasal septum are extremely rare, they should be included in the differential diagnosis when evaluating a septal mass.

The classical histologic appearance of a paraganglioma features an alveolar pattern of well-defined clusters of epithelioid chief cells with round nuclei and eosinophilic cytoplasm. These cells form a "zellballen" pattern of nests separated by vascular stroma and spindle-shaped sustentacular cells [28, 43]. Immunohistochemical staining of paragangliomas generally demonstrates positive markers for NSE, synaptophysin, and chromogranin within the chief cells and S-100 and GFAP within the sustentacular cells [8, 25, 43].

Although the majority of reported nasal paragangliomas are benign, 12 of the cases presented in this review (25.0%) were reported to be malignant, demonstrating intracranial invasion and/or metastasis to the brain, cervical lymph nodes, and bones. It is widely accepted that malignancy cannot be diagnosed by histology alone, but requires evidence of bony invasion or distant metastasis [18, 19, 22]. Certain histological features such as mitotic figures, cellular pleomorphism, necrosis, and vascular invasion can be suggestive of malignancy, though none of these features have been shown to be reliable predictors of malignancy [19, 51]. As such, evaluation with CT imaging and MRI imaging plays a key role in both localization of the primary tumor and identification of local invasion or metastasis.

Almost all of the cases presented in this review were treated surgically. Suggested management of sinonasal paragangliomas involves surgical excision with close follow-up, as several cases of recurrence have been reported [4, 22, 29]. Due to the rich vascularity of these masses, preoperative embolization of the vessels supplying the tumor has been suggested to reduce bleeding during surgery [4, 22, 24]. Many authors suggest the use of radiation therapy to slow the rate of recurrence, although radiation therapy alone has not been shown to be curative [3, 22, 33]. Chemotherapy as a primary treatment for these tumors has been shown to be largely ineffective, though 3 cases reported in this review reported the use of chemotherapy in addition to surgery and radiation therapy in the management of malignant sinonasal paragangliomas [4, 22].

4. Conclusion

We present a rare case of a paraganglioma presenting as a septal mass. To the best of the authors' knowledge, only one other case of nasal septal paragangliomas has been reported. Clinically, these lesions cause symptoms of obstruction, congestion, headache, and epistaxis. Recognizing that paragangliomas can arise from the nasal septum is crucial to accurately diagnose these tumors when evaluating septal lesions. A diagnosis of a paragangliomas can be confirmed based on the histopathologic imaging. These tumors are usually benign but require additional imaging as malignancy cannot reliably be ruled out on the basis of histology alone. Treatment of these tumors requires surgical resection, though radiation therapy has been to show slow growth and decrease recurrence.

Conflicts of Interest

The authors declare that there are no conflicts of interest or financial disclosures.

Acknowledgments

The authors thank Dr. David Yau for providing the histopathology images and Dr. John Go for reviewing the radiology images.

References

[1] C. Offergeld, C. Brase, S. Yaremchuk et al., "Head and neck paragangliomas: clinical and molecular genetic classification," *Clinics*, vol. 67, no. 1, pp. 19–28, 2012.

[2] J. H. Lee, F. Barich, L. H. Karnell et al., "National Cancer Data Base report on malignant paragangliomas of the head and neck," *Cancer*, vol. 94, no. 3, pp. 730–737, 2002.

[3] E. E. Lack, A. L. Cubilla, J. M. Woodruff, and H. W. Farr, "Paragangliomas of the head and neck region: a clinical study of 69 patients," *Cancer*, vol. 39, no. 2, pp. 397–409, 1977.

[4] K. Papaspyrou, H. J. Welkoborsky, H. Gouveris, and W. J. Mann, "Malignant and benign sinonasal paragangliomas," *Laryngoscope*, vol. 123, no. 8, pp. 1830–1836, 2013.

[5] L. Granato, J. D. Prospero, and D. M. Filho, "Nasal paraganglioma: a case report and literature review," *International Archives of Otorhinolaryngology*, vol. 17, no. 1, pp. 92–95, 2013.

[6] U. Kisser, T. Braun, D. Mayr, and A. Leunig, "Paraganglioma of the maxillary sinus," *Auris Nasus Larynx*, vol. 40, no. 5, pp. 506–509, 2013.

[7] H. Morales, M. Castillo, and V. Jewells, "Paraganglioma of the sphenoid sinus: case report and review of literature," *Clinical Imaging*, vol. 31, no. 1, pp. 32–36, 2007.

[8] R. Srivastava, N. Wadhwa, S. Gupta, and U. Razdan, "Nasal polyp—an incidental paraganglioma," *Turkish Journal of Pathology*, vol. 32, no. 3, pp. 196–199, 2016.

[9] W. B. Harkins, "Nonchromaffin paraganglioma of the nasal sinuses," *Laryngoscope*, vol. 67, no. 3, pp. 246–259, 1957.

[10] T. E. Moran, "Nonchromaffin paraganglioma of the nasal cavity," *Laryngoscope*, vol. 72, no. 2, pp. 201–206, 1962.

[11] D. K. Gosavi and A. T. Mohidekar, "Chemodectoma of the nose and sphenoid sinus," *Journal of Laryngology & Otology*, vol. 92, no. 9, pp. 813–816, 1978.

[12] D. Apple and K. Kreines, "Cushing's syndrome due to ectopic ACTH production by a nasal paraganglioma," *American Journal of the Medical Sciences*, vol. 283, no. 1, pp. 32–35, 1982.

[13] L. J. Koegel, H. L. Levine, and S. R. Waldman, "Paraganglioma of the sphenoid sinus appearing as labile hypertension," *Otolaryngology-Head and Neck Surgery*, vol. 90, no. 6, pp. 704–707, 1982.

[14] M. Z. Himelfarb, N. L. Ostrzega, J. Samuel, and E. Shanon, "Paraganglioma of the nasal cavity," *Laryngoscope*, vol. 93, no. 3, pp. 350–352, 1983.

[15] H. J. Straehler-Pohl, "Paraganglioma of the nasal cavity," *Laryngologie, Rhinologie, Otologie*, vol. 64, no. 8, pp. 399–402, 1985.

[16] N. Ueda, A. Yoshida, R. Fukunishi, H. Fujita, and N. Yanagihara, "Nonchromaffin paraganglioma in the nose and paranasal sinuses," *Pathology International*, vol. 35, no. 2, pp. 489–495, 1985.

[17] D. J. Watson, "Nasal paraganglioma," *Journal of Laryngology & Otology*, vol. 102, no. 6, pp. 526–529, 1988.

[18] G. H. Branham, D. R. Gnepp, S. O'McMenomey, and W. H. Friedman, "Malignant paraganglioma—a case report and literature review," *Otolaryngology-Head and Neck Surgery*, vol. 101, no. 1, pp. 99–103, 1989.

[19] J. A. Kuhn and B. L. Aronoff, "Nasal and nasopharyngeal paraganglioma," *Journal of Surgical Oncology*, vol. 40, no. 1, pp. 38–45, 1989.

[20] M. Shimoda, N. Shibuya, and O. Sato, "Nasal cavity paraganglioma with intracranial extension," *Neurologia medico-chirurgica*, vol. 29, no. 2, pp. 132–136, 1989.

[21] A. R. Talbot, "Paraganglioma of the maxillary sinus," *Journal of Laryngology & Otology*, vol. 104, no. 3, pp. 248–251, 1990.

[22] Q. A. Nguyen, P. M. Gibbs, and D. H. Rice, "Malignant nasal paraganglioma: a case report and review of the literature," *Otolaryngology—Head and Neck Surgery*, vol. 113, no. 1, pp. 157–161, 1995.

[23] A. Biswas and R. Pal, "Paraganglioma of nasal gavity," *Indian Journal of Otolaryngology and Head & Neck Surgery*, vol. 52, no. 1, pp. 63-64, 1999.

[24] H. S. Sharma, M. Madhavan, N. H. Othman, M. Muhamad, and J. M. Abdullah, "Malignant paraganglioma of frontoethmoidal region," *Auris Nasus Larynx*, vol. 26, no. 4, pp. 487–493, 1999.

[25] H. J. Welkoborsky, J. Gosepath, R. Jacob, W. J. Mann, and R. G. Amedee, "Biologic characteristics of paragangliomas of the nasal cavity and paranasal sinuses," *American Journal of Rhinology*, vol. 14, no. 6, pp. 419–426, 2000.

[26] M. Scott, D. S. Brooker, and R. I. Davis, "Paraganglioma of the nasal cavity," *Ulster Medical Journal*, vol. 70, no. 2, pp. 149–151, 2001.

[27] J. B. Lecanu, S. Arkwright, P. H. Halimi, J. Trotoux, and P. Bonfils, "Multifocal malignant paraganglioma of the paranasal sinuses: a case report," *Otolaryngology-Head and Neck Surgery*, vol. 126, no. 4, pp. 445–447, 2002.

[28] S. Ketabchi, D. Massi, R. Santoro, and A. Franchi, "Paraganglioma of the nasal cavity: a case report," *European Archives of Oto-Rhino-Laryngology*, vol. 260, no. 6, pp. 336–340, 2003.

[29] D. A. Mouadeb, R. K. Chandra, D. W. Kennedy, and M. Feldman, "Sinonasal paraganglioma: endoscopic resection with a 4-year follow-up," *Head and Neck*, vol. 25, no. 12, pp. 1077–1081, 2003.

[30] B. Lieberum, C. Jaspers, and R. Munzenmaier, "ACTH-producing paraganglioma of the paranasal sinuses," *HNO*, vol. 51, no. 4, pp. 328–331, 2003.

[31] I. Askar, M. F. Oktay, and N. Kilinc, "Use of radial forearm free flap with palmaris longus tendon in reconstruction of total maxillectomy with sparing of orbital contents," *Journal of Craniofacial Surgery*, vol. 14, no. 2, pp. 220–227, 2003.

[32] M. P. Rocha, A. M. Campagnolo, V. S. Macedo, F. B. Scarton, H. P. Rocha, and G. Kuhl, "Nasal paraganglioma: a case report," *Brazilian Journal of Otorhinolaryngology*, vol. 71, no. 2, pp. 237–240, 2005.

[33] B. D. Liess, J. A. Horst, and R. P. Zitsch III, "Sphenoid sinus paraganglioma: first reported case," *American Journal of Otolaryngology*, vol. 28, no. 5, pp. 347–349, 2007.

[34] H. R. Jin, O. J. Lee, and Y. Ahn, "Nasal cavity paraganglioma with malignant transformation: a case report," *Auris Nasus Larynx*, vol. 35, no. 1, pp. 137–139, 2008.

[35] A. J. Fasunla, T. S. Ibekwe, O. A. Afolabi et al., "Sinonasal paraganglioma: a case report," *Oral and Maxillofacial Surgery*, vol. 12, no. 2, pp. 93–96, 2008.

[36] R. Zainine, S. Sahtout, H. Ouertani, M. Sellami, N. Beltaief, and G. Besbes, "Paraganglioma of the nasal cavity," *Journal Medical Tunisie*, vol. 90, no. 2, pp. 178-179, 2012.

[37] J. Michel, D. Taieb, M. Jolibert et al., "Sinonasal paraganglioma with long-delayed recurrence and metastases: genetic and imaging findings," *Journal of Clinical Endocrinology & Metabolism*, vol. 98, no. 11, pp. 4262–4266, 2013.

[38] N. Amiraraghi, M. I. Syed, S. Syed, and A. T. Williams, "Paraganglioma of the skull base presenting as nasal polyps," *Laryngoscope*, vol. 123, no. 3, pp. 577–580, 2013.

[39] V. Arora, P. Verma, P. P. Singh, N. Wadhwa, and K. Bhatia, "Sinonasal paraganglioma: a case report and review of

literature," *Clinical Rhinology An International Journal*, vol. 7, no. 2, pp. 87–89, 2014.

[40] W. Yamaguchi, D. Asaka, K. Wada, T. Okushi, and N. Otori, "A case of paraganglioma of the paranasal sinus operated by endoscopic sinus surgery," *Oto-Rhino-Laryngology Tokyo*, vol. 58, no. 4, pp. 18–23, 2015.

[41] S. Aydin, B. Karabulut, K. S. Orhan, I. Kilicaslan, and K. Deger, "A case of sinonasal paraganglioma with a different morphology: nine-year follow-up," *Turkish Journal of Ear Nose and Throat*, vol. 25, no. 1, pp. 43–45, 2015.

[42] K. C. Ho, G. Meyer, J. Garancis, and J. Hanna, "Chemodectoma involving the cavernous sinus and semilunar ganglion," *Human Pathology*, vol. 13, no. 10, pp. 942-943, 1982.

[43] P. G. Wasserman and P. Savargaonkar, "Paragangliomas: classification, pathology, and differential diagnosis," *Otolaryngologic Clinics of North America*, vol. 34, no. 5, pp. 845–862, 2001.

[44] J. M. Sykes and R. H. Ossoff, "Paragangliomas of the head and neck," *Otolaryngologic Clinics of North America*, vol. 19, no. 4, pp. 755–767, 1986.

[45] I. H. Girgis and S. A. Fahmy, "Nasopharyngeal fibroma: its histo-pathological nature," *Journal of Laryngology & Otology*, vol. 87, no. 11, pp. 1107–1123, 1973.

[46] M. P. Valencia and M. Castillo, "Congenital and acquired lesions of the nasal septum: a practical guide for differential diagnosis," *RadioGraphics*, vol. 28, no. 1, pp. 205–223, 2008.

[47] D. Neskey, J. A. Eloy, and R. R. Casiano, "Nasal, septal, and turbinate anatomy and embryology," *Otolaryngologic Clinics of North America*, vol. 42, no. 2, pp. 193–205, 2009.

[48] A. Shafiee, M. Kabiri, N. Ahmadbeigi et al., "Nasal septum-derived multipotent progenitors: a potent source for stem cell-based regenerative medicine," *Stem Cells and Development*, vol. 20, no. 12, pp. 2077–2091, 2011.

[49] K. Pelttari, M. Mumme, A. Barbero, and I. Martin, "Nasal chondrocytes as a neural crest-derived cell source for regenerative medicine," *Current Opinion in Biotechnology*, vol. 47, pp. 1–6, 2017.

[50] G. Yamin, A. Shabaik, and M. Mafee, "Mass of the anterior nasal septum," *JAMA Otolaryngology–Head & Neck Surgery*, vol. 142, no. 6, pp. 601-602, 2016.

[51] R. I. Linnoila, H. R. Keiser, S. M. Steinberg, and E. E. Lack, "Histopathology of benign versus malignant sympathoadrenal paragangliomas: clinicopathologic study of 120 cases including unusual histologic features," *Human Pathology*, vol. 21, no. 11, pp. 1168–1180, 1990.

46

Skull Base Osteomyelitis from Otitis Media Presenting as the Collet-Sicard Syndrome

Wong-Kein Low[1,2] **and Hui-Ling Lhu**[1]

[1]*Novena ENT-Head & Neck Specialist Centre, No. 04-21/22/34, Mount Elizabeth Novena Medical Centre, 38 Irrawaddy Road, Singapore 329563*
[2]*Duke-NUS Graduate Medical School, 8 College Road, Singapore 169857*

Correspondence should be addressed to Wong-Kein Low; low.wong.kein@gmail.com

Academic Editor: Hidenori Yokoi

Skull base osteomyelitis can involve the jugular foramen and its associated cranial nerves resulting in specific clinical syndromes. The Collet-Sicard syndrome describes the clinical manifestations of palsies involving cranial nerves IX, X, XI, and XII. We present a rare atypical case of skull base osteomyelitis originating from infection of the middle ear and causing the Collet-Sicard syndrome. Caused by *Pseudomonas aeruginosa* and *Klebsiella pneumoniae*, this occurred in an elderly diabetic man subsequent to retention of a cotton swab in an ear with chronic suppurative otitis media. This case report illustrates the possibility of retained cotton swabs contributing to the development of otitis media, skull base osteomyelitis, and ultimately the Collet-Sicard syndrome in the ears of immune-compromised patients with chronically perforated eardrums.

1. Introduction

The jugular foramen (JF) is a clinically important anatomical structure located at the medial end of the skull base. Cranial nerves IX–XI pass through the jugular foramen where cranial nerve XII also lies in close proximity. Various lesions can affect the JF and its associated cranial nerves resulting in specific clinical syndromes. The Collet-Sicard syndrome (CSS) describes the clinical manifestations of palsies involving all four of these cranial nerves.

Typically, skull base osteomyelitis (SBO) or malignant otitis externa originates from the external ear canal and has been well described in the literature [1]. Less is known about atypical types of SBO, which originate from other anatomical structures such as the middle ear [2]. Although both typical and atypical SBO can involve the JF, infectious causes of CSS have been observed to be rare [3].

We present and discuss a case of CSS secondary to middle ear infection in an elderly diabetic patient who had a cotton swab retained in an ear with chronic suppurative otitis media (CSOM).

2. Case Report

An 82-year-old man presented to us for right ear pain and itch for about one week. He had a history of hearing loss for many years with periodic right otorrhea. He had no headaches, and his nose was asymptomatic. He was on oral medications for type 2 diabetes mellitus, hypertension, and hypercholesterolaemia. He had cardiac bypass for ischaemic heart disease 6 months before.

Examination of the left ear showed a healed eardrum perforation. The right ear showed a large retained cotton swab in the medial end of the external ear canal. The external ear canal skin including the bony-cartilaginous junction was not inflamed. On removing the cotton foreign body from the right ear with a pair of microforceps under microscopy, a rapid gush of copious pus was observed emanating from the middle ear through a perforation of the underlying eardrum. The eardrum perforation was large, central in position, and appeared chronic with edges that were scarred (Figure 1). Aural toilet with vacuum suction was performed, and topical ciprofloxacin eardrops were prescribed. The

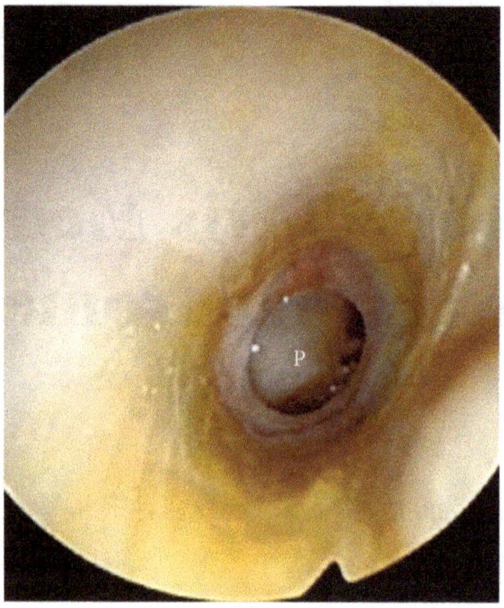

FIGURE 1: The right ear showing a large central eardrum perforation (P).

patient was given a 1-week follow-up review appointment which he defaulted.

The patient returned 1 month later with a new symptom of coughing while eating for 2 weeks associated with right ear pain. The symptom was worse from swallowing solids as compared to liquids, and the patient's intake was increasingly getting reduced.

He was seen earlier by a general practitioner who suspected that he might have a cardiovascular accident. An MRI of the brain was ordered which excluded an infarct of the brain.

The pus in the middle ear seen during the previous consult had resolved. Together with inputs from a neurologist, it was noted that the patient's tongue deviated to the right on protrusion (CN XII) (Figure 2(a)). Gag reflex on the right side was absent (CN IX), and the elevation of the soft palate on the right side was impaired (CN X) (Figure 3(a)). In addition to the reduced mobility of the right vocal cord (CN X), weakness of right sternocleidomastoid muscle (CN XI) was also observed.

Nasoendoscopy showed a slight smooth bulge on the right postnasal space. Videofluoroscopy showed moderate pharyngeal and oral dysphagia with aspiration seen on drinking fluids. A chest X-ray was reported to be normal.

Magnetic resonance imaging (MRI) showed a large mass with central necrosis or suppuration in the right skull base, centering at the right petrous bone and the clivus (Figure 4). It involved the right jugular foramen, the right carotid canal, the right hypoglossal canal, and the nasopharynx. The right jugular bulb and the upper right internal jugular veins were evident on the left side but not on the right. Opacification of the right mastoid air cells was noted. The differential diagnoses considered were severe skull base infection with abscess formation and neoplasm such as nasopharyngeal carcinoma.

Deep punch biopsy of the postnasal space was carried out. Histology revealed inflamed hyperplastic lymphoid tissue with no malignancy. Culture and sensitivity studies showed *Pseudomonas aeruginosa* and *Klebsiella pneumoniae*, both of which were sensitive to cefepime and ciprofloxacin. The cultures were negative for mycobacterium and fungus. Random blood glucose was raised (9.6 mmol/L), and glycated Hb suggested unacceptable glycemic control at 8.2%.

A clinical diagnosis of Collet-Sicard syndrome due to otitis media was made. He had a peripherally inserted central catheter to facilitate intravenous antibiotics. He was treated with intravenous cefepime for 6 weeks and continued with oral levofloxacin and metronidazole thereafter.

He showed progressive improvement clinically. Cranial nerve deficits reverted to normal when he was reviewed after 6 weeks of intravenous antibiotics (Figures 2(b) and 3(b)). The ear pain had resolved, and he was eating normally without symptoms. This was confirmed by biomedical indicators in that the C-protein level was reduced from the pretreatment level (107.40 mL) to <5.00 mL after intravenous treatment. The patient declined to have a repeat post-treatment MRI scan because he felt that he was already getting better.

3. Discussion

SBO commonly originates from the external ear canal with the typical causative pathogen being *Pseudomonas aeruginosa* [1]. In contrast, SBO originating from infections of the middle ear is rare [3]. This could partly be attributed to the fact that *Pseudomonas aeruginosa* is not a cause of acute or serous otitis media [2].

Prasad et al. opined that pus building up under tension in a tympanomastoid sealed with an intact eardrum is a prerequisite for the development of SBO [4]. This may explain why SBO is not commonly seen in CSOM where chronic perforation of eardrums is the norm. This is despite the fact that *Pseudomonas aeruginosa* is one of the commonest organisms causing active infections in CSOM [5].

Our patient was an elderly diabetic with a cotton swab retained in an ear with preexisting chronic eardrum perforation, who subsequently developed SBO. He did not have otitis externa, and the bony-cartilaginous junction of the external ear canal was normal. Upon removal of the cotton swab which was lodged in the medial end of the external ear canal, an abrupt burst of pus was seen emanating from the middle ear. There are a number of possibilities why pus could have accumulated under tension in the middle ear. Firstly, the cotton swab could have acted as a plug in preventing outflow of pus from the middle to external ear. Secondly, as a foreign body, the cotton swab is expected to aggravate any infection in the middle ear. Thirdly, inherent Eustachian tube dysfunction is often associated with a chronically perforated eardrum and, if so, could also have impeded drainage of pus from the middle ear into the nasopharynx. Culture testing of the pus grew *Pseudomonas aeruginosa* which is typically associated with SBO. In addition, the culture results also yielded *Klebsiella pneumoniae*, a microbe which had also been reported to be a cause of SBO albeit rare [6].

According to Climans et al., CSS very rarely results from otitis media [3]. Besides our case, another case of CSS originating from infection of the middle ear occurred in

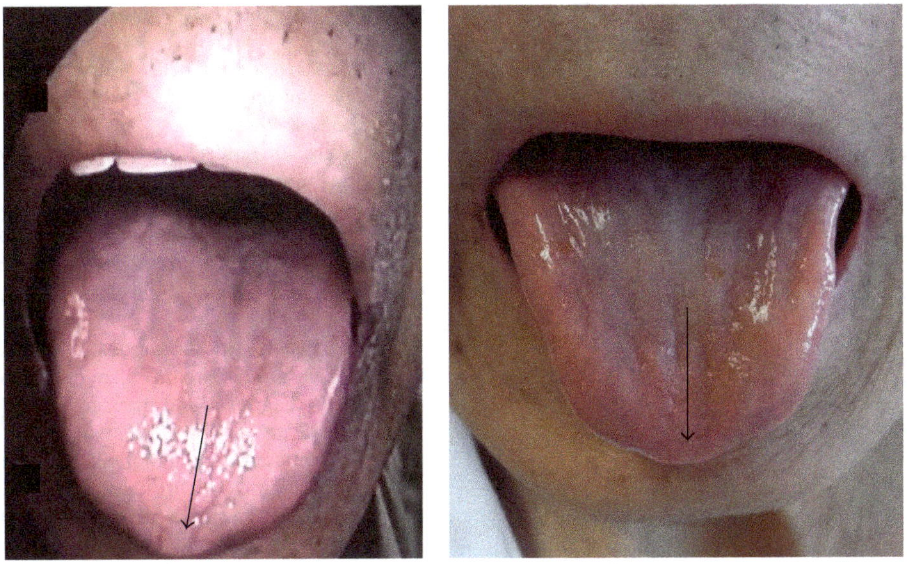

(a) (b)

FIGURE 2: (a) Deviation of the tongue to the right on its voluntary protrusion as illustrated by the direction of the arrow (right CN XII palsy). (b) After treatment, the patient showing symmetrical protrusion of the tongue as illustrated by the direction of the arrow.

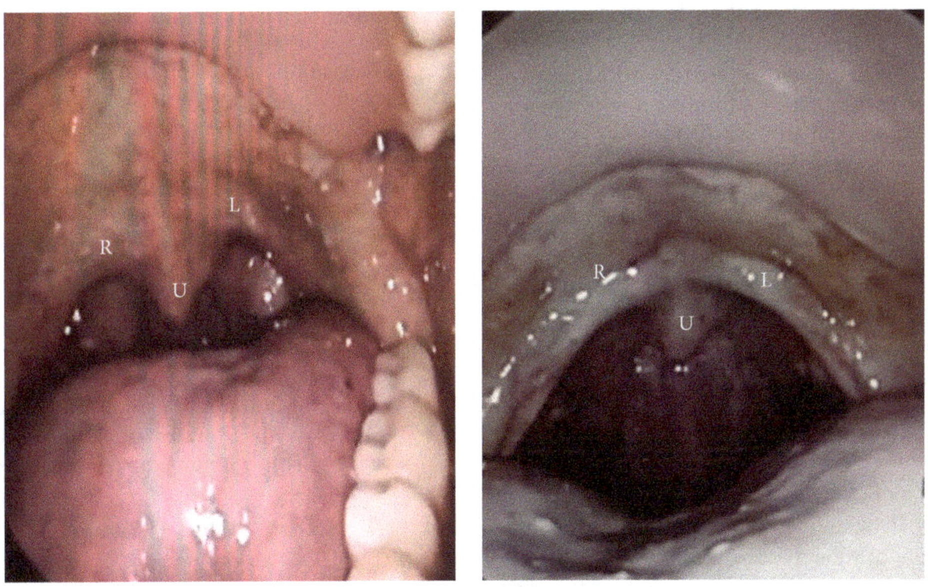

(a) (b)

FIGURE 3: (a) Impaired elevation of the right side of the soft palate (R) as compared to the left (L) with reference to the uvula (U) (right CN X palsy). (b) After treatment, symmetrical elevation of the right (R) and left (L) sides of the soft palate with reference to the uvula (U).

a 56-year-old diabetic man, but the causative pathogens in this case were methicillin-resistant *Staphylococcus epidermidis* and *Corynebacterium* [7].

Delay in diagnosis of CSS is common, partly because of its rarity and partly because of confusion with a primary intracranial event [7]. As illustrated by our case, the neurological manifestations of CSS could be mistaken to be the result of a cardiovascular accident. It is worth noting that cardiovascular accidents involving the brainstem rarely result in isolated palsies of the lower cranial nerves. Such patients are more likely to have additional neurological deficits as a result of involvement of other brainstem structures such as the spinothalamic, spinocerebellar, and pyramidal tracts [8].

Interpretation of the radiological features of CSS could be challenging. Handley et al. reported a case of CSS not caused by SBO but by idiopathic thrombosis of sigmoid-jugular sinus [9]. In our patient, MRI revealed right jugular bulb and upper internal jugular vein obliteration (Figure 4). Although this could suggest venous thrombosis, it could also be due to mere external compression by the surrounding diseased tissues. In any case, even if venous thrombosis has

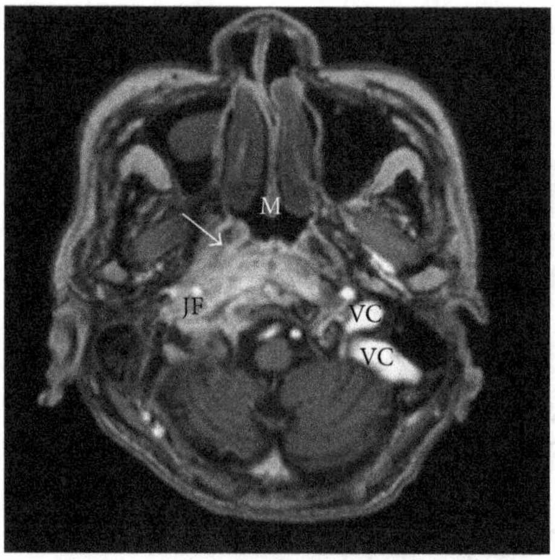

FIGURE 4: MRI scan (axial cut) of the skull base showing a large lesion involving the region of the right jugular foramen (JF). The sigmoid-jugular venous complex (VC) seen on the left side is not apparent on the right side. The lesion extends laterally beyond the jugular foramen and enhances greater than the nasal mucosa (M), and the Eustachian tubal architecture is relatively preserved (arrow).

occurred, the extensive skull base involvement makes it more likely to be a secondary event than as a primary cause of the disease.

The extensive SBO lesion demonstrated by MRI (Figure 4) could also be confused with that of advanced nasopharyngeal carcinoma, a cancer common among Chinese in our local population. Goh et al. suggested that lateral extension, increased T2 signal, lack of architectural distortion, and enhancement greater than or equal to mucosa could be used as differentiating features [10]. As illustrated in Figure 4, SBO has the tendency to extend laterally, to lack architectural distortion, and to demonstrate greater enhancement than mucosa. However, as illustrated by our case, tissue biopsy is ultimately often indicated not only to exclude nasopharyngeal carcinoma but also for culture and sensitivity testing of the causative pathogens.

4. Conclusion

SBO can affect the JF resulting in CSS, a potentially life-threatening condition. Although rare, awareness of SBO as a cause of CSS is important because a delay in its diagnosis is common. Besides the typical type of SBO originating from the external ear canal, atypical types of SBO can originate from other sites such as the middle ear. This case report illustrates the possibility of a retained cotton swab contributing to the development of otitis media, SBO, and ultimately CSS in the ear of an elderly diabetic with a chronically perforated eardrum.

Conflicts of Interest

The authors declare that there are no conflicts of interest regarding the publication of this paper.

Acknowledgments

The support and assistance from Dr. Judy Tan and Dr. Koh Yin Ling are appreciated.

References

[1] M. J. Carfrae and B. W. Kesser, "Malignant otitis externa," *Otolaryngologic Clinics of North America*, vol. 41, no. 3, pp. 537–549, 2008.

[2] S. Merchant and D. M. Vernick, "Osteomyelitis of the temporal bone and skull base in diabetes resulting from otitis media," *Skull Base*, vol. 2, no. 4, pp. 207–212, 1992.

[3] S. A. Climans, M. Melanson, and J. A. Desai, "A case of Collet-Sicard syndrome caused by necrotizing otitis externa," *Canadian Journal of Neurological Sciences*, vol. 40, no. 2, pp. 268–270, 2013.

[4] S. C. Prasad, K. C. Prasad, A. Kumar, N. D. Thada, P. Rao, and S. Chalasani, "Osteomyelitis of the temporal bone: terminology, diagnosis, and management," *Journal of Neurological Surgery Part B: Skull Base*, vol. 75, no. 5, pp. 324–331, 2014.

[5] N. Sharma, A. A. Jaiswal, P. K. Banerjee, and A. K. Garg, "Complications of chronic suppurative otitis media and their management: a single institution 12 years experience," *Indian Journal of Otolaryngology and Head & Neck Surgery*, vol. 67, no. 4, pp. 353–360, 2015.

[6] T. H. Yang, S. T. Kuo, and Y. H. Young, "Necrotising external otitis in a patient caused by *Klebsiella pneumonia*," *European Archives of Oto-Rhino-Laryngology*, vol. 263, no. 4, pp. 344–346, 2006.

[7] T. A. Sibai, P. J. Ben-Galim, S. A. Eicher, and C. A. Reitman, "Infectious Collet-Sicard syndrome in the differential diagnosis of cerebrovascular accident: a case of head-to-neck dissociation with skull-based osteomyelitis," *Spine Journal*, vol. 9, no. 4, pp. e6–e10, 2009.

[8] F. S. Erol, M. Kaplan, A. Kavakli, and M. K. Ozveren, "Jugular foramen syndrome caused by choleastatoma," *Clinical Neurology and Neurosurgery*, vol. 107, no. 4, pp. 342–346, 2005.

[9] T. P. B. Handley, M. S. Miah, S. Majumdar, and S. S. Musheer Hussain, "Collet-Sicard syndrome from thrombosis of the sigmoid-jugular complex: a case report and review of the literature," *International Journal of Otolaryngology*, vol. 2010, Article ID 203587, 5 pages, 2010.

[10] J. P. N. Goh, A. Karandikar, S. C. Loke, and T. Y. Tan, "Skull base osteomyelitis secondary to malignant otitis externa mimicking advanced nasopharyngeal cancer: MR imaging features at initial presentation," *American Journal of Otolaryngology*, vol. 38, no. 4, pp. 466–471, 2017.

Permissions

All chapters in this book were first published in CRO, by Hindawi Publishing Corporation; hereby published with permission under the Creative Commons Attribution License or equivalent. Every chapter published in this book has been scrutinized by our experts. Their significance has been extensively debated. The topics covered herein carry significant findings which will fuel the growth of the discipline. They may even be implemented as practical applications or may be referred to as a beginning point for another development.

The contributors of this book come from diverse backgrounds, making this book a truly international effort. This book will bring forth new frontiers with its revolutionizing research information and detailed analysis of the nascent developments around the world.

We would like to thank all the contributing authors for lending their expertise to make the book truly unique. They have played a crucial role in the development of this book. Without their invaluable contributions this book wouldn't have been possible. They have made vital efforts to compile up to date information on the varied aspects of this subject to make this book a valuable addition to the collection of many professionals and students.

This book was conceptualized with the vision of imparting up-to-date information and advanced data in this field. To ensure the same, a matchless editorial board was set up. Every individual on the board went through rigorous rounds of assessment to prove their worth. After which they invested a large part of their time researching and compiling the most relevant data for our readers.

The editorial board has been involved in producing this book since its inception. They have spent rigorous hours researching and exploring the diverse topics which have resulted in the successful publishing of this book. They have passed on their knowledge of decades through this book. To expedite this challenging task, the publisher supported the team at every step. A small team of assistant editors was also appointed to further simplify the editing procedure and attain best results for the readers.

Apart from the editorial board, the designing team has also invested a significant amount of their time in understanding the subject and creating the most relevant covers. They scrutinized every image to scout for the most suitable representation of the subject and create an appropriate cover for the book.

The publishing team has been an ardent support to the editorial, designing and production team. Their endless efforts to recruit the best for this project, has resulted in the accomplishment of this book. They are a veteran in the field of academics and their pool of knowledge is as vast as their experience in printing. Their expertise and guidance has proved useful at every step. Their uncompromising quality standards have made this book an exceptional effort. Their encouragement from time to time has been an inspiration for everyone.

The publisher and the editorial board hope that this book will prove to be a valuable piece of knowledge for researchers, students, practitioners and scholars across the globe.

List of Contributors

W. X. Yeo and K. K. Tan
Department of Otolaryngology, KK Women's and Children's Hospital, Singapore

Serdal Celik, Osman Kilic and M. Tayyar Kalcioglu
Istanbul Medeniyet University, Faculty of Medicine, Department of Otorhinolaryngology, Goztepe Training and Research Hospital, Istanbul, Turkey

Tulay Zenginkinet
Istanbul Medeniyet University, Goztepe Training and Research Hospital, Department of Pathology, Istanbul, Turkey

Habib G. Zalzal and Steven Coutras
Department of Otolaryngology-Head and Neck Surgery, West Virginia University School of Medicine, Morgantown, WV, USA

Alagesan Chinnasamy
Melbourne Dental School, e University of Melbourne, Melbourne, VIC, Australia

Vidhya Gopinath and Ashish R. Jain
Department of Prosthodontics, Saveetha Dental College and Hospitals, Saveetha University, Chennai, India

Jason Yuen and Samiul Muquit
South West Neurosurgery Centre, Derriford Hospital, Plymouth PL6 8DH, UK

Vinay Varadarajan, Marios Stavrakas and Hisham Khalil
Department of Ear, Nose and Throat, Derriford Hospital, Plymouth PL6 8DH, UK

Waheed Rahman, Nafil Ishaq Arimbrathodi, Faisal Abdulkader, Hussain Al-Enazi, and Zeynel A. Dogan
Department of Otolaryngology, Head and Neck Surgery, Hamad Medical Corporation, Doha, Qatar

Ryan A. Rimmer and Elizabeth E. Cottrill
THomas Jefferson University Hospital, Department of Otolaryngology—Head & Neck Surgery, Philadelphia, PA, USA

C. T. Forde, R. Millard and S. Ali
Department of Otolaryngology, The Royal London Hospital, Whitechapel Road, Whitechapel, London E1 1BB, UK

Ishtyaque Ansari
Department of Neurosurgery, MGM Medical College & Hospital, Aurangabad, India

Ashfaque Ansari, Arjun Antony Graison and Hitendra Joshi
Department of ENT, MGM Medical College & Hospital, Aurangabad, India

Anuradha J. Patil
Department of Plastic Surgery, MGM Medical College & Hospital, Aurangabad, India

Ayako Hashimoto
Department of Otorhinolaryngology, Shizuoka Children's Hospital, Shizuoka, Japan

Tadayuki Kumagai
Department of Pediatrics, Fujieda City General Hospital, Fujieda, Japan

Hiroyuki Mineta
Department of Otorhinolaryngology, Head and Neck Surgery, Hamamatsu University School of Medicine, Hamamatsu, Japan

Yu Saito, Shigeto Itani and Kiyoaki Tsukahara
Department of Otolaryngology, Head and Neck Surgery, Tokyo Medical University, 6-7-1 Nisisinnjuku, Shinjuku-ku, Tokyo 160-0023, Japan

Kazuhiro Nakamura
Department of Otolaryngology, Todachuo General Hospital, 1-19-3 Honthou, Toda-shi, Saitama 335-0023, Japan

Vivian Narana Ribeiro El-Achkar
DDS, PhD Student at Department of Bioscience and Oral Diagnosis, Science and Technology Institute, Universidade Estadual Paulista (UNESP), Sao Jose dos Campos, Brazil

Andressa Duarte
PhD Student at Department of Pathology and Legal Medicine, Ribeirão Preto Medical School, University of São Paulo, Ribeirao Preto, Brazil

Fabiano Pinto Saggioro
PhD, Assistant Physician at Pathology Service of Department of Pathology and Legal Medicine, Ribeirão Preto Medical School, University of São Paulo, Ribeirao Preto, Brazil

Francisco Veríssimo De Mello Filho
MD, PhD, Associated Professor at Department of Ophthalmology, Otorhinolaryngology and Head and Neck Surgery, Ribeirão Preto Medical School, University of São Paulo, Ribeirão Preto, Brazil

Jorge Esquiche León
PhD, Professor at Department of Stomatology, Collective Health and Legal Dentistry, Ribeirão Preto Medical School, University of São Paulo, Ribeirao Preto, Brazil

Alfredo Ribeiro-Silva
MD, PhD, Associated Professor at Department of Pathology and Legal Medicine, Ribeirão Preto Medical School, University of São Paulo, Ribeirao Preto, Brazil

Estela Kaminagakura
DDs, PhD, Associated Professor at the Department of Bioscience and Oral Diagnosis, Science and Technology Institute, Universidade Estadual Paulista (UNESP), Sao Jos´e dos Campos, Brazil

Feride Fatma Görgülü and Ayşe Selcan Koç
Radiology Department, Adana City Research and Training Hospital, University of Health Sciences, Adana, Turkey

Orhan Görgülü
Otorhinolaryngology Department, Adana City Research and Training Hospital, University of Health Sciences, Adana, Turkey

Ashfaque Ansari and Annju Thomas
E. N. T. Department, MGM Medical College and Hospital, Aurangabad, Maharashtra, India

Scott Shapiro and Brian Kellermeyer
Department of Otolaryngology, Head and Neck Surgery, West Virginia University, HSC Room 4520, Morgantown, WV 26506, USA

Jamie L. Schaefer, Sumeet Guptaand John Nguyen
Department of Ophthalmology, West Virginia University, One Medical Center Dr., Morgantown, WV 26506, USA

Mahmoud A. K. Ebrahim
Al-Sabah Hospital, Ministry of Health, Kuwait City, Kuwait

Osamah AlSanea
Department of Surgery Health, Medical Clinic Dammam, Saudi Arabia

Abdulmohsen E. Al-Terki
ENT Clinic, Dasman Diabetes Institute, Kuwait City, Kuwait

Tsutomu Nomura
Department of Otorhinolaryngology, Saitama Medical Center, Saitama, Japan

Megumi Kishimoto, Hirohisa Iwaki and Atsushi Ochi
Department of Otorhinolaryngology, Kameda Medical Center, Kamogawa, Japan

Seiji Kishimoto
Department of Head and Neck Surgery, Kameda Medical Center, Kamogawa, Japan

Francisco Monteiro, Pedro Oliveira and Artur Condé
Department of Otorhinolaryngology, Head and Neck Surgery, Hospital Center of Vila Nova Gaia/Espinho, Rua Conceição Fernandes s/n, 4434-502 Vila Nova de Gaia, Portugal

Elio Bittar Barbosa, Evaldo César Macau Furtado Ferreira and Eulalia Sakano
Department of Ophthalmology and Otorhinolaryngology, Faculty of Medical Sciences, University of Campinas, Campinas, SP, Brazil

Albina Messias de Almeida Milani Altemani and Fernanda Viviane Mariano
Department of Pathology, Faculty of Medical Sciences, University of Campinas, Campinas, SP, Brazil

Emerson Taro Inoue Sakuma
Department of Radiology, Faculty of Medical Sciences, University of Campinas, Campinas, SP, Brazil

Takanori Yamamoto and Keisuke Masuyama
Department of Otorhinolaryngology and Head & Neck Surgery, University of Yamanashi, Yamanashi, Japan

Atsushi Kamijo
Department of Otorhinolaryngology and Allergy Center, Saitama Medical University, Saitama, Japan
Department of Otorhinolaryngology and Head & Neck Surgery, University of Yamanashi, Yamanashi, Japan

Tadao Nakazawa
Department of Pathology, University of Yamanashi, Yamanashi, Japan

Keita Kirito and Kei Nakajima
Department of Hematology and Oncology, University of Yamanashi, Yamanashi, Japan

Norio Komatsu
Department of Hematology, Juntendo University School of Medicine, Tokyo, Japan

Ahmad Al-juboori and Amira Nasser Al Hail
Otorhinolaryngology, Head & Neck Surgery (ORL-HNS) Department, Al Wakra Hospital, Hamad Medical Corporation, Doha, Qatar
Weill Cornell Medical College, Ar-Rayyan, Qatar

Kohei Yamahara, Yuki Katsura and Satoshi Ikegami
Department of Otolaryngology, Head and Neck Surgery, Shizuoka City Shizuoka Hospital, Shizuoka City, Shizuoka 420-8630, Japan

Yuki Egawa
Department of Pathology, Shizuoka City Shizuoka Hospital, Shizuoka City, Shizuoka 420-8630, Japan

Kana Lee
Department of Otolaryngology, Shin-Suma General Hospital, Kobe, Hyogo 654-0048, Japan

Eugene Omakobia, Ahmad Orabi
Department of ENT, Calderdale Royal Hospital, Halifax, UK

Richard Knights
Department of Histopathology, Calderdale Royal Hospital, Halifax, UK

Fernando Mendoza-Moreno, Ángel Rodriguez-Pascual, Marina Pérez-González, Laura Jiménez-Alvárez, Isabel Furtado-Lobo, Manuel Díez-Alonso and Fernando Noguerales-Fraguas
1Department of General and Digestive Surgery, Príncipe de Asturias Teaching Hospital, Alcalá de Henares, Madrid, Spain

María Rocío Díez-Gago
Department of Emergency Medicine, Príncipe de Asturias Teaching Hospital, Alcalá de Henares, Madrid, Spain

Dionisios A. Klonaris, Alexander D. Karatzanis, Stylianos G. Velegrakis, Emmanuel P. Prokopakis and George A. Velegrakis
Department of Otorhinolaryngology, University of Crete Medical School, Heraklion, Crete, Greece

Eleni D. Lagoudakis
Department of Pathology, University of Crete Medical School, Heraklion, Crete, Greece

Wyatt J. Weinheimers Randal Otto and Philip G. Chen
Department of Otolaryngology Head Neck Surgery, University of Texas Health at San Antonio, 7703 Floyd Curl Dr, MC 7777, San Antonio, TX 78229, USA

Justin G. Rowley
UT Long School of Medicine, University of Texas, Austin, TX 78712, USA

John Floyd
Department of Neurosurgery, University of Texas Health at San Antonio, 7703 Floyd Curl Drive, MC 7843, San Antonio, TX 78229, USA

Smriti Panda, Rajeev Kumar and Prem Sagar
Department of Otorhinolaryngology and Head and Neck Surgery, All India Institute of Medical Sciences, New Delhi, India

Vikram Raj Gopinath
Department of Pathology, All India Institute of Medical Sciences, New Delhi, India

Shori Tajima, Takashi Anzai, Rina Matsuoka, Hiroko Okada, Takuma Ide, Mitsuhisa Fujimaki, Shota Kaya, Shin Ito and Katsuhisa Ikeda
Department of Otorhinolaryngology, Juntendo University Faculty of Medicine, Tokyo, Japan

Daisuke Maki, Kenji Okami, Koji Ebisumoto, and Akihiro Sakai
Department of Otolaryngology, Head and Neck Surgery, Tokai University, Kanagawa, Japan

Lama S. Alalula
College of Medicine–King Saud bin Abdulaziz University for Health Sciences, Riyadh 11426, Saudi Arabia

Abdullah S. Arafat, Riyadh A. Alhedaithy and Mohammed Elkrim
Division of Otolaryngology–Head and Neck Surgery, Department of Surgery, King Abdulaziz Medical City, National Guard Health Affairs, Riyadh, Saudi Arabia

Hideki Tanaka, Kiyoaki Tsukahara, Isaku Okamoto, Rio Kojima, Kazuhiro Hirasawa and Hiroki Sato
Department of Otorhinolaryngology, Head and Neck Surgery, Tokyo Medical University, Tokyo, Japan

Leison Maharjan, Yogesh Neupane and Bibhu Pradhan
Department of ENT-HNS, Institute of Medicine (IOM), Kathmandu, Nepal

Marwan Alqunaee
Otorhinolaryngology, Head and Neck Surgery Resident, Kuwait Institute of Medical Specialization, Kuwait City, Kuwait

Abdullah Aldaihani
Department of Surgery, Adan Hospital, Hadiya, Kuwait

Mohammed AlHajery
Department of ENT, Zain and Al Sabah Hospitals, Kuwait City, Kuwait

Seijiro Hamada, Keishi Fujiwara and Akihiro Homma
Department of Otolaryngology Head and Neck Surgery, Faculty of Medicine and Graduate School of Medicine, Hokkaido University, N15W7, Kita-Ku, Sapporo 0608638, Japan

Hiromitsu Hatakeyama
Department of Otolaryngology Head and Neck Surgery, Yokohama City University Medical Center, 4-57 Urafune-cho, Minami-ku, Yokohama 2320024, Japan
Department of Otolaryngology Head and Neck Surgery, Faculty of Medicine and Graduate School of Medicine, Hokkaido University, N15W7, Kita-Ku, Sapporo 0608638, Japan

Daniel C. O'Brien and Jason McChesney
Department of Otolaryngology Head and Neck Surgery, University of West Virginia, Morgantown, WV, USA

Garrett Jones
Department of Medical Education, University of West Virginia, Morgantown, WV, USA

Maggie Yell
Department of Pathology, Anatomy, and Laboratory Medicine, University of West Virginia, Morgantown, WV, USA

Kentaro Kikuchi, Fumio Ide and Kaoru Kusama
Division of Pathology, Department of Diagnostic and erapeutic Sciences, Meikai University School of Dentistry, 1-1 Keyakidai, Sakado, Saitama 350-0283, Japan

Shota Takizawa, Seiji Suzuki and Hideaki Sakashita
Second Division of Oral and Maxillofacial Surgery, Department of Diagnostic and erapeutic Sciences, Meikai University School of Dentistry, 1-1 Keyakidai, Sakado, Saitama 350-0283, Japan

Tie-Jun Li
Department of Oral Pathology, Peking University School of Stomatology, 22 South Zhongguancun Avenue, Haidian District, Beijing 100081, China

Yassmeen Abdel-Aty
Mayo Clinic Arizona, Department of Otolaryngology Head and Neck Surgery, 5777 E Mayo Blvd, Phoenix, AZ 85054, USA

Michael P. Bellew
Department of Medical Education, Assistant Professor of Neurosurgery, UCF College of Medicine, 6850 Lake Nona Blvd, Orlando, FL 32827, USA
Florida Hospital Orlando, 601 East Rollins Street, Orlando, FL 32803, USA

Aziz Mustafa, Burhan Toçi and Hajdin Thaçi
ENT Clinic, University Clinical Center of Kosova, Prishtina, Kosovo

Bujar Gjikolli
Radiology Clinic, University Clinical Center of Kosova, Prishtina, Kosovo

Nehat Baftiu
Anesthesiology/Reanimation Clinic, University Clinical Center of Kosova, Prishtina, Kosovo

J. Vilain, J.-C. Degols and S. Ledeghen
ENT Department, Clinique Saint-Pierre, 9 Av Reine Fabiola, 1340 Ottignies LLN, Belgium

Mahmoud A. K. Ebrahim
Farwaniya Hospital, Ministry of Health, Kuwait City, Kuwait

Mishal M. AlMutairi
Zain Hospital, Ministry of Health, Kuwait City, Kuwait

Khaled M. Hindi
Kuwait Institute Medical Specialties, Kuwait City, Kuwait

Jassem M. Bastaki
Al-Sabah Hospital, Ministry of Health, Kuwait City, Kuwait

Karuna Dewan, Andrew Erman, Jennifer L. Long, and Dinesh K. Chhetri
Department of Head and Neck Surgery, David Geffen School of Medicine at UCLA, Los Angeles, CA 90095, USA

Numan Kökten, Lokman Uzun and M. Tayyar Kalcıoğlu
Department of Otolaryngology, Istanbul Medeniyet University Medical Faculty, Goztepe Training and Research Hospital, Istanbul, Turkey

Ayşe Serap Karadağ
Department of Dermatology, Istanbul Medeniyet University Medical Faculty, Goztepe Training and Research Hospital, Istanbul, Turkey

Tülay Zenginkinet
Department of Pathology, Istanbul Medeniyet University Medical Faculty, Goztepe Training and Research Hospital, Istanbul, Turkey

Evaldas Padervinskis and Saulius Vaitkus
Department of Otorhinolaryngology, Academy of Medicine, Lithuanian University of Health Sciences, Eiveniu 2, LT-50161 Kaunas, Lithuania

Nora Siupsinskiene
University of Klaipeda, Herkaus Manto 84, LT-92294 Klaipeda, Lithuania
Department of Otorhinolaryngology, Academy of Medicine, Lithuanian University of Health Sciences, Eiveniu 2, LT-50161 Kaunas, Lithuania

Irina Arechvo
Department of Ear, Nose and .roat Diseases, Republican Vilnius University Hospital, Siltnamiu 29, LT-04130 Vilnius, Lithuania

Rimante Lapinskaite
Raseiniu Hospital, Ligonines 4, LT-60127 Raseiniai, Lithuania

Silvija Ryskiene
Department of Radiology, Academy of Medicine, Lithuanian University of Health Sciences, Eiveniu 2, LT-50161 Kaunas, Lithuania

Antonio Dionízio De Albuquerque Neto, André Vitor Alves Araújo, Daniel Assunção Cerqueira, Lorenzzo De Angeli Cesconetto, Nilton Provenzano and Eder Magno Ferreira de Oliveira
Oral and Maxillofacial Surgery, Dr. M´ario Gatti Municipal Hospital, Campinas, SP, Brazil

Hiroki Sato, Shoko Yoshimasu, Isaku Okamoto, Akira Shimizu, Yasuaki Katsube, Hideki Tanaka and Kiyoaki Tsukahara
Department of Otorhinolaryngology, Head and Neck Surgery, Tokyo Medical University, Tokyo, Japan

James H. Kim
Keck School of Medicine of the University of Southern California, Los Angeles, CA, USA

Nathan Tu
University of Southern California LAC+USC Medical Center Department of Otolaryngology, Los Angeles, CA, USA

Bozena Barbara Wrobel
Associate Professor of Clinical Otolaryngology Head and Neck Surgery, Keck School of Medicine, Los Angeles, CA, USA

Hui-Ling Lhu
Novena ENT-Head & Neck Specialist Centre, No. 04-21/22/34, Mount Elizabeth Novena Medical Centre, 38 Irrawaddy Road, Singapore 329563

Wong-Kein Low
Novena ENT-Head & Neck Specialist Centre, No. 04-21/22/34, Mount Elizabeth Novena Medical Centre, 38 Irrawaddy Road, Singapore 329563
Duke-NUS Graduate Medical School, 8 College Road, Singapore 169857

Index

R

S

T

V

W

www.ingramcontent.com/pod-product-compliance
Lightning Source LLC
LaVergne TN
LVHW060557210926
848485LV00005B/1328